The Five Senses
and Beyond

The Five Senses and Beyond

The Encyclopedia of Perception

JENNIFER L. HELLIER, EDITOR

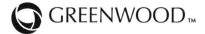 GREENWOOD™

An Imprint of ABC-CLIO, LLC
Santa Barbara, California • Denver, Colorado

Copyright © 2017 by ABC-CLIO, LLC

Library of Congress Cataloging-in-Publication Data

Names: Hellier, Jennifer L., editor.
Title: The five senses and beyond : the encyclopedia of perception /
    Jennifer L. Hellier, editor.
Description: Santa Barbara, California : Greenwood, [2017] |
    Includes bibliographical references and index.
Identifiers: LCCN 2016021791 (print) | LCCN 2016023799 (ebook) |
    ISBN 9781440834165 (hardback) | ISBN 9781440834172 (eisbn) |
    ISBN 9781440834172 (ebook)
Subjects: LCSH: Perception—Encyclopedias. | Senses and sensation—Encyclopedias.
Classification: LCC BF311 .F53 2017 (print) | LCC BF311 (ebook) |
    DDC 152.103—dc23
LC record available at https://lccn.loc.gov/2016021791

ISBN: 978-1-4408-3416-5
EISBN: 978-1-4408-3417-2

21 20 19 18 17   1 2 3 4 5

This book is also available as an eBook.

Greenwood
An Imprint of ABC-CLIO, LLC

ABC-CLIO, LLC
130 Cremona Drive, P.O. Box 1911
Santa Barbara, California 93116-1911
www.abc-clio.com

This book is printed on acid-free paper ∞
Manufactured in the United States of America

Contents

Preface

Understanding how the different sensory systems integrate information from the outside world to the brain for perception has been questioned and studied since the time of the ancient Greeks. With today's new technologies and research, neuroscientists have uncovered many physiological mechanisms of the senses and have learned how some can be associated with neurological deficits or disorders. Research has also developed new treatments to alleviate sensory deficits and in some cases to prevent further damage. Thus, the purpose of this encyclopedia is to provide a wide-ranging reference of the five main sensory systems and is written at a level easily accessible for high school and college students as well as the layperson. The encyclopedia provides insights into the discipline of neuroscience, covering both normative and neurological disorders and factors that promote general nervous system health. By addressing both ends of the spectrum, the encyclopedia presents a more holistic and comprehensive perspective of the fast-growing discipline of neuroscience.

This encyclopedia helps the reader understand how research is integral to understanding both normal and abnormal sensory function. *The Five Senses and Beyond: The Encyclopedia of Perception* contains more than 200 entries and pulls together topics that illuminate (1) the five basic senses and special senses, (2) anatomy and physiology related to the senses, and (3) organizations and individuals important to sensory research. To help the reader understand the basics of the brain and sensory systems, there are entries about brain anatomy and physiology, as well as how neurons "talk" to each other in brain circuits to provide normal function. There are various entries that discuss abnormal or dysfunctional sensory systems, which may develop into disorders or diseases. Finally, selected entries include references to research designs and experimental procedures commonly used to study sensory systems with examples from current and relevant clinical research as well as short biographies of famous scientists who furthered the knowledge of neuroscience and neurology. All entries include cross-references and further readings to aid in additional study.

The encyclopedia also includes 15 hands-on activity sidebars that give readers the chance to learn about the senses and their anatomy firsthand. From testing for eye dominance to discovering the interrelatedness between smell and taste to modeling brain anatomy with clay, these activities make the material more interactive.

The contributors to this work are all uniquely qualified to speak with authority regarding at least one aspect of the brain, the nervous system, and its disorders.

The contributors include (1) neuroscientists who are immersed in cutting-edge research to better understand both normative and abnormal activities of the brain and the nervous system; (2) neurologists and family physicians who routinely diagnose and treat neurological diseases; and (3) public health professionals who work endlessly to educate the public about preventing neurodevelopmental disorders.

Acknowledgments

This project was a joy to work on as it allowed me to share my love of neuroscience research with everyone. However, I could not have completed this project without the help of my assistants Riannon Atwater and Renee Johnson. Both jumped in at the beginning with enthusiasm and worked endlessly with me on this reference. I thank Riannon and Renee for their dedication, time, and effort.

I thank Maxine Taylor, senior acquisition editor, for initiating this project and selecting me to be the lead editor. Her guidance and excellent editing skills have made me a better writer. I truly enjoyed working with Maxine during these past two years.

Lastly and most importantly I must thank my immediate and extended family for understanding how I needed to work during the weekends to make this a successful reference and for supporting me throughout this endeavor. I especially thank my husband, Chuck, and my two amazing sons, Jack and Sam.

Introduction

The nervous system helps an organism understand the environment around it and helps the organism respond and interact within its world. The most fundamental portion of the nervous system is its sensory system. This system consists of the five main senses—audition (hearing), gustation (taste), olfaction (smell), touch, and vision (sight)—as well as complex senses such as balance, interoception (also written as enteroception; sensory information from the walls of hollow internal organs), and proprioception (limb position).

Anatomical Organization of a Sensory System

The system consists of a network of neurons that work together to sense and then to process this information. The network of neurons will be described in three different divisions called first-order neurons, second-order neurons, and third-order neurons.

To begin with the sensing portion of the system, it involves a somatic (body) receptor that is within the skin, bones, muscles, joints, eyes, and ears. These specialized receptors will pick up sensory information and begin a nerve impulse. The receptor is part of the sensory neuron, which is considered the first-order neuron or primary afferent neuron for sensory information. This neuron comes from the periphery and will travel the afferent pathway (toward the central nervous system). For most of the sensory neurons, their cell body (or soma) is located in the dorsal root ganglion (a group of cell bodies outside of the central nervous system) just lateral of the spinal cord. For sensation to the head, neck, and face, these nuclei (a group of cell bodies inside of the central nervous system) are found in the brainstem and are named for the cranial nerve that carries the sensory and/or motor information to the central nervous system.

The second-order neuron is an interneuron. This secondary neuron will receive information from the first-order neuron's synapse, where neuronal information is transferred from one neuron to another. Some of these second-order neurons may send their axons to cross over to the other side of the spinal cord or brainstem before carrying the information to the thalamus, which is a deep relay structure within the brain. All second-order neurons will synapse in the thalamus, except for the sense of smell.

Lastly, the third-order neuron is located in the thalamus, which is made up of several different nuclei. The second-order neuron synapses on the third-order neuron. Here the sensory information is transferred and then carried to the correct sensory area of the cerebrum, such as the primary visual cortex for vision and the somatosensory cortex for pain, temperature, touch, and proprioception.

In the brain the somatosensory system involves the thalamus, reticular formation, and the postcentral gyrus, which is found posterior to the central sulcus in the parietal lobe of the cerebral cortex. Along the surface of the postcentral gyrus, the body is mapped from the midline to the temporal lobe. This means that a specific body region is located in a specific region of the postcentral gyrus. This map is called a homunculus, meaning "little man." The purpose of the thalamus is to act as the relay center from the spinal cord or brainstem to the homunculus. This is the same as the reticular formation, but the reticular formation acts as a relay for the spinal cord or brainstem to the thalamus. The postcentral gyrus is the main processing center of the somatosensory system. It processes the sensory impulses received from the thalamus. If a reaction is necessary, such as to move away from a heat source, this sensory information in the cerebral cortex will be transferred to the motor cortex to respond.

Sensory System Pathways

The somatosensory system has specific ascending pathways that are dependent on the information carried and how they ascend. It is important to note that the terms "tract" (a group of fibers or axons) and "pathway" may be interchangeable, and that these tracts are named by where they are located in the central nervous system and/or where they originate and then terminate. One of the pathways is the anterolateral tract. In these spinothalamic pathways, the first step is the first-order neuron. It carries the sensory impulse for touch, pressure, pain, and temperature. The neuron's axon enters the spinal cord and synapses in the posterior gray horns. The secondary neuron then decussates (crosses) the impulse by the ventral white commissure to the contralateral (opposite) side where it ascends to the thalamus. The thalamus then directs the signal to the correct area.

There are three distinct pathways within the anterolateral tract. They are the (1) lateral spinothalamic tract, (2) anterior spinothalamic tract, and (3) spinoreticulothalamic tract. The lateral spinothalamic tract is a pathway that carries pain and temperature information. The cell body of the secondary neuron is located in the dorsal horn of the spinal cord. It will decussate via the ventral white commissure and then ascend within the lateral funiculus. Upon reaching the posterolateral nucleus of the thalamus, it will then project the impulse to the postcentral gyrus of the cerebrum. The anterior spinothalamic pathway is much like the lateral pathway except it carries crude touch sensory information. Additionally, instead of ascending through the lateral funiculus the anterior spinothalamic tract will ascend through the anterior funiculus. Finally, the spinoreticulothalamic tract is different as its cell bodies are located in the substantia gelatinosa, a more anterior and slightly medial region of the dorsal horn. These then decussate to the spinoreticular tract and ascend to the reticular formation in the brainstem. From there the impulse is sent to the thalamus. This is different from all the ascending pathways because it synapses into the reticular formation in the brainstem rather than going straight to the thalamus.

Another pathway is the posterior column or lemniscus pathway of the spinal cord. This pathway carries highly localized information to the central nervous system. One part of this pathway, the fasciculus gracilis, sends impulses that perceive fine touch, proprioception, vibration, and pressure from the inferior half of the body (legs and trunk) to the central nervous system. The first-order neuron synapses in the nucleus gracilis, where it will then decussate and ascend to the thalamus. The other part of the posterior column—the fasciculus cuneatus—carries similar information to the central nervous system, but these are sensory impulses from the arms and upper body. The fasciculus cuneatus will go through the nucleus cuneatus before decussating and ascending to the thalamus.

Since these pathways involve multiple relay stations, they can be vulnerable to injury. If there were damage to an area anywhere along these pathways, it could lead to the loss of sensation. However, these paths act as a type of anastomosis of the nerves and will provide backup routes for pain and temperature impulses, as these sensations are important for survival. For example, if the spinal cord were damaged on one side, the person would still be able to feel pain and possibly temperature. However, if the spinal cord were damaged completely through, the person might not be able to sense anything.

Special Senses

Balance and equilibrium are senses perceived by the vestibular system, which detects the position and movement of the head. The main organs of the vestibular system—the semicircular canal system and the otoliths—are located within the inner ear on both sides of the head, just posterior to the cochlea of the auditory system. Each component is responsible for detecting different types of movement. The semicircular canals detect rotational movement, and the otoliths detect gravity and linear acceleration. The vestibular system is closely tied to the visual centers of the brain that control eye muscle movement as well as areas of the autonomic nervous system within the cerebellum that maintain subconscious muscle tension. When the vestibular system is malfunctioning and the subconscious muscle tension is abnormal, it may cause symptoms like motion sickness, vertigo, or uncontrolled eye movements.

Interoception is associated with autonomic motor control and provides humans with the sense of hunger, fullness (satiety), thirst, pain, and the need to breathe (air-hunger). These signals travel through the spinothalamic and vagal tracts and are represented in the brain at the dorsal posterior insula (located in the deep temporal lobe), the somatosensory cortex, and the orbitofrontal cortex. In humans, the sense of emotional awareness is represented in the right anterior insula. Interoceptive ability has been shown to vary between persons, as some individuals are more sensitive to visceral signals compared to others. Furthermore, it has been shown that the behavior to fulfill the signals (e.g., hunger, thirst) also varies between persons.

Proprioceptive stimuli are internal forces that are made by the position or movement of a body part. Proprioception is different from exteroception, which perceives the outside world; and it is also different from interoception, which perceives pain, hunger, and the movement of internal organs. Instead, proprioception uses static forces on the joints, muscles, and tendons, which keep the limb in position against the force of gravity, to denote the position of the limb. The movement of the limb is due to the changes in these forces. Proprioception is important in posture and balance, and its receptors are located in joint capsules, joint ligaments, skeletal muscles, and tendons.

Types of Sensory Receptors

Sensory receptors have been categorized into five groups: mechanoreceptors, chemoreceptors, thermoreceptors, photoreceptors, and nociceptors. Some of these different receptor types are found throughout the body or in almost every sensory system.

Mechanoreceptors are receptors that respond to a physical stimulus such as mechanical pressure or distortion. These receptors are important for discerning between different sensations such as light touch, touch, positional change (balance), and pressure. Perhaps the most notable stimuli that mechanoreceptors respond to are sound waves that physically bend the stereocilia of the hair cells in the cochlea to transmit sound as a nerve impulse.

Chemoreceptors are receptors that respond to chemical stimuli in the environment. The two prominent classes of chemoreceptors are those involved in the olfactory and gustatory systems. Chemicals such as odorants or tastants will bind to receptors in the nose (olfactory sensory neurons) or on the tongue (taste cells located in taste buds) and transmit a signal to the brain to be perceived.

Thermoreceptors are specialized sensory receptors that determine temperatures that are generally not painful (not too hot and not too cold). Thermoreceptors do not have a specific form, like a hair cell or olfactory sensory neuron, but are considered to be free nerve endings or free nonspecialized endings. These receptors are found throughout the skin, cornea (the covering of the eye), and the bladder. There are two fiber types used to sense temperature. Unmyelinated C-fibers sense warm to hot temperatures and lightly myelinated A delta fibers sense cool to cold temperatures. Nociceptors can act as thermoreceptors to determine pain from temperature, such as when a person burns his or her hand.

Photoreceptors are specialized sensory receptors that convert visible white light into the sense of vision. Specifically, these receptors absorb photons of light and transduce that absorption into a membrane potential, which activates the neuron. There are two main types of photoreceptors: cones and rods. Cone cells perceive color and need bright light to be activated. In contrast, rod cells are activated with dim lighting, as they are more sensitive to light. Rod cells are used for night and peripheral vision and have no role in color vision.

Nociceptors are specialized sensory receptors that determine when a stimulus is painful. These receptor types are generally called free nerve endings or free nonspecialized endings. Nociceptors send their signal to the brain and spinal cord so that the body can appropriately respond, such as let go of a hot handle. Nociceptors are found in all locations of the body, both internally (such as the gut, heart, joints, and muscles) and externally (like the cornea, mucosa, and skin—also known as cutaneous nociceptors). This is because pain is an important signal that should not be ignored.

Jennifer L. Hellier

Further Reading

Craig, A. D. (Bud). (2003). Interoception: The sense of the physiological condition of the body. *Current Opinion in Neurobiology, 13*(4), 500–505.

Dougherty, Patrick, & Chieyeko Tsuchitani. (2015). Somatosensory pathways. In *Neuroscience Online, an electronic textbook for the neurosciences* (Chap. 4). John H. Byrne (Ed.). Open-access educational resource provided by the Department of Neurobiology and Anatomy at the University of Texas Medical School at Houston. Retrieved from http://neuroscience.uth.tmc.edu/s2/chapter04.html

Dougherty, Patrick, & Chieyeko Tsuchitani. (2015). Somatosensory processes. In *Neuroscience Online, an electronic textbook for the neurosciences* (Chap. 5). John H. Byrne (Ed.). Open-access educational resource provided by the Department of Neurobiology and Anatomy at the University of Texas Medical School at Houston. Retrieved from http://neuroscience.uth.tmc.edu/s2/chapter05.html

Kandel, Eric R., James H. Schwartz, Thomas M. Jessell, Steven A. Siegelbaum, & A. J. Hudspeth (Eds.). (2012). *Principles of neural science* (5th ed.). New York, NY: McGraw-Hill.

Stevenson, Richard J., Mehmet Mahmut, & Kieron Rooney. (2015). Individual differences in the interoceptive states of hunger, fullness and thirst. *Appetite, 95*, 44–57. http://dx.doi.org/10.1016/j.appet.2015.06.008

A

ACCOMMODATION

Animals are highly visual beings and the eyes are needed to maintain focus of an object at both close and far distances. This action of changing optical power over various distances is called accommodation. Accommodation uses both the optic nerve (cranial nerve II) and the oculomotor nerve (cranial nerve III) to maintain the focus of the image on the fovea, which is the part of the retina that has the greatest resolution. Accommodation can be controlled (conscious action), but is more often a reflex (unconscious action). Thus it is called the accommodation reflex. Many animals, particularly mammals, birds, and reptiles, will change the optic power of their eye by altering the shape of the elastic lens. This is accomplished by using the ciliary body within the eye. The ciliary body is a tissue within the eye and near the lens. It is made up of the ciliary muscle and ciliary processes. As humans age, the elasticity of the lens decreases, which in turn makes the lens rigid. This means adults who are generally older than 50 years of age will have more difficulty in accommodating. Thus, most older adults will need to wear glasses to adjust their near vision for reading.

Anatomy and Physiology

The accommodation reflex allows the eye to change its focus from a near object to one that is far away and vice versa. This reflex is extremely fast and most people do not even realize that it is occurring. The speed of accommodation, however, slows down as a person ages because the lens becomes less flexible. The accommodation reflex changes the shape of the lens and pupil size during the action. The ciliary muscles alter the lens shape by changing the amount of muscle contraction, which in turn keeps the focus of the object on the retina. The ciliary muscles can make the lens flatten out for distance focus and then change to a very convex shape for close focus. Since it is a reflex, it is controlled by the autonomic nervous system, particularly the parasympathetic division. The reflex has three parts: pupil accommodation, lens accommodation, and convergence.

Pupil accommodation occurs with the changes in the amount of light entering the eye. For a single point of light in the distance, the pupil must dilate (enlarge) so that the greatest amount of light can enter, which produces a clear image on the retina (the photosensitive lining of the eye). At the same time, the ciliary muscle must relax, allowing the lens to have a long focal length. This process is the lens accommodation. However, when a single point of light enters the eye up close, the result is constriction of the pupil (gets smaller). This will divert light rays from entering the peripheral portions of the retina, allowing the image to be in focus. At the same time the ciliary muscle contracts so that the lens will have a shorter focal length. The optic nerve (the output of the retina) then takes this light and image information to the brain, specifically to the occipital lobe (the most posterior portion of the cerebrum). This is where vision is interpreted as well as the action of accommodation. The signal is then sent to the Edinger-Westphal nucleus in the midbrain and to the oculomotor nerve. The Edinger-Westphal nucleus is the accessory parasympathetic nucleus of cranial nerve III. Activation of the oculomotor nerve contracts and relaxes the ciliary muscle as well as the medial rectus and sphincter pupillae muscles of the eye.

Convergence is the process of both eyes moving to the center at the same time. This process is also called adduction. The left eye moves medially to the right and the right eye moves medially to the left. This helps in focusing objects just in front of the face, such as a computer monitor. Thus, for up-close vision, the eyes will adduct, the ciliary muscles will contract, increasing the curvature of the lens, and the pupils will constrict. For a video showing accommodation, please use this link: https://www.youtube.com/watch?v=p_xLO7yxgOk

Jennifer L. Hellier

See also: Cranial Nerves; Hubel, David H.; Nerves; Optic Nerve; Visual Motor System; Visual System

Further Reading

Blumenfeld, Hal. (2013). *Pupillary responses (CN II, III)*. Neuroexam.com. Retrieved from http://www.neuroexam.com/neuroexam/content.php?p=19

Liang, Barbara. (2012). *The 12 cranial nerves*. Retrieved from http://www.wisc-online.com /objects/ViewObject.aspx?ID=AP11504

Schachar, Ronald A., Barbara K. Pierscionek, Ali Abolmaali, & Tri Le. (2007). The relationship between accommodative amplitude and the ratio of central lens thickness to its equatorial diameter in vertebrate eyes. *British Journal of Ophthalmology, 91*(6), 812–817.

ACTION POTENTIAL

Action potentials are discrete electrical signals that are transmitted along the length of axons and propagate information within the nervous system. These signals are generated as a result of a transient change in membrane permeability: from a state where it is more permeable to potassium (K^+) than sodium (Na^+), to a reversal of these permeability properties. During the action potential, an influx of Na^+ is responsible for rapid depolarization and an efflux of K^+ causes repolarization or hyperpolarization. These changes in membrane permeability are due to the opening and closing of voltage-gated ion channels. The speed at which action potentials are conducted is based on the radius of the axon, the presence of a myelin sheath, and the number of ion channels.

When the neuron is at rest, there is an excess of positive charge on the outside of the cell (positive potential) and an excess of negative charge on the inside of the cell (negative potential). This creates the resting membrane potential, which is measured by recording the voltage inside the cell relative to the outside in the extracellular fluid. For most neuron types, resting membrane potential is usually –70 mV; however, it may be between –40 and –90 mV depending on the brain region. An electrical potential difference exists across the plasma membrane of cells and is created by differences in the concentration of charged ions between the cytosol and interstitial fluid. The equilibrium potential, the electrical potential generated across the membrane, can be predicted with the Nernst equation. The two major ions involved in maintaining a resting potential and generating an action potential are K^+ and Na^+.

At rest, Na^+ ions slowly leak into the cell as a result of two forces: a Na^+ concentration gradient and the electrostatic force of anions inside the cell. The membrane is relatively permeable to K^+ ions that have the tendency to move down their concentration gradient: from the inside to the outside of the cell. Two negatively charged anions are also important to establish the membrane potential: chloride (Cl^-) and organic anions.

An ionic pump, the Na^+ and K^+ ATPase (or Na^+/K^+ pump), is a membrane-bound protein that maintains the concentration gradient for Na^+ and K^+. This pump creates a natural imbalance in the concentration of K^+ and Na^+ on either side of the plasma membrane. Adenosine triphosphate (ATP) provides the energy to actively pump three Na^+ ions out of the cell while two K^+ ions are pumped into the cell. This results in an intracellular concentration of K^+ that is 20 times higher than the extracellular concentration of K^+. The concentration gradient of Na^+ runs in the opposite direction, with a concentration that is 10 times higher outside the cell compared to the Na^+ concentration inside the cell. Overall, this results in a net increase in positive charges on the outside of the cell.

Voltage-gated sodium channels (VGSC) embedded within the phospholipid membrane play an important role in the generation of an action potential. The VGSC is selectively permeable to Na^+ ions but is normally closed. Na^+ ions have a great desire to be inside the cell as a result of two electrochemical forces: Na^+ wants to equilibrate its concentration between the outside and inside of the cell, and it wants to neutralize the charge difference between the inside and outside of the cell. Depolarization of the membrane stimulates the opening of VGSC, allowing Na^+ to rush into the cell. The initial depolarizing event must change the membrane potential by about 15–30 mV for the event to occur. This is known as the threshold of excitation.

At peak depolarization, Na^+ channels close and voltage-dependent ion channels that are only permeable to K^+ open. The opening of these channels increases potassium permeability, allowing K^+ ions to rapidly travel outside the cell down its concentration gradient. This is known as repolarization. As K⁺ continues to travel outside of the cell, the membrane becomes slightly hyperpolarized or more negative. While the membrane is hyperpolarized, another action potential cannot be generated. Following the completion of an action potential, all ion channels return to their resting state and the activity of the Na⁺/K⁺ pump returns the membrane potential to its normal resting state.

Action potentials are self-propagating, meaning that depolarization of a small region of the membrane triggers the opening of nearby Na⁺ channels. In this way, a wave of depolarization travels along the nerve. Once an action potential is triggered in one region of the membrane, the voltage Na⁺ channels become temporarily inactivated, preventing it from doubling back. This is referred to as the refractory state. Action potentials are referred to as "all-or-none" events, meaning that all action potentials are identical when it comes to the magnitude of the membrane depolarization. In contrast, the initial membrane depolarization is a graded response.

Danielle Stutzman

See also: Axon; Membrane Potential: Depolarization and Hyperpolarization; Nerves

Further Reading

Fletcher, Allan. (2011). Action potential: Generation and propagation. *Anaesthesia & Intensive Care Medicine, 12*(6), 258–262.

Fry, Chris H., & Rita I. Jabr. (2010). The action potential and nervous conduction. *Surgery (Oxford), 28*(2), 49–54.

ADAPTIVE TECHNOLOGY: *See* Assistive Technology

ADRENALINE

Adrenaline or epinephrine is a molecule that functions as both a hormone and a neurotransmitter. Epinephrine is a type of monoamine (made of one amino acid, one base unit of protein) that functions in the autonomic nervous system (ANS), more specifically in the sympathetic branch of the ANS. The sympathetic nervous system (SNS) is responsible for the "fight-or-flight" response. In a sympathetic response, the nervous system directs blood away from the internal organs responsible for digestion and urination, and away from the skin. The heart, lungs, and skeletal muscles receive more blood, and the pupils are dilated (enlarged) so that the organism is better able to respond to a threat. Epinephrine is stimulatory on the SNS and promotes the fight-or-flight response. The adrenal medulla (a gland located on top of both kidneys) is what secretes most of the epinephrine found in the human body. However, epinephrine also acts as a neurotransmitter within the nervous system. Since epinephrine is nonspecific and acts as an agonist (because it is stimulatory on postsynaptic neurons), it can be used to treat a large number of severe allergies (anaphylactic) such as allergies to food, insect stings, animals, or drugs.

Synthesis and Mechanism of Action

Epinephrine is mainly synthesized and secreted by the adrenal medulla. Not only does it act as an agonist on postsynaptic neurons (and other effector cells such as muscles, blood vessels, etc.), but it also can function as a hormone to have a metabolic effect and as a bronchodilator on those organs that do not have direct SNS innervation. This helps to coordinate the effect of the SNS with other actions in the body to have a more efficient and synchronized response to threats.

The adrenals secrete epinephrine into the bloodstream (without the use of ducts) where it travels around the body and stimulates certain postganglionic fibers. Since epinephrine acts as both a hormone and a neurotransmitter, it functions on almost all tissues of the body. The receptor in each tissue type is part of what determines the result of the effect of epinephrine stimulation on a tissue. There are multiple types of adrenergic receptors (these are postsynaptic receptors that recognize and bind to both epinephrine and an oxidized variant, norepinephrine) to which epinephrine can bind. Epinephrine is nonspecific when binding to these receptors, thus it has multiple effects on the nervous system. It can stimulate pathways that inhibit the pancreas from secreting insulin and stimulates glycolysis (release of glycogen) in the liver and muscles. Epinephrine can also stimulate increased lipolysis by adipose tissue (release of fatty acids from fat storage). The increase in serum levels of glycogen and fat allows for a more ready supply of energy for the cells and muscles to use in response to a threat.

Medical Applications

Adrenaline given intramuscularly through an injection can be used to treat multiple medical conditions including, most notably, anaphylaxis and cardiac arrest. The injection of epinephrine in cardiac arrest patients works to increase peripheral resistance, thus keeping most of the blood in and around the heart. This allows for better gas diffusion in the lungs, which in turn increases the amount of oxygen available for the heart and other tissues. Currently, the benefits of using epinephrine in the treatment of a patient experiencing cardiac arrest are being debated. Some think that the administration of epinephrine can actually have adverse effects on the patient. In anaphylaxis, epinephrine is the drug most commonly used to reduce the immune response to extreme allergy. Specifically, epinephrine is important for reducing the swelling (inflammatory edema) and inflammation that is associated with severe allergies. By reducing the swelling in anaphylaxis, the patient is able to overcome the allergic response.

It is important to note, however, that there may also be adverse effects of getting an injection of epinephrine. Some of these effects are heart palpitations, tachycardia, arrhythmia, anxiety, panic attack, pulmonary edema, tremor, hypertension, and headache. This is just a short list of the possible side effects of intramuscular or intravenous injections of epinephrine. It is important that any injections of epinephrine be carefully monitored by a health care professional to ensure that overdosage and adverse effects are avoided as much as possible.

Riannon C. Atwater

See also: Autonomic Nervous System; Noradrenaline

Further Reading

Clark, Josh. (2007). How can adrenaline help you lift a 3,500-pound car? *HowStuffWorks.com*. Retrieved from http://entertainment.howstuffworks.com/arts/circus-arts/adrenaline-strength.htm

Klabunde, Richard E. (2012). Norepinephrine, epinephrine and acetylcholine—synthesis, storage, release and metabolism. In *Cardiovascular pharmacology concepts*. Retrieved from http://www.cvpharmacology.com/norepinephrine.htm

MedlinePlus. (2012). *Epinephrine injections*. Retrieved from http://www.nlm.nih.gov/medlineplus/druginfo/meds/a603002.html

AFFERENT TRACTS

Nerves and tracts travel in two basic directions within the central nervous system (CNS), toward—which is called afferent—and away from—which is called efferent. This makes up the two general types of pathways within the CNS, which are essential for proper functioning throughout the body. Afferent and efferent tracts can be remembered by A for "*a*fferent connections *a*rrive" and E for "*e*fferent connections *e*xit." For afferent tracts, the general function is to bring sensory information from the body to the brain.

Anatomy and Function

Afferent tracts carry sensory information to the brain, where the sensory information is then interpreted. This sensory information tells an animal important information about its surroundings, such as the temperature or if a predator is nearby. It also gives the animal information about its internal organs that are necessary for survival, such as whether its stomach is empty and it needs to eat. The traditional sensory or afferent information includes sight, smell, sound, taste, and touch. However, there are other sensory modalities, which include acceleration and balance, kinesthetic sense, pain, proprioception, temperature, time, and visceral senses (interoception).

The afferent pathways from the sensory neurons to the brain generally include three neurons: a first-order neuron, a second-order neuron, and a third-order neuron. The first-order neuron receives a stimulus and sends the signal to the spinal cord. Within the spinal cord the neuron passes the information on to a second-order neuron, which will carry the information up the spinal cord to the thalamus. In the thalamus the signal will be passed to a third-order neuron that will take the signal to a specific region of the brain that will process the information.

Specific Afferent Tracts

Within the spinal cord, afferent tracts are also called ascending tracts. These tracts are divided into groups that carry similar sensory information. Some of these tracts are the gracile fasciculus, cuneate fasciculus, and spinothalamic. These tracts are named for where the neuron's cell body is located and where it will synapse on to the next neuron. These pathways can vary on which side of the spinal cord the signal travels after being received in the body. Some of the pathways enter the spinal cord and travel on the contralateral side to the brain. Other pathways enter the spinal cord and travel on the ipsilateral side and then cross in the brain.

Pain, however, is considered to be one of the most important sensory systems; this is because an animal must know if its body is hurt and how to self-preserve. Thus, pain afferent tracts are brought to both sides of the spinal cord. When pain occurs, the afferent tracts on the ipsilateral side of the pain will carry the information toward the brain as well as send the information to the contralateral side of the spinal cord, so it too can send the pain information to the brain. This allows pain to have a "backup" system to ensure that the pain information reaches the brain for interpretation.

The gracile fasciculus (Latin meaning "thin bundle") receives signals from the mid-thoracic and lower parts of the body. Below the sixth thoracic vertebra, the gracile fasciculus makes up the posterior column of the spinal cord. This pathway carries vibration, visceral pain, deep touch, discriminative touch, and proprioception signals for the lower limbs and lower trunk of the body. After the sixth vertebra the posterior column of the spine becomes split between the gracile fasciculus in the medial portion and the cuneate fasciculus in the lateral portion of the column. The cuneate fasciculus (Latin meaning "wedge-shaped bundle") is responsible for signals from the upper limbs and chest. The cuneate fasciculus is larger than the gracile fasciculus because in mammals (and particularly in humans) the forelimbs or arms carry much more sensory information than the hind limbs or legs. This is because the hands are used to grasp small items and have more sensory receptors than most body regions. The types of signals that the cuneate fasciculus pathway carries are the same as those of the gracile fasciculus. From the sixth thoracic vertebra up, the posterior column is divided unequally between the cuneate fasciculus and the gracile fasciculus. These two pathways lead to the ipsilateral side of the medulla oblongata of the brainstem. From the medulla oblongata the gracile and cuneate pathways cross and form the medial lemniscus, which leads to the contralateral thalamus. From here, third-order neural fibers lead to the cerebral cortex of the brain where the sensory information will be processed.

The spinothalamic tract is another major tract of the afferent nervous system. This tract along with some smaller tracts form the anterolateral system in the spinal cord. This tract is responsible for carrying signals for pain, temperature, pressure, tickle, itch, and light or crude touch. Within the anterolateral system, the first-order neurons end in the posterior horn of the spinal cord where the second-order neurons carry the signals to the contralateral side of the spinal cord and up the cord to the thalamus. The signals are then passed on to third-order neurons that take the information to the cerebral cortex to be processed.

Stephen Mazurkivich and Jennifer L. Hellier

See also: Discriminative Touch; Nociception; Sensory Receptors; Somatosensory Cortex; Somatosensory System; Taste System; Touch; Vestibular System

Further Reading

Spilman, Bernard. (2003). Ascending spinal tracts. In *Neurokinesiology: A new path to human health.* Retrieved from http://neurokinesiology.nuxit.net/Neurological_Background/ascending_spinal_tracts.html

AGE-RELATED HEARING LOSS

Age-related hearing loss (ARHL), also called presbycusis, describes the gradual progressive loss of hearing that people experience as they age. Twenty-five percent of people aged 65–74 and 50 percent of people 75 and older have disabling hearing loss (NIDCD, 2010). However, the majority of older adults suffer from a lesser, nondisabling degree of hearing loss. ARHL often affects hearing in both ears and leads to difficulty hearing and understanding speech in noisy environments. Current treatments focus on restoring hearing through the use of hearing aids.

History

Hearing loss from various causes has been described throughout history, with several attempted techniques to improve hearing. In the 1600s, hollow cones called ear trumpets were placed in the ear to help amplify sound waves and improve hearing. Electronic hearing aids became available in the late 1800s, with constant improvement in the technology throughout the 20th century.

Tuning Fork Test

Health care providers may use a tuning fork to test a patient's hearing ability; that is, to determine if a patient has a specific type of deafness or difficulty in hearing certain tones. There are two specific tests that use a tuning fork: the Rinne test and the Weber test. These examinations are named after the otologist or physician that created the assay: Drs. Heinrich Adolf Rinne (1819–1868) and Ernst Heinrich Weber (1795–1878), respectively. Using a tuning fork gives a physician a quick and easy tool to determine the patient's general level of hearing or deafness.

The tuning fork contains two prongs of equal length and a handle. It is usually made of different metals such as aluminum, magnesium alloy, or steel. The health care provider will strike the prongs against their hand or a table. This will cause the prongs to vibrate at a certain frequency—preferably 512 Hertz (Hz)—based on the properties of the metal, and the tuning fork will produce a specific tone.

If the vibrating tuning fork is placed on the skull behind an ear, the physician is testing the conduction of sound through bones. If the vibrating fork is placed near an ear, the physician is testing the conduction of sound through air. This is called the Rinne test, which determines if the patient has deafness due to bone or air conduction. To test if a patient has a hearing loss in only one ear—termed asymmetrical hearing loss—the doctor will use the Weber test.

Materials:

Volunteer
512 Hz tuning fork (can be purchased on Amazon.com) or other metallic instrument

Directions:

Rinne test: Gently hit the tuning fork on a table or the palm of your hand. This will make the tuning fork vibrate. Place the end of the handle of the vibrating fork on any bony prominence near and behind the ear. Ask the person to tell you when they no longer hear the tone. Note the duration of time from the start of the test to when the person cannot hear the tone. Next, move the vibrating tuning fork tines perpendicular to the front of the ear canal, about 1 centimeter away. Ask the person to tell you when they no longer hear the tone and note the time. Compare the time differences between each location. Repeat this same test with the other ear.

Weber test: Place the vibrating tuning fork handle on the skull in the middle of the forehead, the middle of the top of the head, or along the midline of the face. Ask the person if the sound is louder in the left ear, right ear, or if both ears hear the tone at the same volume.

Jennifer L. Hellier

Types and Symptoms

ARHL describes the process where people gradually lose hearing as they age. ARHL is often experienced first in the higher pitches. There are several changes in the inner ear related to aging that can explain the decreased sensitivity to sound and decreased ability to understand speech.

In a normal ear, sound waves enter the external ear canal and reach the eardrum, which will then vibrate. These vibrations are transferred through the small bones in the middle ear to the cochlea. The cochlea is fluid filled; the vibrations reaching the cochlea are detected by specialized hair cells as a wave. The hair cells in the cochlea transmit information as a nerve signal to the brain.

Several types of structural changes can cause age-related hearing loss. Hair cells in the cochlea can be damaged, so that they can no longer receive information to transmit to the brain. Damage to the hair cells results in hearing loss for pitches in the higher frequencies. Alternatively, changes in the blood supply to the cochlea can decrease hearing. Hearing loss from cochlear wall damage results in loss of hearing across a range of tones from low to high. Lastly, ARHL can result from changes in the nerve link from the cochlea to the brain. Often this type of hearing loss causes problems understanding speech.

Symptoms of ARHL are a gradual decrease in the ability to hear. This hearing loss is often first noticed in high-pitched sounds, but can include a variety of pitches. Patients may report difficulty in hearing conversations in noisy environments, understanding speech, or confusing words or sounds. Partners may report communication frustrations.

Treatment

A medical professional will determine the cause of hearing loss. This investigation will include taking a history of symptoms and considering current and past medication use. The health care professional will also examine the ear for mechanical problems such as wax buildup. Once all causes have been investigated, a patient may be diagnosed with ARHL.

Treatment for ARHL involves providing the patient with the best amplification possible. In order to determine which type of hearing aid is appropriate, audiologists perform detailed testing to identify the range of hearing affected and the degree of loss. Current digital hearing aids are programmable to accommodate hearing loss in various ranges and are able to automatically adjust to various sound environments.

Outcomes

ARHL is degenerative. Hearing loss will continue to worsen over time, often at a slow and steady rate. Currently there are no known ways to slow or stop these age-related changes. Hearing aids are available, however, that can restore hearing in the ranges that have been lost, allowing patients to communicate more easily and engage in most activities.

Among patients who seek treatment, most have a positive outcome in terms of restoring hearing and the ability to engage in activities involving hearing. It should be noted, however, that many patients who could benefit from assistive technologies to improve their hearing do not seek help.

Future

As our population ages, more patients will be managing ARHL. Public education could raise awareness of ARHL and the availability of hearing aids to improve hearing.

In addition to developing better assistive devices for communication, research may reveal other therapies that could delay or reverse ARHL. Current areas of research relevant to ARHL include use of antioxidants to reverse or delay hearing loss, stem cell therapy in the cochlea, and cochlear implants. Research preventing or reversing ARHL will improve quality of life and decrease social isolation for those impacted.

Lisa A. Rabe

See also: Auditory Hallucinations; Auditory System; Cochlea; Cochlear Implants; Deafness; Ear Protection

Further Reading

Huang, Tina. (2007). Age-related hearing loss. *Minnesota Medicine, 90*(10), 48–50.
NIDCD: National Institute on Deafness and Other Communication Disorders. (2014). Quick statistics. Retrieved from http://www.nidcd.nih.gov/health/statistics/Pages/quick.aspx

AGEUSIA

Ageusia is the loss of taste functions in the tongue. These functions include but are not limited to detecting sweetness, sourness, bitterness, and saltiness. The tongue can only detect texture and differentiate between those functions. Because of this, most of our sense of taste actually comes from the sense of smell. Ageusia is diagnosed by an otolaryngologist (ear, nose, and throat specialist) by measuring the lowest concentration of taste quality one can detect or recognize.

Causes

The loss of taste can be a side effect or a primary sign or symptom of a disease process. Thus, ageusia is caused by a number of issues including but not limited to (1) neurological damage, (2) endocrine system problems, (3) cancers of the mouth and tongue, (4) side effects of medications in cardiac and extracardiac vascular diseases, or (5) other causes. Bell's palsy, familial dysautonomia, and multiple sclerosis are diseases that are commonly associated with neurological damage to the cranial nerves that supply the tongue and provide the sensation of taste, thus causing ageusia. These nerves are the glossopharyngeal—or cranial nerve IX—and chorda tympani nerve, which is a branch of the facial nerve—or cranial nerve VII. Specifically, the chordatympani nerve passes through and innervates the front two-thirds of the tongue while the glossopharyngeal nerve passes through and innervates the back third of the tongue.

Disorders of the endocrine system such as Cushing's syndrome, hypothyroidism, and diabetes mellitus have also been known to cause ageusia. These are generally due to an imbalance of hormones, either over- or underexposure. These hormone levels are necessary to maintain homeostasis of the body. In Cushing's syndrome, there is a prolonged exposure to cortisol, which can also lead to issues including but not limited to high blood pressure, abnormal obesity, and weak muscles. Conversely, hypothyroidism is when a person's thyroid is underactive, resulting in a decreased production of thyroid hormone by the thyroid gland. Hypothyroidism can lead to a person having increased weight gain, fatigue, dry skin and hair, and a poor ability to tolerate cold. Multiple sclerosis is a demyelinating disease in which the myelin—insulation and covering of nerve cell axons—in the brain and spinal cord are damaged, resulting in slower and/or lost transmission of nerve signals. When damaged, parts of the nervous system cannot communicate with each other, causing symptoms such as loss of sensitivity, muscle weakness, and feeling tired. Other causes of ageusia include but are not limited to tobacco use, denture use, cancer, and renal failure.

Treatment

The treatment of ageusia is solely dependent on the source of the disease. If it is due to tobacco use, then a primary care provider can help a person work on quitting or reducing nicotine intake. If it is due to an endocrine or a neurological problem, then common treatments are changing a person's medication(s), diet, and/or lifestyle. Sometimes surgery may be effective in treating ageusia, but it should be an option only when all other treatments have been thoroughly tried. If ageusia is caused purely by a person's older age, then no known medical treatments are available. It is a permanent disorder and all that can be done is to learn how to cope with the reduced or loss of taste. Health care providers can help a patient learn how to prepare foods that have more color and spices in order to stimulate any remaining taste ability along with visual stimulation of the food. This has been shown to help individuals with ageusia still obtain healthy nutrition through eating food.

Renee Johnson

See also: Dysgeusia; Familial Dysautonomia; Taste Bud; Taste System

Further Reading

Ksouda, Kamilia, Hanen Affes, Boutheyna Hammami, Zouheir Sahnoun, Rim Atheymen, Serria Hammami, & Khaled Mounir Zeghal. (2011). Ageusia as a side effect of clopidogrel treatment. *Indian Journal of Pharmacology, 43*(3), 350–351. http://dx.doi .org/10.4103/0253-7613.81498. Retrieved from http://www.ncbi.nlm.nih.gov/pmc /articles/PMC3113393/

Maheswaran, T., P. Abikshyeet, G. Sitra, S. Gokulanathan, V. Vaithiyanadane, & S. Jeelani. (2014). Gustatory dysfunction. *Journal of Pharmacy & Bioallied Sciences, 6*(Suppl. 1), S30–33. http://dx.doi.org/10.4103/0975-7406.137257. Retrieved from http://www .ncbi.nlm.nih.gov/pmc/articles/PMC4157276/

AGNOSIA

Try to identify the following object based on a description of its parts: four wheels, four doors, a front and rear windshield, headlights, taillights, seatbelts, and a steering wheel. Clearly, what is being described is a car. Now imagine being able to look at a car and identify all of those separate parts, and be able to understand the car's purpose, but not be able to identify the object as a whole. This curious disorder is referred to as agnosia.

First coined by Austrian neurologist Sigmund Freud (1856–1939) in 1891, agnosias are disorders of recognition in patients who have fully intact primary sensations, meaning patients are not blind, deaf, or have any other sensory deficits. Criteria for diagnosis of agnosia include failure to recognize an object, normal perception of the object excluding an elementary sensory disorder, ability to name the object once it is recognized, and absence of generalized dementia.

Agnosias usually only affect one sensory modality, for example, one may not be able to identify a cookie by sight, but will be able to identify it by taste and smell. They are defined in terms of the specific sensory modality affected and generally fall into the categories of visual, auditory, or tactile.

Visual Agnosias

Visual agnosias are the best studied form of this disorder and are associated frequently with forms of brain injury such as a lesion, stroke, and/or brain trauma. Visual object agnosia falls into two categories: apperceptive visual object agnosia and associative visual object agnosia.

Apperceptive agnosia is exemplified in the situation described in the introduction. Patients can pick out features of an object correctly, but are unable to appreciate the whole object, they literally only see the trees, not the forest. The right parietal cortex has been identified as important to visual processing of objects; however, this syndrome has also been identified in patients with bilateral occipital lesions, where vision is primarily located.

Associative agnosia has to do with recognition of appropriately perceived objects. Patients with associative agnosia may be able to copy or match drawings of an object they cannot name, or identify it using other senses, such as seen in the cookie example. This deficit is usually associated with bilateral posterior hemisphere lesions involving the fusiform or occipitotemporal gyri. Additionally patients with this form of agnosia often have other related recognition deficits such as color agnosia (cannot name or identify a color by sight, but this is not to be confused with being color-blind), prosopagnosia (see the following paragraph), and alexia (inability to see words or to read because of a brain defect).

Prosopagnosia is an interesting form of this disorder in which patients are unable to recognize faces, even of family and friends, and instead must focus on specific details associated with individuals. In severe cases of prosopagnosia, a patient may not even recognize his or her own face. Clearly in this patient population small changes to things such as hair color and aging can be problematic.

Auditory Agnosias

Similar to visual agnosia, auditory disorders range from primary auditory syndromes of cortical deafness to partial deficits or recognition of specific types of sounds. These disorders are also associated with bilateral cerebral lesions involving the temporal lobes, as this region contains the primary auditory cortex. Auditory agnosias can be divided into pure word deafness, pure auditory nonverbal agnosia, phonagnosia, and pure amusia.

Pure word deafness involves the inability to comprehend spoken words, but with the ability to hear and recognize nonverbal sounds. The area of the brain most often associated with this disorder is Wernicke's area in the left hemisphere. Patients with this disorder may also experience paraphasic speech, meaning they use unintended or inappropriate words in an attempt to communicate. For example, they may say "purple" when they were meaning to say "friend."

Auditory nonverbal agnosia refers to patients who have preserved hearing and language comprehension but have lost the ability to identify nonverbal sounds. For example, a patient may not be able to identify animal sounds, or sounds associated with specific objects such as an alarm.

Phonagnosia is similar to prosopagnosia; however, instead of not being able to recognize faces, these patients have difficulty recognizing familiar people by their voices. Failure to recognize a familiar voice may involve a right parietal lobe locus corresponding to the specific area for recognition of faces. Related to this defect is auditory affective agnosia, or failure to recognize emotional intonation of speech.

Amusia is the loss of musical abilities after focal brain lesions. Recognition of melodies and musical tones is a right temporal lobe function, whereas analysis of pitch, rhythm, and tempo involves the left temporal lobe. Famously, the composer Maurice Ravel (1875–1937) suffered a progressive aphasia, which took his ability to read or write music, but not his capacity to listen and appreciate it.

Taste Agnosias

Patients with lesions of the parietal cortex may have preserved the ability to feel pinpricks, temperature, vibration, and proprioception, but fail to identify objects in the contralateral hand or recognize numbers or letters written by the opposite side of the body. These deficits are called astereognosis (if both hands are affected, it results in the inability to identify an object by active touch and without any other sensory input) and agraphesthesia (the inability to know what number or letter is drawn on their skin by an examiner) and tend to represent deficits of cortical sensory loss rather than full tactile agnosias.

Stephanie Dunlap

See also: Color Blindness; Sacks, Oliver Wolf

Further Reading

Farah, Martha. (2004). *Visual agnosia.* Cambridge, MA: MIT Press.
Kirshner, Howard S. (2002). Agnosias. In *Behavioral neurology: Practical science of mind and brain.* Boston, MA: Butterworth Heinemann.
National Institute of Neurological Disorders and Stroke (NINDS). (2007). *NINDS agnosia information page.* Retrieved from http://www.ninds.nih.gov/disorders/agnosia/agnosia.htm

AMBLYOPIA

Amblyopia, or lazy eye, causes decreased vision in a child's eye despite normal eye structure. Three to 5 percent of children are affected by amblyopia. When a child is young, several conditions can cause an eye to send a blurry image to the brain. Then, during visual development, a child's brain gets used to receiving a blurry image; even if the underlying cause of vision impairment is addressed, the brain may not be able to interpret the clear visual image, resulting in reduced vision. If not treated, amblyopia causes a permanent decrease or loss of vision in the affected eye. With treatment, most children have improved vision.

History

Hippocrates (460–377 BCE) used the term amblyopia to describe diminished visual acuity. The treatment at that time focused on the whole person rather than the eye, because the eye problem was viewed as a symptom of a larger problem in the body. Many cultures subsequently have records of treating amblyopia by attempting to strengthen the eyes directly.

By the 1700s in France, the field of ophthalmology was growing with hospitals and specialists dedicated to the eye. Georges-Louis Leclerc, Comte de Buffon (1707–1788), a French naturalist, described occlusion (patching) therapy. Patching therapy involves applying a patch to the stronger eye in order to strengthen the weaker eye. Working on a theory similar to patching, eye drops have also been used to block the vision in the stronger eye. Many therapies have been described for amblyopia, but the use of patching remains constant throughout history.

Types and Symptoms

Several underlying causes result in amblyopia. Strabismic amblyopia is caused by a misalignment of the eyes. Strabismus (also called crossed eye or eye turn) happens when the eye muscles fail to align the eyes symmetrically. The brain receives two different images from the eyes, and to resolve the images and see a single image, the brain ignores one image. Deprivation amblyopia results when the brain is not receiving input from an eye. Cataracts, for example, can decrease vision and lead to deprivation amblyopia as can other physical causes including drooping eyelids. Refractive amblyopia results when there is a significant difference between the prescription needed to correct each eye, causing the brain to suppress the eye sending the blurrier image.

Treatment

Treatment for amblyopia involves several steps and may take a year or longer to correct. The first step in treating amblyopia is to identify patients affected. Children with one eye functioning normally may not report vision difficulties. After the cause of amblyopia has been identified, appropriate treatment will be started. Correcting the misalignment of the eyes treats strabismic amblyopia. Eye muscles can be shortened or lengthened surgically. Nonsurgical treatments such as drug injections can weaken the muscles pulling the eye. Deprivation amblyopia is corrected by removing the visual block; treatments include cataract surgery, or addressing the cause of the drooping eyelid. Correcting the refractive difference between the eyes with glasses treats refractive amblyopia.

After the underlying condition causing the amblyopia has been corrected, the brain learns to interpret signals from both eyes. Patching the strong eye allows the brain to accept and interpret signals from the weaker eye, improving vision. Vision therapy may be designed to help the weaker eye improve, and unlike patching can be designed to encourage both eyes to work together.

Outcomes

Early diagnosis is key to preventing vision loss secondary to amblyopia. Because of the difficulty of detecting some forms of amblyopia and the finding that there is a window during which treatment is more successful, vision screening is recommended at each well child check with referrals to a pediatric eye specialist if needed. Many schools in the United States also offer vision screenings.

Treatment of amblyopia can reverse or reduce vision loss. Treatment of children younger than six years of age is often effective, with success rates cited of restoring near normal visual acuity in 50–75 percent of children. Recent literature (Scheiman et al., 2005) showed that treating older children also had benefits: up to 47 percent of children treated with glasses, patching, and eye drops for 2–6 hours per day showed more than a two-line improvement on an eye chart (a measure of improved visual acuity) after treatment.

Future

Additional research will reveal therapies appropriate for treating amblyopia and refine the amount of treatment time patients need to achieve maximal results. As more is understood about how the brain works, treatments will continue to focus on the brain and brain plasticity and may be offered to older patients, too.

Lisa A. Rabe

See also: Cataracts; Diplopia; Eye Protection; Ptosis; Strabismus

Further Reading

Scheiman, Mitchell M., Richard W. Hertle, Roy W. Beck, Allison R. Edwards, Eileen Birch, Susan A. Cotter, . . . & Susanna M. Tamkins. (2005). Randomized trial of treatment of amblyopia in children aged 7 to 17 years. *Archives of Ophthalmology, 123*(4), 437–447.

AMERICAN SIGN LANGUAGE

For persons who are deaf or hard of hearing, it can be difficult to communicate with hearing individuals as well as with other deaf people. Thus, sign languages were developed for this reason. A sign language is a type of communication generated by different hand motions that may be combined with facial expressions or body positions. However, not all sign languages are the same throughout the world, meaning that a hand gesture with a facial expression in one region of the world may have another meaning in a different country. In 2015, there were 141 known sign languages in use in multiple countries and regions, including the United Kingdom, Africa, Japan, France, and North America, to name a few. In the United States and English-speaking parts of Canada, the primary language for the deaf is American Sign Language or ASL.

Language acquisition is crucial to learn within the first two years after birth so that a child's communication skills are developed. This is the same for learning American Sign Language. The earlier a deaf child is taught American Sign Language, the better his or her communications skills will be as well as his or her emotional development. Studies have shown that deaf children born to hearing-impaired parents who sign American Sign Language will learn ASL at the same rate as hearing children will learn spoken language. However, 9 out of 10 deaf children are born to hearing parents. Thus, if the parents do not know sign language, the deaf child's communication development can be significantly delayed.

History

It is estimated that American Sign Language was developed more than 200 years ago by intermixing local sign language with Langue des Signes Française (or French Sign Language). However, the American School for the Deaf has since standardized gestures with facial expressions to represent words and developed standard American Sign Language letters for fingerspelling English words that do not have a sign, thus making American Sign Language a complex and rich language. Today, American Sign Language and French Sign Language are different languages, although some components are still similar. Nonetheless, a person signing American Sign Language would not be able to understand a person using French Sign Language and vice versa.

American Sign Language vs. Spoken Language

Spoken language is the process of forming and saying sounds to produce words by moving the mouth and tongue. Pushing air through different shapes of the mouth and/or tongue produces unique sounds for each letter or letter combination. However, deaf people cannot hear these sounds and lip reading can be difficult, particularly in rapid speech. Since some words can be read, it was recognized that the best way for a deaf person to communicate with others is through sight.

In spoken language, there are specific language rules for sentence structure and grammar. This is similar in American Sign Language; however, ASL does not follow the same rules as English but does have the fundamental features of a language—subject, verb, object components; word order; punctuation, and so on. For example, in spoken language to ask a question, a person will raise the pitch of his or her voice at the end of the sentence. In American Sign Language to show that a question is being asked, the signer will raise the eyebrows, widen the eyes, and tilt the body forward.

Lastly, spoken languages tend to have several dialects depending on the location of a community—a southern drawl, nasal pronunciations, and so on. American Sign Language has similar dialect and regional affectations. Specifically, a sign for a word may have a slightly different form or shape of the hand or gesture in one region compared to the standardized gesture. The rhythm of signing either faster or slower is another way to identify an American Sign Language dialect.

Jennifer L. Hellier

See also: Auditory System; Cochlea; Cochlear Implants; Deafness

Further Reading

Lewis, M. Paul, Gary F. Simons, & Charles D. Fennig (Eds.). (2015). Deaf sign language. In *Ethnologue: Languages of the World* (18th ed.), SIL International. Retrieved from http://www.ethnologue.com/subgroups/sign-language

Meir, Irit, Wendy Sandler, Carol Padden, & Mark Aronoff. (2010). Emerging sign languages. In *The Oxford Handbook of Deaf Studies, Language, and Education*, Vol. 2. Oxford Handbooks Online. Eds. M. Marschark & P. Spencer. Retrieved from http://sandlersignlab .haifa.ac.il/html/html_eng/pdf/EMERGING_SIGN_LANGUAGES.pdf

National Institute on Deafness and Other Communication Disorders (NIDCD). (2015). American Sign Language. Retrieved from https://www.nidcd.nih.gov/health/american -sign-language

AMERICANS WITH DISABILITIES ACT

The Americans with Disabilities Act (ADA) of 1990 is a law that prohibits discrimination against people with disabilities in employment, transportation, public accommodation, communications, and governmental activities. It also mandates the establishment of TDD (Telecommunications Device for the Deaf)/telephone relay services (United States Department of Labor, 2015). The 101st U.S. Congress enacted the ADA, which was signed by President George H. W. Bush (1924–) on July 26, 1990. In 2008, President George W. Bush (1946–) signed the ADA Amendments Act of 2008, which included some changes from the original act of 1990 and became effective on January 1, 2009.

History

During the late 1980s, voices to enact federal legislation to give more civil rights to Americans with disabilities gained support. Exclusion and segregation due to a person's disability or disabilities came to be viewed as discrimination against this population in the United States. The disability community fought in the courts, streets, and media in order to broaden their civil rights in areas such as education and employment. In 1988, Connecticut Republican senator Lowell P. Weicker (1931–) and California Democratic representative Anthony Lee "Tony" Coelho (1942–) introduced the first version of the ADA to the 100th Congress in April 1988 during the presidency of Ronald Reagan (1911–2004). Subsequently a joint hearing was held before the Senate Subcommittee on Disability Policy and the House Subcommittee on Select Education. In 1989, Senators Thomas Richard Harkin (1939–, Democrat, Iowa) and David Ferdinand Durenberger (1934–, Republican, Minnesota) along with Representatives Tony Coelho and Hamilton Fish IV (1926–1996, Republican, New York) introduced the new ADA bill to the 101st Congress, and it was passed into law.

Titles

The ADA of 1990 contains five titles that describe the rights and regulations protecting individuals with disabilities in the United States. Title I of the ADA prohibits private employers, state and local governments, employment agencies, and labor unions from discriminating against qualified individuals with disabilities in job application, hiring, compensation, training, and other terms, conditions, and privileges of employment. The individual with a disability is a person who has a physical or mental impairment that can substantially limit one or more major life activities. However, if the individual is capable of handling the essential functions of the job, then he or she cannot be discriminated against in selection, accommodation, and other terms and conditions. Title I also covers medical examinations and inquiries, and testing for drug and alcohol abuse. More regulations were added to the original act, such as Title II, which prohibits discrimination in public transportations. Title III of the ADA protects individuals with disabilities from discrimination in public accommodations such as services and facilities in education, restaurants, and recreational places. Title IV of the ADA ensures that telecommunication companies in the United States have equipment services designed for individuals with hearing impairment, and other disabilities concerned with using the telecommunication services. Lastly, Title V of the ADA contains other miscellaneous provisions that protect individuals with disabilities, including but not limited to insurance, relationship to other laws, and definitions of "reasonable accommodations and modifications."

ADA Amendments Act of 2008

The ADA was amended in terms of defining "disability" and extended the scope of its protection to more people. The current text of the ADA includes these amendments made from the ADA Amendments Act of 2008, which became effective on January 1, 2009. Originally a public law format, the ADA was republished in the United States Code, which classifies laws based on subject matter. Thus, the ADA's titles are coded in different sections of the United States Code. Specifically, Titles I, II, III, and V can be found in the United States Code under Title 42, chapter 126, starting at section 12101, while Title IV is filed under Title 47, chapter 5.

Significance of the Act

The Americans with Disabilities Act of 1990 ensured that individuals with disabilities are not discriminated against in terms of services, privileges, opportunities, and safety in public areas, private and public employment, transportation, and telecommunications. Previously, individuals with disabilities had disadvantages in using public services as well as getting employed or reaping benefits from companies and unions. With this act, it became illegal to discriminate against people with disabilities.

Paul Hong

See also: Blindness; Color Blindness; Congenital Insensitivity to Pain; Deafness; Meniere's Disease; Phantom Pain; Seizures

Further Reading

Mayerson, Arlene. (1992). The history of the Americans with Disabilities Act: A movement perspective. *Disability Rights Education & Defense Fund.* Retrieved from http://dredf .org/news/publications/the-history-of-the-ada/

United States Department of Labor. (2015). *Disability resources.* Retrieved from http://www .dol.gov/dol/topic/disability/

United States Department of Labor. (2015). *Disability resources: Americans with Disabilities Act.* Retrieved from http://www.dol.gov/dol/topic/disability/ada.htm

AMYGDALA

The amygdala is a relatively small structure composed of several nuclei located deep within the temporal lobe. The name amygdala is derived from the Greek word *amygdale*, which means "almond," denoting its general size and shape. Although its Latin name is corpus amygdaloideum, it is also called the amygdala nuclei, amygdaloid region, and corpus amygdalae. The amygdala is considered a component of the limbic system; however, the criteria for determining what is part of the limbic system are not uniformly accepted among scientists. Nonetheless, the amygdala has been clearly associated with certain emotions, especially fear. This association with emotions has determined its classification as a limbic system component.

History

The first scientists to formally recognize the amygdala in the early 19th century named it for its size and shape since its function was still unknown. Until recently, researchers had only vague notions about the amygdala and were not interested in exploring its function. Early studies suggested that it was tied to vigilance and attention, much like an alarm system. More recent research has confirmed this as one of its many functions and has explored further connections that allow it to participate in a wide range of behaviors such as fear conditioning and decision making. The simplest summary of the amygdala's function is its ability to recognize and respond to fear stimulus. Further research, however, is continuing to expand knowledge of its function and connections with other regions of the brain, and many researchers are finding that its function extends beyond simple emotion.

Anatomy and Physiology

The number of nuclear groups associated with the amygdala varies depending on how neurologists choose to split up the 13 interconnected nuclei. To date, the number of groups may range from about three to six. Without a standard set of terms that all scientists agree upon and refer to in their studies, literature on the amygdala can be tricky to decipher. Scientists have not yet agreed upon anything because neuroimaging technology is not precise enough for the complexity of the connections of the amygdala. This makes it difficult to separate nuclei into clearly bordered regions. Most authors subdivide it into three portions: (1) the basolateral nuclear group, which is the largest portion; (2) the centromedial group, the second largest portion; and (3) the cortical nucleus, also known as the olfactory amygdala for its connections with the olfactory bulb and olfactory cortex.

The stria terminalis and the ventral amygdalofugal pathway are two main fiber bundles connecting the amygdala to other parts of the brain. The stria terminalis enables the amygdala to activate the hypothalamus, which activates the autonomic nervous system, or the "fight-or-flight" response. The ventral amygdalofugal pathway connects the amygdala to the brainstem, affecting hormones and behavior such as eating, drinking, and sex. The basolateral group of the amygdala is directly connected to the insular cortex, orbital cortex, and frontal lobe. There are also projections to the hippocampus, a part of the brain responsible for storing memories. Some research has also suggested that it affects which memories are stored by categorizing the importance of a memory. Neuroimaging studies indicate that the amygdala helps to recognize both basic and complex facial emotions through access to emotional memory in the hippocampus.

Individual neurons within the amygdala have been found to have specific functions. Some neurons respond separately to sight, sound, smell, taste, and touch stimuli. Some also respond specifically to faces. The most abundant type is the visual responder neurons, which may explain why the strongest neural activity in the amygdala occurs in response to fearful faces. Studies in which only selective parts of a person's face, such as the eye or mouth region, were revealed show that the amygdala responds more strongly to expression in the eye region than any other part of the face.

The amygdala, particularly the central nucleus, has been shown to play a role in detecting and resolving ambiguity, that is, when a situation can be interpreted in more than one way. For example, because fearful expressions recruit a stronger response from the amygdala than angry expressions, scientists hypothesize that fearful expressions signal ambiguity in a situation—they present a sign of imposing threat without giving very much information about the threat. Angry expressions cause a response in the amygdala to a lesser degree because anger in the eyes is less ambiguous than fear in the eyes.

Once the amygdala is activated by a frightening stimulus, it begins the process of attention. Amygdala experiments with cats have shown that after a loud noise, the cat ceases all activities, perks up its ears, and orients itself in the direction of the noise. This series of actions is termed "attention response" or "arrest response." The researchers conducting this experiment hypothesized that this is the amygdala's attempt to resolve the ambiguity of the noise, urging the cat to see if there is a threat by finding out where the noise came from.

Alyssa M. Wienecke

See also: Autonomic Nervous System; Brain Anatomy; Limbic System; Olfactory System

Further Reading

Cohen, Lisa J. (2011). *The handy psychology answer book: Your smart reference.* Detroit, MI: Visible Ink Press.

Díaz-Mataix, Lorenzo, Lucille Tallot, & Valerie Doyère. (2014). The amygdala: A potential player in timing CS-US intervals. *Behavioral Processes, 101*, 112–122. http://dx.doi. org/10.1016/j.beproc.2013.08.007

ANESTHESIA

Anesthesia is a pharmacologically induced and reversible loss of responsiveness. It is used in surgery or other procedures to block pain sensations in patients. The word anesthesia is derived from Greek meaning "without sensation" and is used to describe the state of analgesia (meaning painless or numbness). These effects can be from a single drug or a combination of drugs that provides a very specific combination of effects depending on the surgical needs.

History

During ancient Greek and Roman periods, some plants (like opium) were known to provide euphoric effects as well as make a person unconscious. It was this knowledge that 12th-century Arab physicians used to develop the first documented inhaled anesthetic. It was said that a sponge soaked in a dissolved solution of opium, mandragora, hemlock juice, and other substances would be dampened and placed under the nose of the patient just prior to surgery. However, the amounts had to be regulated as too much of the solution could cause death.

In the following centuries, volatile liquids and gases were developed for inhalational anesthetics including ether (previously known as "sweet vitriol"), nitrous oxide (also known as "laughing gas"), and chloroform. It is well documented that English physician John Snow (1813–1858) used chloroform in 1853 to anesthetize Queen Victoria during the birth of her eighth child, Prince Leopold. Dr. Snow is also noted as one of the first physicians to calculate the doses needed for successful surgical anesthesia for chloroform and ether as well as developing the equipment used to volatilize liquids into inhaled gases.

Types of Anesthesia

Volatile liquids, inhaled gases, and some manmade drugs are used as anesthetics. Specifically, the goal of an anesthetic is to provide a reversible loss of responsiveness, meaning putting a person, body part, or body region "to sleep" that will eventually wake up. The reversible loss of responsiveness may include the loss of muscle reflexes, the loss of sensation, and a decreased stress response. Some anesthesia may induce all of the above.

Within medicine, there is a specialty called *anesthesiology* in which the physician is an expert at putting patients to sleep for the surgery and then waking them up at the end of the procedure. An anesthesiologist may also be called an anesthetist, meaning a person who professionally administers anesthesia. Because of the delicate procedure of inducing a reversible loss of responsiveness, anesthesiologists must constantly monitor patients' breathing, heart rate, blood pressure, and body temperature so that they will not have complications while under anesthesia.

Today there are four main types of anesthesia: local, regional, general, and dissociative. Local anesthesia is mostly used when a specific location on the body needs to have no sensation. For example, local anesthesia is used by dentists to fill a cavity in a tooth, by podiatrists to remove a toenail, or by dermatologists to remove a mole on the skin.

Regional anesthesia is used to block sensation to a region of a body, such as the lower half of the body. Regional anesthesia is used during an epidural or a spinal block. The anesthetic is injected within the spinal column space below the spinal cord, which blocks the transmission of nerve signals to the spinal cord. This is the preferred method of anesthesia during a Caesarean section (C-section) for complicated childbirths.

General anesthesia is performed when a person undergoes major surgery as it renders a person unconscious with no sensation. This occurs by inhibiting the sensory and motor functions of the peripheral and central nervous systems as well as blocking the sympathetic division of the autonomic nervous system. General anesthesia would be used during knee surgery as well as during heart surgery.

Finally, dissociative anesthesia is used when the higher brain regions need to be disassociated from the lower brain regions, causing the person to feel detached from the environment. These types of drugs are also called hallucinogens because they alter the perception of sight and sound while putting the person in a dreamlike state. Hallucinogens may be used in combination with other drugs to help induce general anesthesia.

Modern Anesthesiology

Today, anesthesiologists must understand how to use the complex equipment needed for the different types of anesthetics as well as how to properly calculate doses for the correct level of anesthesia for the patient. Since a person can die from the anesthesia, the American Society of Anesthesiologists (ASA) has established minimum guidelines for monitoring patients under anesthesia to reduce the chance of death. These include measuring the electrographic activity of the heart, heart rate, blood pressure, breathing rates (inspired and expired gases), saturation of oxygen within the blood, and body temperature.

Patricia A. Bloomquist

See also: Autonomic Nervous System; Central Nervous System; Discriminative Touch; Nociception; Peripheral Nervous System; Peripheral Neuropathy

Further Reading

Smith, Eckehard A., Astrid G. Stucke, & Edward J. Zuperku. (2012). Effects of anesthetics, sedatives, and opioids on ventilatory control. *Comprehensive Physiology*, 2(4), 281–367.

ANOPHTHALMIA

Anophthalmia is a rare disorder in which a child is born without an eye or eyes. The absence of both eyes is more common. It is characterized by a complete lack of ocular tissue, and affected children typically have small eye sockets. This disorder develops during pregnancy and can occur along with other birth defects or by itself. It is believed to occur during development, resulting when the anterior neural tube fails to develop. There are many possible causes of anophthalmia, but many times the exact cause is unknown. Possible causes include mutations, both genetic and random, abnormalities of the chromosomes, and environmental factors such as drugs, radiation, and chemicals. The National Eye Institute reported an occurrence rate of 0.18 per 10,000 births in the United States (National Eye Institute, 2009).

Types

There are three classifications of anophthalmia: primary, secondary, and degenerative. In primary anophthalmia, the part of the brain responsible in forming the eye fails, resulting in no eye tissue whatsoever. In secondary anophthalmia, some eye tissue or very small eyes were present as the eye started developing but stopped developing for unknown reasons. In degenerative anophthalmia, the eye began forming, but at some point degenerated for unknown reasons. One explanation for this could be a lack of eye blood supply (Verma & Fitzpatrick, 2007).

Diagnosis

Anophthalmia can be diagnosed in several ways. A prenatal diagnosis can be made using a transvaginal ultrasound. After the baby is born, imaging using CT (computed tomography) and/or MRI (magnetic resonance imaging) of the head and eye sockets, physical examination of the eye sockets and surrounding areas, genetic testing, and ultrasound can all be used to make a diagnosis. Some of the physical characteristics, both of the eyes and generally, of children born with anophthalmia include absence of extraocular muscles, deformed eyelids, possible absence of the lacrimal glands, cleft lip or palate, possible hearing loss, and some irregularities of the heart.

Treatment

The treatment for anophthalmia focuses on treating the bony growth of the child's face. The eye sockets play an important role in the bony and soft tissue growth and development of the face. Without proper treatment, the bones in the face will not grow properly and will lead to facial deformity. A child's face grows at a fast rate, so treatment must be started as soon as possible. Treatment involves the use of conformers, which are plastic devices that are placed in the child's eye sockets to help the bones in the face to develop correctly. Conformers enlarge the orbit and assist the face in developing to normal proportions. They also help to stimulate bone growth. As a child grows and develops, he or she will need different sized conformers. The number of conformers depends on each individual child, as no child grows at the same rate. Once the child is old enough and growth is maintained, a prosthetic eye may be used. This can help with overall appearances.

A child born with anophthalmia will need to see many different doctors for different treatments and overall care. The doctors will most likely include an ophthalmologist, an ocularist, and an oculoplastic surgeon. Surgical treatment may be recommended in some cases. Surgical procedures may include placement of inflatable expanders, eyelid surgery, or surgery for the eye sockets. Other treatments will include early and special intervention programs to help the child cope and learn to deal without vision, or limited vision. The first few years of a child's life are critical for development. Children with anophthalmia may experience developmental delays and may have learning difficulties or behavioral issues.

Risk Factors

Genetics may play a role in anophthalmia. Genetic testing may be a helpful diagnostic tool. Currently, research is being performed to help identify which genes are involved in eye development. Many genes have been identified that play a role, and it has been shown that changes, or mutations, can cause atypical eye development. Many times, there is no family history of anophthalmia. One syndrome that has been described is sometimes associated with anophthalmia. It is known as SOX2 (SRY [Sex Determining Region Y]-Box 2) syndrome, and people who have this syndrome are often born with anophthalmia. It has also been shown that 10–15 percent of people with anophthalmia affecting both of their eyes have SOX2 syndrome (Genetics Home Reference, 2016). SOX2 syndrome is autosomal dominant, but many times the disorder is caused by a new mutation and is not inherited. People with SOX2 syndrome may have other problems associated with the syndrome, other than anophthalmia. These can include seizures, a blocked esophagus, delayed growth, and genital abnormalities, which occur most often in males.

Shannen McNamara

See also: Blindness; Microphthalmia; National Organization for Rare Disorders; Optic Nerve; Visual System

Further Reading

Genetics Home Reference. (2016). *SOX2 anophthalmia syndrome.* Retrieved from http://ghr
   .nlm.nih.gov/condition/sox2-anophthalmia-syndrome
International Children's Anophthalmia Network (ICAN). (n.d.). *General information.* Re-
   trieved from http://www.anophthalmia.org/general_information/
National Eye Institute (NEI). (2009). Anophthalmia and microphthalmia. Retrieved from
   https://nei.nih.gov/health/anoph
Verma, Amit S., and David R. Fitzpatrick. (2007). Anophthalmia and microphthalmia.
   Orphanet Journal of Rare Diseases, 2, 47. http://dx.doi.org/10.1186/1750-1172-2-47

ANOSMIA

Anosmia is the inability to smell, whether the instance is acute (temporary) or chronic (permanent). Any deviation in people's ability to smell can adversely impact their quality of life and influence what and how much they eat, whom they talk to, and where they may go.

Disease

Olfactory dysfunction (reduced ability to smell) and anosmia (complete inability to smell) can have profound effects on a person's quality of life. In fact, a sudden onset of anosmia can affect a person's ability to cope emotionally and may lead to severe clinical depression, increasing the risk for suicide. A loss in olfactory function can arise from a variety of reasons with the most frequent causes being (1) upper respiratory tract infection (like a cold or a stuffy/runny nose), which can kill olfactory sensory neurons; (2) head trauma, which can sever olfactory sensory neurons axons; and (3) nasal and paranasal sinus disease, which can block airflow in the nasal passage. In a minority of cases, olfactory loss can arise from the inhalation of toxic chemicals, intranasal or intracranial tumors, and from congenital defects. Certain endocrine and psychiatric disorders have also been associated with a decrease or loss of olfactory function.

In some cases, a single nostril can lose the sense of smell. This may occur by an injury or minor trauma to the side of the head. The loss of smell to one side is called unilateral anosmia.

Signs, Symptoms, and Treatment

The loss of smell can be caused by multiple factors. Inflammation of the mucosal layer of the nasal passageway is the most common sign of acute anosmia. Inflammation can be caused by the common cold, flu, or allergies and may be resolved by anti-inflammatory medications, sleeping in a humidified room, and nasal sprays. There are three types of nasal sprays: decongestant, saline, and steroid. Decongestant nasal sprays work by reducing the blood vessel size in the mucosal layer of the nose that cause "stuffiness." These can be purchased over the counter (without a prescription) but should not be used for more than three days in a row. Continual use can become "addictive" and reduce the spray's effectiveness, resulting in a person's cold or flu worsening. Saline nasal sprays thin the mucus within a stuffy nose, allowing it to be easier to blow your nose and remove the mucus buildup. These do not contain medicine—like decongestant nasal sprays—and can be used as often as needed. Finally, a health care provider may prescribe a steroid nasal spray for a patient to improve stuffiness caused by allergies. These should only be used as prescribed.

Chronic causes of anosmia are lesions to the olfactory system and polyps that develop in the nose. Lesions to the smell centers of the brain (especially the temporal lobes) or to the olfactory sensory neurons can cause permanent damage to the sense of smell. In congenital anosmia, a rare disease, an infant is born without the ability to smell. This can be life-threatening as the infant will have difficulty smelling its mother's milk, which is necessary for survival. Polyps within the nose block the nasal turbinates, which in turn reduces airflow into the nasal passage. Nasal polyps are generally noncancerous and are thought to develop from chronic inflammation of the mucosal layer. Nasal polyps are often associated with allergies and/or asthma. Such polyps can be surgically removed if they are large enough to block the nasal passage and cause chronic sinusitis.

Jennifer L. Hellier

See also: Dysosmia; Interrelatedness of Taste and Smell; Olfactory Mucosa; Olfactory Nerve; Olfactory Sensory Neurons; Olfactory System; Phantosmia

Further Reading

Mayo Clinic. (2014). Loss of smell (anosmia). Retrieved from http://www.mayoclinic.org/symptoms/loss-of-smell/basics/definition/sym-20050804

National Institute on Deafness and Other Communication Disorders (NIDCD). (2013). NIH senior health: Problems with smell. Retrieved from http://nihseniorhealth.gov/problemswithsmell/aboutproblemswithsmell/01.html

National Institute on Deafness and Other Communication Disorders (NIDCD). (2014). Smell disorders. Retrieved from http://www.nidcd.nih.gov/health/smelltaste/smell.asp

ASSISTIVE TECHNOLOGY

Assistive technology (AT), often used synonymously with the term adaptive technology, is an overarching term that encompasses assistive, adaptive, and rehabilitative devices for individuals with disabilities. AT promotes autonomy by allowing users to accomplish tasks that would otherwise be impossible or extremely difficult to manage. Specific items, equipment, software, and products are used to increase, maintain, or improve the functional capabilities of individuals with disabilities. AT also includes the process used in selecting, locating, and using such devices.

History

As early as 950 BCE, examples of AT can be found. The "Cairo Toe" was discovered attached to the foot of a mummy buried in an Egyptian tomb at Luxor. Made of wood and leather, this is believed to be an ancient prosthesis. Discovered in an ancient Roman grave, a bronze leg from 300 BCE was a known mobility support device. As early as 1286, during the European Renaissance, traders introduced convex lenses developed from writings by Muslim scholars such as Ibn al-Haytham (965–1040). Ambroise Pare's (1510–1590) 16th-century book *Dix Livres de la Chirurgie* earned him the reputation of the father of modern surgery, with his detailed and advanced designs of mechanical prostheses. As human needs increased, our industriousness grew and the development of early AT gave us devices such as rudimentary ear trumpets, wheeled chairs, bifocals, dentures, braille, hearing aids, guide dogs, and text to speech communication tools. Today, devices are being developed at a rapid pace. With technological advances and rapidly expanding markets, AT has become widespread and increasingly available.

Legislation for Assistive Technology

In the United States, the Rehabilitation Act of 1973 (Public Law 93–112) was signed into law, prohibiting discrimination against individuals with disabilities in regard to employment and academic program admission. In 1975, the Education for All Handicapped Children Act (Public Law 94–142) was enacted. This monumental decision paved the way for millions of children with disabilities, ensuring that children with disabilities have access to education. Now known as the Individuals with Disabilities Education Act (IDEA), it guarantees every child with a disability access to a free, appropriate, public education (FAPE) in the least restrictive environment.

AT devices and services were first defined in federal law in the Individuals with Disabilities Education Act of 1990 (Public Law 101–476) as: "Any item, piece of equipment or product system, whether acquired commercially off the shelf, modified, or customized, that is used to increase, maintain, or improve the functional capabilities of children with disabilities" (Assistive Technology Industry Association, n.d.). These definitions remained unchanged until 2004 with the passage of the Individuals with Disabilities Education Improvement Act (Public Law 108–446) when an exemption to the definition of an assistive technology device was added to clarify a school system's responsibility to provide surgically implanted technology such as cochlear implants. The definition of an assistive technology device is very broad and gives Individualized Education Plan (IEP) teams the flexibility that they need to make decisions about appropriate devices for individual students.

Types of Assistive Technology

AT has grown to include a wide spectrum of equipment and products. Those with mobility impairments now have access to devices such as wheelchairs, transfer devices, walkers, and prostheses. These allow for independent mobility and the ability to perform daily living activities, such as feeding, toileting, dressing, grooming, and bathing. Tools and techniques to improve independence for those with visual impairments include products such as screen readers, screen magnifiers, braille and braille embossers, desktop video magnifiers, and screen magnification software. Individuals who are deaf or hard of hearing utilize a variety of assistive technologies that provide them with improved accessibility to information in numerous environments. Products such as hearing aids, assistive listening devices, and amplified telephone equipment allow for improved communication. People experiencing cognitive impairments have the opportunity to implement products that aid with attention, memory, self-regulation, navigation, emotion recognition and management, planning, and sequencing activity. Memory aids and educational software assist with reading, learning, comprehension, and organizational difficulties.

Future

AT has come a long way from the basic support devices created to make life with a disability easier. The complexity and variety of today's devices allow for individualized support and independence. Researchers are now conducting studies on the types of AT used and the influence such products have on major life activities. These projects hope to increase the capacity of the independent living community to work with its members and stakeholders to collect research data on access and use of AT to improve the lives of people with disabilities. Enabling individuals to participate more fully in all aspects of life while increasing opportunities for independence, education, employment, and social interaction remains the goal and driving force behind the continued progress of AT.

Lin Browning

See also: Americans with Disabilities Act; Blindness; Braille; Cochlear Implants; Deafness

Further Reading

Assistive Technology Industry Association (ATIA). (n.d.). What is assistive technology? How is it funded? Retrieved from http://www.atia.org/i4a/pages/index.cfm?pageid=3859

Bluebird Care. (n.d.). Assistive technology from ancient times to modern times! *Bluebird care: Care at home and in the community.* Retrieved from http://bluebirdcare.ie/assistive-technology-ancient-modern-times/

U.S. Department of Education. (n.d.). Building the legacy: IDEA 2004. Retrieved from http://idea.ed.gov/

ASSOCIATION FOR CHEMORECEPTION SCIENCES

The Association for Chemoreception Sciences (AChemS) is a professional society for basic science and clinical researchers studying normative and disease processes in the chemoreception and chemosensory sciences, such as found in the olfactory and taste systems. The mission of AChemS has been divided into five core areas: (1) to advance the understanding of chemosensory mechanisms by bringing to one forum the variety of different scientific disciplines currently being used to approach the chemical senses; (2) to encourage basic, clinical, and applied research in the chemical senses; (3) to promote an appreciation, beyond the chemosensory community itself, of the need and impact of chemosensory research; (4) to act as an identifiable organ representing the interests of the chemosensory research community; and (5) to act as an identifiable directory for those requiring particular types of chemosensory expertise.

History

In 1978, Dr. Maxwell M. Mozell, a renowned professor in neuroscience and physiology at State University of New York Health Science Center, founded AChemS. Mozell received a planning grant from the National Science Foundation (NSF) to initiate the formation of the association. With the help of 10 colleagues, who studied the chemical senses, the group planned its first research meeting, which was held in Sarasota, Florida, in April 1979. The annual meeting continued to be held in Sarasota until it became too large for the venue in 2010. The meeting is still held in Florida but is located at hotels and conference centers that are large enough to accommodate the higher number of meeting attendees and poster presentations. The annual meeting has evolved into the United States' major forum for presenting advances in chemical senses research.

Publications

In addition to the annual meeting, AChemS sponsors a bimonthly journal, *Chemical Senses*, which is published by Oxford University Press. *Chemical Senses* publishes original research that includes all aspects of chemosensory biology, including taste, smell, vomeronasal, and trigeminal chemoreception in both vertebrates and invertebrates. An important part of the journal's coverage is devoted to techniques and the development and application of new methods for investigating chemoreception and chemosensory structures. Such research ranges from behavioral studies to molecular approaches to electrophysiology of chemosensory neurons. Mozell was the executive editor of the journal *Chemical Sciences* from 1992 to 1998. Today, the current editor-in-chief is German scientist Wolfgang Meyerhof.

Funding Opportunities

In the United States, most chemoreception research is supported by the National Institutes of Health (NIH), which is part of the U.S. Department of Health and Human Services. NIH's mission is "to seek fundamental knowledge about the nature and behavior of living systems and the application of that knowledge to enhance health, lengthen life, and reduce illness and disability." The institute that provides competitive grants for chemosensory research is the National Institute on Deafness and Other Communication Disorders (NIDCD). The areas of research supported by the NIDCD include but are not limited to biophysics and mechanics of sensory cells; cell biology of sensory cells and neurons; development, plasticity, and regeneration; functional and molecular imaging; genetics; hearing and balance; ion channels, receptors, and molecular signaling; taste and olfaction; tumor biology; and, voice, speech, and language.

The NIH is the main federal agency that oversees how medical research is performed, particularly clinical trials. The NIH provides guidelines and training to make sure that research is executed ethically toward people and animals. Clinical trials examine new ways to prevent, detect, or treat diseases. They are designed to allow researchers and patients to examine whether a particular type of treatment or medication is more or less effective than a placebo (no treatment) and also to determine if the treatment is safe. Thus, clinical trials are evidence-based research that helps health care providers deliver effective treatments to patients. The general public as well as health care providers are encouraged to look up multiple health topics on the NIH website and receive up-to-date, current research information. Topics include obesity, diabetes, cancer, and nutritional facts labels.

Jennifer L. Hellier

See also: Anosmia; Olfactory System; Taste System

Further Reading

Association for Chemoreception Sciences. (2014). About AChemS. Retrieved from http://www.achems.org/i4a/pages/index.cfm?pageid=3277

National Institute on Deafness and Other Communication Disorders (NIDCD). (2015). Research. Retrieved from http://www.nidcd.nih.gov/research/Pages/Default.aspx

National Institutes of Health. (2015). Turning discovery into health. Research & training. Retrieved from http://www.nih.gov/science/education.htm

ASTIGMATISM

Astigmatism is a visual condition that causes blurred vision. For most people, the cornea of the eye has a spherical shape so that when light hits the tissue in the back of the eye, or the retina, the vision is clear and even. Individuals with astigmatism have a retina with an irregular shape that causes steep or rounded areas in the cornea, such as the shape of a football. These irregularities in the cornea cause it to have a harder time properly focusing light to the retina, which results in blurred vision. Similar to nearsightedness and farsightedness, astigmatism is a type of refractive error that causes light to bend at a certain angle. Although they may not know it, many people have varying forms of astigmatism from mild to severe. Genetics plays a role because astigmatism is inherited and may decrease or worsen over time as the individual grows. Irregular astigmatism occurs when a degenerative disease called keratoconus causes the cornea to become thinner and more cone-shaped, resulting in protrusion of the cornea. Other causes of astigmatism may result from eye injuries.

Symptoms

For people with mild cases of astigmatism, symptoms are hard to distinguish and treatment may be limited to correcting the blurriness with prescription contact lenses or eyeglasses. Those with severe cases may report being unable to see fine details either nearby or far away and suffer from headaches, weariness, and variable vision. This may be due to added tension on the eyes from prolonged reading, staring at a computer or phone screen, or looking off into the distance.

Types

The three types of astigmatism include myopic astigmatism, hyperopic astigmatism, and mixed astigmatism. Myopic astigmatism occurs when the meridians of the eye, or the flattest parts of the eye, are nearsighted while hyperopic astigmatism occurs when the meridians are farsighted. Meridians are imaginary lines separated into one-degree units to determine where the most and the least curved sections of the cornea are present. The lines or curves bisect the sphere of the eyeball. The 90-degree angle is the vertical meridian of the eye while the 180-degree angle is the horizontal meridian. The meridians are classified as regular, at a 90-degree angle, or as irregular, not perpendicular. In myopia, light is focused in front of the retina due in part to the additional thickness of the eye. This results in nearby objects being seen as clear and objects far away being seen as blurry. Hyperopia results when the light rays are focused behind the surface of the retina, resulting in objects that are nearby seen as blurry and objects that are far away seen as clear. Mixed astigmatism involves one meridian being nearsighted while the other meridian is farsighted. Presbyopia occurs as the individual ages and the soft crystalline lens of the eyes loses its flexibility and starts to harden. This loss of flexibility results in the inability to focus light accurately, so nearby objects tend to appear more blurry.

Diagnosis and Treatment

Astigmatism is diagnosed through routine eye exams by an optometrist or ophthalmologist. Eye doctors perform a series of tests that involve having the patient read letters and numbers on a chart as well as using a keratometer to measure the amount of curvature to the surface of the cornea. Doctors may use a keratoscope device that includes a video camera to map the planes on the cornea's surface to measure the variations on the surface. Usually eye doctors conduct a retinoscopy test that includes switching back and forth between various lenses while examining the eye with light shining at it.

From there, the doctor can determine the prescription to correct the blurred vision with noninvasive methods of prescribing either prescription glasses or contact lenses, or orthokeratology, a process that involves wearing rigid contact lenses to reshape the curve of the cornea. On an eyeglass prescription, cylinder or CYL indicates the lens power for astigmatism. Cylinder refers to the lens power so that one meridian has no added power to correct the lens curvature while the other meridian has the maximum power. If the individual decides to forgo the eyeglass methods, toric contact lenses are another but a more expensive means of correcting astigmatism. Invasive methods include eye surgery, laser in situ keratomileusis, or LASIK, which utilizes a laser to remove small amounts of tissue from the inner layer of the cornea while the outer layer is folded back during the procedure and then properly replaced after the procedure. Another invasive technique is photorefractive keratectomy (PRK), which corrects the cornea by removing tissue from both the inner and outer layers.

Simi Abraham

See also: Diplopia; Hyperopia; Myopia; Presbyopia; Retina; Visual Fields; Visual System

Further Reading

American Optometric Association. (n.d.). Astigmatism. *Astigmatism*. Retrieved from http://www.aoa.org/patients-and-public/eye-and-vision-problems/glossary-of-eye-and-vision-conditions/astigmatism?sso=y

Mayo Clinic. (2014). Astigmatism. *Treatments and Drugs*. Retrieved from http://www.mayoclinic.org/diseases-conditions/astigmatism/basics/treatment/con-20022003

ATTENTION DEFICIT HYPERACTIVITY DISORDER

Attention deficit disorder (ADD), also known as attention deficit hyperactivity disorder (ADHD), affects nearly 5 percent of children in the United States. Children with ADD struggle with paying attention and staying focused on everyday jobs like cleaning their room or completing homework. Additionally, these children may be overly sensitive to external stimuli such as touch. It was thought that adults outgrew the symptoms of ADD; however, research now suggests that some adults can retain their symptoms of ADD. This leads the adult to struggle with organizational tasks and the condition can even proceed to destructive behaviors such as addiction and substance abuse. The topic of ADD is riddled with controversy due to the tendency to misdiagnose active, yet healthy children with this disorder. Although medication is available, many experts suggest that prescribing medication to children who actually do not have ADD is highly destructive and may cause problems as the brain continues to develop.

History

Although ADD or ADHD is a disorder that has only recently been introduced into the daily vernacular, children and adults affected by the disorder have long been observed throughout the history of the world. The first recorded incident of ADD was in 1904, when the British medical journal *The Lancet* published a short poem about a boy with the disorder. Specifically, the verse titled "The Story of Fidgety Philip" told the story of a young boy who just seemed to have too much energy to sit still. His antics often got him in trouble, resulting in the disgrace of his parents. These same characteristics have often been re-created in other fictional characters such as "Dennis the Menace" by Hank Ketcham.

In 1970, C. Kornetsky proposed the catecholamine hypothesis of hyperactivity to describe ADD/ADHD. Catecholamine is a group of neurotransmitters that include norepinephrine, adrenaline, and dopamine. Kornetsky hypothesized that the lack of or a decreased amount of naturally occurring catecholamines is what caused ADD, therefore by prescribing drugs such as Ritalin, artificial catecholamines were added back into the brain. It is important to notice that a consensus has yet to be reached about what causes ADD. Although some say that it is caused by a chemical imbalance, there is evidence that suggests that it is not the only factor. Furthermore, scientists have shown that ADD is not caused by a decrease in a single neurotransmitter system, but that ADD or ADHD is a complex disease that may have many components.

Types and Symptoms

Symptoms of ADD are sometimes confused with hyperactivity and an inability to focus in young children. The ADD Association stresses the importance of proper testing with a qualified and certified health care provider such as a psychiatrist or physician. ADD is appropriately diagnosed if children and adults display the triad of ADD symptoms. The first symptom is distractibility, or an inability to focus on any idea for too long a time. The second symptom is impulsivity, or the inability to control oneself. This includes displaying a lack of patience or the inability to wait for gratification. The last characteristic and diagnostic behavior of ADD is hyperactivity, or excessive activity. Simply having these qualities, however, is not enough to diagnose someone with ADD. These behaviors must appear in a patient before the age of seven and be present for at least a period of six months. The symptoms must also disrupt two or more areas of a person's life, including school, work, home, or social life. Other common symptoms include failure to pay attention to details, not listening when spoken to, constantly fidgeting, and excessive activity. The severity of these symptoms differs for each person, and in fact about one-third of all people diagnosed with ADD do not have symptoms of hyperactivity and lack of focus.

It is also important to note that ADD is not caused by food allergies, certain dyes in food, or a lack of activity caused by watching too much television or playing video games. Nonetheless, excess sugar and a lack of activity can cause normal children to exhibit what seems like symptoms of ADD. Thus, family members, teachers, and society must not jump to the conclusion that a child or adult has ADD simply because he or she cannot sit still.

Treatments and Outcomes

Although there is not a cure for ADD or ADHD, there are a multitude of treatment options for individuals with the syndrome. Some of them include medication and others include a series of steps for the patient to manage or control the symptoms of ADD. Often, parents help their children choose and try to implement both regimens into their everyday activities.

The first treatment is medication (a stimulant), which is needed to help with the chemical imbalance in the brain. The stimulant can come in a multitude of forms and a number of compounds; the most common is Adderall. These medications do have side effects, with the most common being a decreased appetite and trouble sleeping or falling asleep. Other less common side effects include tics, which are sudden and repetitive motions usually of the face. In general, when children are taken off the medication, these tics will disappear. Another side effect that can occur, although it is rare, is a state of mind where the individual lacks emotion. This is sometimes dramatized in television shows and movies. Once again, when taken off the medication these side effects for the most part go away.

Other treatments that have helped individuals manage their symptoms include dietary changes, exercise, psychotherapy, and support and understanding from friends and family. Many times, patients with ADD feel out of place and incapable of doing anything. Low self-esteem can only compound the effects of ADD.

Cynthia M. Joseph

See also: Excitation; Neurological Examination

Further Reading

Centers for Disease Control and Prevention. (2013). *Attention-deficit/hyperactivity disorder (ADHD)*. Retrieved from http://www.cdc.gov/NCBDDD/adhd/facts.html

National Institute of Mental Health. (2008). *Attention deficit hyperactivity disorder (ADHD)*. Retrieved from http://www.nimh.nih.gov/health/publications/attention-deficit-hyperactivity-disorder/complete-index.shtml

AUDITORY HALLUCINATIONS

Auditory hallucinations occur when a person hears sound without external auditory stimulation. This phenomenon is sometimes referred to as paracusia, although paracusia also refers to other disorders involving impaired hearing. Five to 28 percent of the population suffers from auditory hallucinations (de Leede-Smith & Barkus, 2013). Symptoms of auditory hallucinations range from hearing voices to hearing music. Depending on the cause, auditory hallucinations can be treated in a variety of ways with varying success.

History

Auditory hallucinations have been reported throughout human history. Perhaps people who were revered as being in contact with God, or the gods, were experiencing auditory hallucinations. Socrates (ca. 470–399 BCE) may have experienced auditory hallucinations that he referred to as his "daemon" or his "voice of reason." During the Dark Ages trepanning (drilling a hole in the skull) was used to treat auditory hallucinations. Later in history, those hearing voices might have been tried as witches. Throughout history, auditory hallucinations could land a person in an insane asylum or a sanatorium.

Types and Symptoms

Auditory hallucinations are often associated with schizophrenia and related disorders, yet may occur in mental health disorders such as bipolar disorder, depression with psychotic features, and posttraumatic stress disorder. Auditory hallucinations, however, may have causes other than mental illness.

A variety of medical conditions can cause auditory hallucinations. Patients with temporal lobe epilepsy, for example, may have damage to the temporal cortex of their brain. Some of these patients have auditory hallucinations, and the hallucinations may be a predictor of an impending seizure. Other medical conditions including stroke and migraine can cause auditory hallucinations, as can tumors and infectious diseases. Various forms of stress are also associated with auditory hallucinations including sleep deprivation and drug use.

Dementia patients experience many changes in their ability to perceive their environment. One of the changes some experience is auditory hallucinations. These patients are complex; the patient may be taking medications that contribute to auditory hallucinations, or may be experiencing strokes or migraines that cause auditory hallucinations.

Other auditory hallucinations do not involve hearing voices. Instead, patients hear a range of sounds, from buzzing and tones to complex sounds including music and singing. Single tones including ringing, buzzing, and humming are referred to as tinnitus, whereas complex sounds involving music and singing are called musical ear syndrome (Bauman, 2013).

Treatments

Auditory hallucinations associated with mental health disorders, such as voices heard by patients with schizophrenia, are disruptive to patients' lives. These hallucinations are treated with a combination of medication and therapy. Treatments are not always effective, so additional treatments are being developed, including transcranial magnetic stimulation (TMS), a technique using low-frequency magnetic fields to reduce brain activity in areas of the brain generating the "voices."

Auditory hallucinations can be associated with a variety of medical conditions including epilepsy, brain tumors, dementia, drug use, and infectious causes. In order to treat these hallucinations the underlying medical cause must be addressed. Treatments vary widely and may range from surgery to remove a tumor to medical treatment of an infection.

Patients with tinnitus often seek treatment for this condition if it becomes disruptive to their day-to-day lives. The cause of tinnitus must be investigated; many underlying medical conditions cause tinnitus including age-related hearing loss, earwax, and medications. Once the cause has been identified, treatments range from addressing the cause to prescribing hearing aids, introducing white noise, and retraining the brain to mask the tinnitus.

Patients with musical ear syndrome may not seek treatment if the music is not disruptive to everyday life. In the case of patients with hearing loss, some would miss the music if it were to stop. "I mean, where else can you hear beautiful music without wearing hearing aids, assistive devices, iPods, headphones or other paraphernalia?" (Bauman, 2013).

Outcomes of Treatment

The outcome of the treatment of auditory hallucinations depends on the identification and treatment of the underlying cause.

Future Directions

Mechanism of auditory hallucinations remains largely unknown. Future research focusing on the mechanism of these hallucinations will aid in treatments. The auditory hallucinations associated with tinnitus, dementia, and epilepsy may each have a different mechanism than those associated with mental illness. It is important to realize that the presence of auditory hallucinations does not, on its own, indicate mental illness, but auditory hallucinations should be discussed with a health care provider.

Lisa A. Rabe

See also: Age-Related Hearing Loss; Tinnitus

Further Reading

Bauman, Neil. (2013). Musical ear syndrome. *Tinnitus Today*, Spring 2013. Retrieved from http://ata.org/sites/ata.org/files/pdf/TT_Spring2013_Final.pdf

de Leede-Smith, Saskia, & Emma Barkus. (2013). A comprehensive review of auditory verbal hallucinations: Lifetime prevalence, correlates and mechanisms in healthy and clinical individuals. *Frontiers in Human Neuroscience, 7*(367). http://dx.doi.org/10.3389/fnhum.2013.00367

AUDITORY PROCESSING DISORDER

The brain may have problems processing auditory information resulting in an auditory processing disorder, previously called central auditory processing disorder. Auditory processing disorder is a generic term for all hearing disorders that have a mismatch between the normal function of the peripheral auditory organs and structures and the brain's ability to interpret or discriminate sounds. It is a heterogeneous group of auditory-specific disorders exhibiting one or more deficits in (1) auditory processing of sound localization and lateralization, (2) discriminating sounds, (3) auditory pattern recognition, and (4) temporal resolution, masking, integration, and ordering. Furthermore, a person with an auditory processing disorder will have difficulty in picking out sounds and/or words in noisy environments.

Anatomy and Physiology

Persons with an auditory processing disorder generally have normal anatomical structures of the outer, middle, and inner ear. These structures also function normally for the sense of hearing. It is the structures in the brain that have problems integrating the auditory signal into perceived sounds. Thus, these patients have problems in recognizing sounds as well as interpreting what the sound is, particularly when there are background noises. These difficulties are magnified when identifying speech sounds. Persons with auditory processing disorder generally have problems understanding rapid speech or degraded speech and following oral instructions. To compensate for the disorder, individuals may try to fill in the missing words.

Causes

Auditory processing disorder is usually noticed in young infants and children. Caregivers and teachers may see that the child is regressing during development, particularly in language comprehension. Studies have shown that causes of auditory processing disorder are ectopic cells in the primary auditory cortex and genetic seizure disorders, to name a few. The primary auditory cortex (located in the left temporal lobe) is essential for performing basic and higher functions in hearing. Ectopic or misplaced cells in the primary auditory cortex will have malformations in circuitry, resulting in abnormal processing. Furthermore, function of the primary auditory cortex depends on the sounds encountered early in life, and if the circuitry is not properly working, this can result in an auditory processing disorder. Other causes have been associated with autosomal dominant epilepsy or seizures that affect the left temporal lobe, resulting in auditory processing problems.

Diagnosis

There are several disorders that have deficits similar to those of auditory processing disorder. Thus, it can be difficult to properly diagnose. The most common similar disorders are language processing disorders as well as attention deficit hyperactivity disorder (ADHD). To obtain a diagnosis, speech-language pathologists, psychologists, health care providers, and teachers all work together to perform a comprehensive assessment. Diagnosis requires specific outcomes of behavioral tests, measuring brainstem auditory evoked potentials (BAEP), and auditory tests. However, it can be difficult to determine auditory processing disorder in infants and children as they have limited language ability, may be unable to pay attention to the test, and may not be able to cope with testing demands.

Intervention

To date, interventions for persons with auditory processing disorder include improving (1) the quality of the acoustic signal—such as ensuring that speech is clear and not degraded, (2) the listening environment by decreasing background noise, (3) auditory skills, and (4) language skills.

Jennifer L. Hellier

See also: Auditory System; Auditory Threshold; Brainstem Auditory Evoked Potentials; Tonotopic Map; Vestibulocochlear Nerve

Further Reading

Chermak, Gail D. (2002). Deciphering auditory processing disorders in children. *Otolaryngologic Clinics of North America, 35*(4), 733–749.

Micallef, Lara A. (2015). Auditory processing disorder (APD): Progress in diagnostics so far. A mini-review on imaging techniques. *Journal of International Advanced Otology, 11*(3), 257–261. http://dx.doi.org/10.5152/iao.2015.1009

Vermiglio, Andrew J. (2016). On diagnostic accuracy in audiology: Central site of lesion and central auditory processing disorder studies. *Journal of the American Academy of Audiology, 27*(2), 141–156. http://dx.doi.org/10.3766/jaaa.15079

AUDITORY SYSTEM

The auditory system is a sensory system that is responsible for the sense of hearing. The ability to hear allows animals to be able to detect sounds in their surroundings without direct contact or without seeing the source of the sound. All mammals including humans have bilateral auditory systems, meaning that there are two sets of auditory structures (ears) on opposite sides of the head. The bilateral orientation of the auditory system helps to localize sound direction by using time delay. Specifically, the time of the arrival of the sound at each ear occurs at slightly different epochs, which is used to find the location of the sound. Overall the auditory system allows mammals to detect, locate, and interpret a plethora of sounds. The auditory system comprises several organs and structures, all of which collect and concentrate sound waves through each anatomical segment to the cochlea (see below) where the waves are converted into electrical impulses. The electrical impulses produced by the cochlea are then sent to auditory processing centers in the brain and are subsequently interpreted as sound.

Anatomy and Physiology

The auditory system is divided into three anatomical segments: the outer ear, middle ear, and inner ear. The outer segment of the ear acts like a cone and captures sound waves; the middle segment of the ear concentrates and directs the vibrations to the inner segment of the ear, which converts the wave into electrical impulses. The neural impulses that are created in the inner ear are then sent to the brain and interpreted as sound in the auditory cortex. As mentioned, the first segment is the outer ear, which is the only portion of the auditory system that is visible externally. On each side of the head there are cartilaginous skin folds that are commonly recognized as the ear. The scientific name for this structure is the pinna, which is Latin for "wing." At the center of the cone-shaped pinna is the external auditory meatus, which is the opening to the auditory canal. The auditory canal is a small tube that is about 2.5 centimeters long and extends from the external auditory meatus to the internal auditory meatus. Within the auditory canal earwax, or cerumen, is produced by modified sweat glands to help protect the canal from various infections and parasite infestations. The structure found at the end of the auditory canal is a thin tissue layer called the tympanic membrane, more commonly known as the eardrum, which is attached to the internal auditory meatus.

The eardrum is slightly conical shaped and taut, similar to the head of a drum that is stretched over the drum's opening. The eardrum is attached to the internal auditory meatus and is the first structure of the middle ear. The three smallest bones in the body, the ossicles, are directly after the eardrum. Each of the three ossicles is connected to one another; in order they are the malleus, incus, and stapes. Two small muscles attach the malleus and incus to the walls of the middle ear. These muscles help dampen the vibrations of the ossicles and prevent damage to the middle ear. A small tube, also a part of the middle ear, called the auditory tube or eustachian tube, extends from the middle ear down to the back of the throat or nasopharynx. The auditory tube helps equalize the pressure between the middle ear and the outer ear and prevent eardrum damage. It is this tube that is responsible for the "ear popping" experience when changing altitudes. The "pop" occurs at the eardrum when the pressure between the outer ear and the middle ear equalizes.

The final segment of the ear is the inner ear; it begins at the oval window, which is found attached to the footplate of the stapes. A thin membrane covering the oval window separates the middle and inner ear. Within the inner ear is the organ responsible for converting the mechanical sound waves into an electrical impulse, the cochlea. There are two noticeable landmarks on the external surface of the cochlea adjacent to each other, the oval window and the round window. Externally the cochlea looks like the shell of a snail; internally it consists of three fluid-filled cavities. Within one of the cavities is the organ of Corti, which contains specialized sensory receptors called hair cell receptors. These hair cells convert sound waves into electrical impulses that are sent to the brain to be interpreted into sound.

Collectively hearing can be divided into two processes: transmission and transduction. Transmission is the collection of sound waves from the outer ear to the inner ear, whereas transduction is the conversion of sound waves to electrical impulses. In the process of transmission, sound is captured by the pinna and then funneled toward the auditory canal. As the sound vibrations travel down the auditory canal they are concentrated, then at the end of the canal the waves strike the tympanic membrane. The eardrum vibrates in response to the airwave at the same frequency as the sound. This vibration is then transferred to the ossicles of the middle ear; the small muscles attached to the ossicles tighten in response to the vibrations and dampen any loud or unexpected sounds. Next the vibration reaches the oval window via the footplate of the stapes where the vibrations are transferred to the fluid-filled cavities of the cochlea. In the cochlea the basilar membrane vibrates at the same frequency as the fluid of the cochlea. The organ of Corti, with its hair cell receptors, lies on top of the basilar membrane. Hair cells are so named because they contain tiny hair-like projections on their top surface called cilia. The cilia of the hair cells are embedded into a shelf-like membrane called the tectorial membrane, which does not move. It is important to note that the hair cells are "trapped" between two different membranes, one that moves with the fluid of the cochlea and the other that does not move at all. Thus, when a sound wave causes the basilar membrane to move, the hair cells move as well. However, since the cilia are stuck in place, the base of the cilia bends back and forth. It is this back and forth movement of the cilia that produces transduction of sound. The bending force on the cilia changes the resting membrane voltage of the hair cell, causing the voltage to be more positive, which then creates an action potential at the cochlear nerve. The cochlear nerve joins the vestibular nerve to form the eighth cranial nerve (vestibulocochlear nerve or cranial nerve VIII). Auditory signals produced in the cochlea are sent to several areas of the brain for processing such as the auditory cortex, thalamus, and the brainstem. The auditory cortex, located within the temporal lobe of the brain, interprets the signal as the conscious perception of sound, whereas in the brainstem, signals are used in reflexes and feedback in the auditory system.

Diseases

In a normal functioning auditory system, sound transmission and sound transduction are not impeded. This means that a human with normal hearing should be able to hear sounds within the 20 to 20,000 Hz (hertz) range. There are several disease processes and pathologies that can reduce this range of hearing permanently; however, some disease processes may change the normal range of human hearing only temporarily. Diseases that perpetually affect the ability to hear are referred to as deafness. Typically, deafness is caused by damage at or near the cochlea where sound is transduced. Hearing loss is categorized as either conductive deafness or neural deafness. Issues that impede the conduction of sound waves typically cause conductive deafness such as sinus congestion, earwax buildup, middle ear infection, or even eardrum perforation. Conductive deafness can easily be treated by various medical interventions. Sinus infections and ear infections can often be cleared with antibiotic treatment, and once treated the normal hearing range should return. Chronic ear infections caused by buildup of fluid in the middle ear can damage the cochlea if not treated. The typical treatment for chronic ear infections is surgical placement of artificial auditory tubes, which help drain excess fluid. Eardrum perforations generally occur directly from a perforating instrument, like a cotton-tipped swab being inserted too deeply, or indirectly via a blow to the head or other head trauma. When the eardrum is perforated an individual will experience sharp pain and mild conductive hearing loss. The membrane can heal on its own with full recovery of hearing; however, some severe tears require surgical repair before hearing returns to normal.

Lynelle Smith

See also: Cochlea; Cochlear Implants; Deafness; Inferior Colliculus; Sound Localization; Thalamus; Tonotopic Map; Vestibulocochlear Nerve

Further Reading

Bear, Mark F., Barry W. Connors, & Michael A. Paradiso. (2007). *Neuroscience exploring the brain* (3rd ed.). Baltimore, MD: Lippincott Williams & Wilkins.
Morlet, Thierry. (2011). *Auditory neuropathy spectrum disorder.* Retrieved from https://www.akronchildrens.org/cms/kidshealth/157f026c1db11d09/index.html
Nevals Digital Hearing. (n.d.). *How does hearing work?* Retrieved from http://www.lushnewmedia.com/nevalsdigitalhearing/about_hearing.htm

AUDITORY-TACTILE SYNESTHESIA

Certain sounds can cause ordinary people to experience sensations in their body. Think of the sound of chalk on a blackboard and the cringing sensation that accompanies it. This is similar to one of the rarest forms of synesthesia called auditory-tactile synesthesia. Synesthesia is the cross-integration of senses due to cross-connectivity within the brain. This can include the association of two or more senses at the same time. Some synesthetes with this form of synesthesia experience the sound of instruments while at the same time feeling them someplace on their bodies, feelings like brushing or tickling. Typically, individuals affected by auditory-tactile synesthesia associate sounds with particular tactile (touch) feelings.

Types of Auditory-Tactile Synesthesia

Auditory-tactile synesthesia seems to have two forms: individuals who have had it since birth and individuals who acquire it later in life. For those individuals who have had this form of synesthesia since birth, it can be thought of as merely a different, more enhanced way of experiencing the environment. Usually these experiences are automatic, involuntary, and consistently unique to the individual. Acquired auditory-tactile synesthesia usually occurs as a result of some sort of neurological damage to the brain, especially the thalamus, although sensory deprivation and hallucinogenic or psychedelic drug usage can also induce it. This form of auditory-tactile synesthesia typically has resultant unpleasant and intense tingling sensations.

Connection of Hearing and Touch

It is hypothesized that abnormal or cross-modal connectivity results in inappropriate structural links between the sensory modalities of touch and hearing. Stroke-induced masking of somatosensory thalamic input might allow short-term, already existing connections between the adjacent regions of the brain. Both feeling and hearing depend on the transduction of physical events into frequency-based neural codes, which suggests that the two systems may be linked in every individual. Synesthesia might be an enhanced form of these cross-cortical links that the brain utilizes every time it integrates audition and vision. Physiologically, auditory, and somatosensory processing begins with receptor organs that are similar in structure and function. Both touch and audition rely upon the displacement of mechanoreceptors (neuroreceptors that respond to physical deformation) to translate physical events into nerve signals. For touch, the cell membrane of mechanoreceptors lying within the skin detect any sort of physical deformation and can determine the amount of pressure and length of touch. Within the ear, hair cells are responsible for converting vibrations that enter the inner ear into neural messages that can then be passed on to the brain in order to create sound. Both are also frequency-dependent and tuned to different frequencies. One way that auditory-tactile synesthesia may come about is damage to the brain. Damage to the regions directly involved in the integration of tactile stimuli or auditory stimuli tends to encourage compensation by the brain near the lesion. This can result in crossover of the modalities.

Applications of Auditory-Tactile Synesthesia

It is speculated that the sense of hearing may have evolved from the sense of feeling. Research with twins demonstrates that touch sensitivity is correlated with hearing acuity and can be heritable. Additionally, recent research shows evidence that the middle ear bones (the stapes, incus, and malleus) may have evolved from certain jaw bones. A practical and exciting application of induced visual tactile synesthesia is work in patients with phantom limbs. The phantom limb is resurrected visually in a virtual reality box containing a mirror. The intact hand's reflection is superimposed on the phantom limb, thus making it appear as if the phantom hand were moving when the normal hand moves. More than half of the patients studied had the kinesthetic sensation of the involved hand, and most of these patients obtained relief from the painful spasms of the phantom limb.

Carolyn Johnson Atwater

See also: Auditory System; Mirror-Touch Synesthesia; Synesthesia; Touch

Further Reading

Afra, Pegah, Michael Funke, & Fumisuke Matsuo. (2009). Acquired auditory-visual synesthesia: A window to early cross-modal sensory interactions. *Psychological Research and Behavioral Management, 2,* 31–37. Retrieved from http://www.ncbi.nlm.nih.gov/pmc/articles/PMC3218766/

Carpenter, Siri. (2001). Everyday fantasia: The world of synesthesia. *American Psychological Association*, 32(2). Retrieved from http://www.apa.org/monitor/mar01/synesthesia.aspx

Naumer, Marcus J., & Jasper J. F. van den Bosch. (2009). Touching sounds: Thalamocortical plasticity and the neural basis of multisensory integration. *Journal of Neurophysiology, 102*(1), 7–8. Retrieved from http://jn.physiology.org/content/102/1/7

Schnabel, Jim. (2008). The sounds of silent movies: Flickering images can trigger perception of sound. *Nature*. http://dx.doi.org/10.1038/news.2008.1014. Retrieved from http://www.nature.com/news/2008/080805/full/news.2008.1014.html

AUDITORY THRESHOLD

The lowest or minimal level of a pure tone that an average human ear can detect in a quiet room is called the auditory threshold. This threshold level, however, can vary depending on the frequency of the tone, whether it is a low or high frequency. Since sound is a wave, the auditory threshold is truly measuring a change in pressure sensation in an individual's ear. Audiologists are health care professionals who use specific tools to test a person's hearing abilities and his or her auditory threshold. Certain tools are used for different age groups, particularly since infants and young children may not understand the directions to show that they hear a sound or tone.

Types of Auditory Tests

There are two methods to measure an individual's absolute threshold of hearing: minimal audible field and minimal audible pressure tests. The main difference between these tests are that the minimal audible field tests both ears at the same time—binaural hearing—while minimal audible pressure tests one ear at a time—monaural hearing. In a minimal audible field test, the person sits in a sound booth (field) with stimuli being presented via loudspeakers. The person steps out of the booth and the level of sound is measured at the position of the person's head. In minimal audible pressure test, the individual puts on headphones and stimuli are presented though the headphones. This process measures sound pressure in the person's ear canal using a small probe microphone. Generally, minimal audible field thresholds are lower than the minimal audible pressure threshold because binaural hearing is more sensitive than monaural hearing. This could be due to the person with the headphones also hearing internal noises such as heartbeat or swallowing that could mask the pressure stimuli.

Classical Auditory Testing

To understand how the test is performed, the patient is told that a sound will be produced and how to respond when he or she hears the tone. In this yes/no paradigm, during each interval of the hearing test a sound is either present or absent. The individual then responds, stating whether he or she heard the stimulus. The hearing test continues with a predetermined sequence including a catch trial where no tone is presented.

The most common test for absolute threshold of hearing is the method of limits. In this paradigm, the tester controls the levels of stimuli but there are no catch trials. The tone progresses through multiple series of ascending or descending intensities. In the ascending trial run, the tone is presented well below the person's expected auditory threshold. The tone is then slowly increased until the individual responds. The opposite occurs in the descending trial run. In this test the tone is well above the anticipated auditory threshold. When the person responds correctly to the stimulus, the tone is decreased by a specified amount and presented again. This paradigm continues until the individual no longer responds to the presented stimuli. After several ascending and descending trials, the person's absolute hearing threshold is calculated as the average intensity between the last audible tone and the first inaudible level.

Patricia A. Bloomquist and Jennifer L. Hellier

See also: Auditory Hallucinations; Auditory Processing Disorder; Auditory System; Brainstem Auditory Evoked Potentials; Cochlea; Cochlear Implants; Vestibulocochlear Nerve

Further Reading

Gorga, Michael P., Tiffany A. Johnson, Jan K. Kaminski, Kathryn L. Beauchaine, Cassie A. Garner, & Stephen T. Neely. (2006). Using a combination of click- and toneburst-evoked auditory brainstem response measurements to estimate pure-tone thresholds. *Ear and Hearing*, 27(1), 60–74. Retrieved from http://www.ncbi.nlm.nih.gov/pmc/articles/PMC2441480/

Nave, R. (2016). Threshold of hearing. *HyperPhysics at Georgia State University*. Retrieved from http://hyperphysics.phy-astr.gsu.edu/hbase/sound/earcrv.html

Van Dun, Bram, Harvey Dillon, & Mark Seeto. (2015). Estimating hearing thresholds in hearing-impaired adults through objective detection of cortical auditory evoked potentials. *Journal of the American Academy of Audiology, 26*(4), 370–383. http://dx.doi.org/10.3766/jaaa.26.4.5

AURA

There are two different experiences both described as auras: the ability to see colors around individuals and those experiences that are typically thought to be precursors to neurological issues such as epilepsy. Auras visible around individuals have recently been linked to synesthesia and are often viewed by individuals who are synesthetes. Auras are also highly associated with a large number of neurological conditions such as migraine, epilepsy, lesions within the brain, and swelling in the brain. These auras are classified based on the experience the patient goes through and change depending on the region of the brain that is affected. Patients with auras describe them as a precursor or a warning.

Historical Views

Metaphysics defines the energy field that emanates from everything, person or object, as the aura. Auras are visualized as an outline of color and represent soul vibrations, the reflections of surrounding energy fields, or chakra emergence. These electromagnetic fields may be viewed by the naked eye. Anthropologist Carlos Castaneda (1925–1998) referred to auras as "luminous cocoons." Auras vibrate to different sounds, light frequencies, and colors with the color spectrum reflecting one's emotional, mental, physical, and spiritual state. The ability to see auras has held an important place in mysticism throughout the ages.

Science, on the other hand, holds a completely different view of auras. The existence of electromagnetic fields is a scientifically proven fact, but the ability to see these fields with the naked eye is highly debatable. It is more likely that people who can see auras have the gift of synesthesia. Seeing auras is an example of the historical presence of synesthesia and the use of New Age beliefs and superstitions to explain and understand this condition.

Research completed on a Spanish faith healer has determined that he has mirror-touch synesthesia and face-color synesthesia. This means that he experiences the sensation of being touched when he sees others being touched and experiences color when his brain processes faces. These synesthetic conditions coupled with a high empathy level mean that he has special pain and emotional reading skills. His synesthetic conditions translate into his perceived special abilities as a faith healer.

Evidence

There are reasons for seeing auras: migraines, a visual system disorder, retinal fatigue and other natural visual processes, a certain form of epilepsy, or a brain disorder. Equipment exists that is capable of measuring extremely minute energy levels, but no one has detected an aura using this equipment. However, bioelectrophotography and quantum physics research might open up new hypotheses regarding auras and the human energy field. A Russian scientist has been examining the impact of human thought on the surrounding environment. He postulates that the human body and consciousness are constantly emitting energy that is captured via bioelectrophotography as light around the body. This energy emission is the aura. At the Princeton Engineering Anomalies Research (PEAR) Laboratory, researchers have concluded that there is a very subtle capacity of the mind to influence the output of random event generators (REGs) in a relationship that is not physical in nature. Another type of photography used to explain auras is Kirlian photography, invented in 1939 by Semyon Davidovitch Kirlian (1898–1978), which reveals visible auras around the objects photographed. Kirlian believed that these photographs actually depicted the life force or aura surrounding all things.

Types of Auras

There are two main ways that auras brought on by a neurological condition can be classified: sensory and experiential. Within the category of sensory auras there are many subtypes based on the experience. These include somatosensory (these auras are characterized by abnormal and often uncomfortable sensations about the body such as tingling, pain, numbness, etc.), auditory (involving the auditory system, mostly buzzing, banging, etc., but in severe cases can be voices), visual (involving the visual system), gustatory (involving taste), olfactory (involving the olfactory system), epigastric (characterized by symptoms coming from the upper abdomen such as nausea, discomfort, emptiness, cramping, churning, etc.), and cephalic (auras described as lightheadedness and headache).

Experiential auras are based on illusions or hallucinations that produce an altered and incorrect view of the external and internal environments. These can also be broken down into subcategories: affective auras (based in altered emotions), mnemonic auras (characterized by memory alterations such as déjà vu—a sense that the experience has happened before—and jamais vu—a sense that the experience is highly unfamiliar even though it is recognized), hallucinatory auras (imagined complex sensory experiences), and illusory auras (incorrectly processed sensory experiences). In all cases, these auras can be a precursor to epileptic episodes and can occur in individuals without neurological defects. Each aura arises from overstimulation in different regions of the brain, and typically this overstimulation is associated with the same stimulation causing epilepsy.

Carolyn Johnson Atwater

See also: Brain Anatomy; Mirror-Touch Synesthesia; Seizures; Synesthesia

Further Reading

PsyBlog. (2013). Synesthesia could explain how some people see "auras." Retrieved from http://www.spring.org.uk/2013/10/synesthesia-could-explain-how-some-people-see -auras.php

AUTONOMIC NERVOUS SYSTEM

The nervous system can be structurally divided into the central (CNS) and peripheral nervous systems (PNS). It is further divided into two functional systems, the somatic nervous system and the autonomic nervous system (ANS). The ANS is also called the involuntary nervous system because it affects the activity of the internal organs (viscera) and smooth muscle. The ANS is divided into two parts based on the different functions they serve: the parasympathetic and sympathetic systems. These two systems work together and in opposing actions to maintain homeostasis of the body and its viscera.

Anatomy

The ANS is made up of sensory and motor nerve fibers as well as ganglia. Each part of the ANS consists of a two-neuron chain with the first neuron originating in the brain or spinal cord. These preganglionic neurons are named as such because their cell bodies are located within the CNS or before the ganglion of the ANS. The second neuron is located in a ganglion outside of the CNS, and thus it is referred to as a postganglionic neuron.

The parasympathetic system promotes normal homeostatic or vegetative functions of the body. The cell bodies of its preganglionic neurons are located in two separate regions in the brainstem and at the end of the spinal cord. Specifically, these neurons are located in the medulla oblongata in the nuclei of cranial nerves III, VII, IX, and X, and in the sacral region of the spinal cord. These preganglionic neurons send their axons out toward the target organ where the postganglionic cell bodies are located. Generally, postganglionic neurons are located in ganglia very close to or within the target organ.

The sympathetic system is part of the emergency response system that speeds up the heart, increases blood pressure, and generally diverts blood away from the organs and out to the extremities. These actions are referred to as the "fight-or-flight response." The preganglionic cell bodies for the sympathetic system are found in one area, and the preganglionic cell bodies in the parasympathetic systems are found above and below these neurons. Thus, the preganglionic neurons of the sympathetic system are located in the lateral horn of the spinal cord, specifically at the levels of T1 through L3. The cell bodies of the postganglionic neurons are located in two regions. The ganglia that are next to the main branches of the abdominal aorta are called the prevertebral ganglia. These axons run to the organs located in the abdominal and pelvic regions. The other ganglia are part of the sympathetic trunk and run from the skull to the coccyx. These are called the paravertebral ganglia, which have axons running to the eye, nose, mouth, respiratory tract, and heart.

The axons of the preganglionic sympathetic neurons exit the spinal cord by passing through the ventral root and separate from the spinal nerve to form the white ramus communicans. They then join a distinct chain of sympathetic ganglia called the vertebral or paravertebral ganglia that are arranged along either side of the vertebral column. At the level of the paravertebral ganglia, there are several options for the axons to exit. They can synapse with the postganglionic neuron, ascend or descend in the sympathetic trunk, then synapse with a postganglionic neuron at a different level, pass through the trunk and synapse with a prevertebral ganglia, or pass through without synapsing on anything until they reach the organ. This latter option is specific for the adrenal gland, which makes and secretes hormones to regulate the fight-or-flight response.

The postganglionic sympathetic axons from the paravertebral ganglia leave as gray rami communicans and join the spinal nerves on their way out to the body. These axons synapse with postganglionic neurons at the most superior paravertebral ganglia, then travel with blood vessels to the head and neck, or they travel to organs in the thorax, such as the heart, lungs, and esophagus. From the prevertebral ganglia, these postganglionic sympathetic axons travel with blood vessels out to the abdominal and pelvic organs. They terminate and act on glands, blood vessels, and smooth muscle.

Physiology

The efferent nervous activity of the ANS is regulated by autonomic reflexes. In many of the reflexes, sensory information is transmitted to control centers in the CNS. These include the hypothalamus and the brainstem and are involved in the overall homeostatic regulation of the body. Most of the sensory input arriving from the abdominal and thoracic viscera is transmitted to the brainstem by the afferent fibers of the vagus nerve (cranial nerve X). Other cranial nerves also bring a rich supply of sensory input to the hypothalamus and brainstem. By integrating these signals, the hypothalamus and brainstem are able to monitor and regulate important body processes including blood pressure, respiration, blood/oxygen/CO_2

levels, body temperature, heart rate, hunger, and thirst. The hypothalamus and brainstem are controlled by higher centers in the brain like the cerebral cortex and limbic systems, so integration of body processes is monitored at multiple levels of the CNS.

Robin Michaels

See also: Central Nervous System; Cranial Nerves; Peripheral Nervous System

Further Reading

Moore, Keith L., Anne M. R. Agur, & Arthur F. Dalley (Eds.). (2010). *Essential clinical anatomy* (4th ed.). Baltimore, MD: Williams and Wilkins.

AXEL, RICHARD

American researcher, molecular biologist, and neuroscientist Richard Axel is a professor at Columbia University and a 2004 Nobel Prize winner for Physiology or Medicine. Axel's work has demonstrated the intricate workings of smell, or olfaction. Axel also holds the titles of Professor of Biochemistry and Molecular Biophysics and of Pathology at Columbia University's College of Physicians and Surgeons, and Investigator at the Howard Hughes Medical Institute.

Born in the summer of 1946 in the Brooklyn borough of New York City, New York, as the first child of Polish immigrants, Richard Axel grew up with few intellectual aspirations. Recognized as gifted by his grade school principal, Axel was encouraged to attend Stuyvesant High School in 1963. It was here that he began his fascination with perception and how the brain represents the external world. On a scholarship to Columbia University, Axel met Bernard Weinstein (1930–2008), became his assistant, and fell in love with molecular biology, going on to study genetics at the graduate level. Upon being made a full professor at Columbia in 1978, Axel continued to explore perception and brain functioning.

Axel, along with microbiologist Saul J. Silverstein and geneticist Michael H. Wigler (1947–), discovered a technique of cotransformation, a process that allows foreign DNA to be inserted into a host cell to produce certain proteins. Axel filed for patents covering this technique, and they became a fundamental process in recombinant DNA research. The use of these techniques by pharmaceutical and biotech companies has earned the University of Columbia significant licensing revenue.

As Axel progressed in his field, he was particularly struck by observations from animal behavior, noticing that what an organism detects in its environment is only part of what is around it and that part varies in different organisms. Axel proposed that the brain functions not by recording an exact image of the world, but by creating its own selective picture. Further, what the brain interprets as reality therefore reflects the representation that the brain has built. Because the brain requires genes to build, it is the genes that determine what is perceived. Axel's work became focused on understanding these genes to provide insight into how the external world is represented in the brain.

Together with Linda Buck (1947–), a creative fellow in the lab, Axel's research turned to exploring how the chemosensory world is represented in the brain. The complexity of olfaction was an intriguing model for the molecular biologist. Assuming that olfaction involved a large family of genes, Buck and Axel worked together to identify an approach that indeed identified the genes encoding the receptors that recognize the vast array of odorants in the environment.

It was this work for which Axel and Buck were awarded the Nobel Prize in Physiology or Medicine. In addition to making contributions as a scientist, Axel has also mentored many leading scientists in the field of neurobiology. Seven of his trainees have become members of the National Academy of Sciences, and currently six of his trainees are affiliated with the Howard Hughes Medical Institute's investigator and early scientist award programs.

Lin Browning

See also: Buck, Linda; Olfactory System; Society for Neuroscience

Further Reading

Nobel Media AB. (2014). Richard Axel—Facts. *Nobelprize.org*. Retrieved from http://www.nobelprize.org/nobel_prizes/medicine/laureates/2004/axel-facts.html

The Royal Society. (2016). *Richard Axel*. Retrieved from https://royalsociety.org/people/richard-axel-11019/

AXON

An axon is a single, dedicated, long cellular process of a neuron that transmits electrical signals from the neuron to its target cell. In general, most neurons have just a single axon that extends out from the main body of the neuron. The axon consists of the cell membrane with cytoplasm and microtubule fibers running the length of the projection. The particular location where the axon extends from the soma (cell body) is called the axon hillock. It is this area where the cell body is connected to the axon.

In addition to an axon, neurons have numerous other shorter cell processes called dendrites that extend out of the soma. Axons are distinguishable from dendrites as both projections are structurally and functionally very different. While dendrites are specialized to receive signals from other neurons and transmit them toward the soma, axons are specialized to conduct the signals from the soma to the branched terminal ends of the axon. These terminal ends are called the axon terminals or boutons, while the electrical signals are called action potentials.

In both the peripheral and central nervous systems (PNS and CNS, respectively), axons may be myelinated or unmyelinated. Myelin is a coating of "insulation" surrounding axons. Glial cells, a specialized group of support cells, myelinate these axons. Specifically, glial cells that myelinate axons in the PNS are called Schwann cells, while glial cells in the CNS are called oligodendrocytes. The cytoplasm and plasma membrane of these glial cells flatten into a thin sheet, which wraps around a segment of an axon at regular intervals to form myelin sheaths. These cells protect, support, and insulate axons so that action potentials may skip the myelinated regions of the axon, making the conduction of signals through the entire length of axon fast and efficient. Small, unmyelinated gaps in the myelin sheath, present at regular intervals throughout the length of the axon, are called the nodes of Ranvier. These structures ensure the signal reaches the terminal end of the myelinated axon without degradation. Nonmyelinated axons do not have the myelin sheath, hence the action potential must travel down the entire length of the axon membrane, which results in a slower transmission speed of the action potential compared to its myelinated counterpart.

History and Function

The axon was first described and distinguished from dendrites by a German neuroanatomist, Otto Friedrich Karl Deiters (1834–1863). Since then, numerous studies were conducted to decipher its exact function and mechanism. In 1952, details of the axon's functionality and its physiology were elucidated by Alan Hodgkin (1914–1998) and Andrew Huxley (1917–2012). These two scientists used giant axons of squids to measure the electrical signals transmitted through the axon. The squid giant axon served as an excellent experimental model due to its large size (up to 1 millimeter in diameter), length, and ease of access. Hodgkin and Huxley's work resulted in a comprehensive mathematical model of the action potential and its electrical mechanism that is known today as the Hodgkin-Huxley model. For their work, Hodgkin and Huxley were awarded the Nobel Prize in 1963. In 1978, Louis-Antoine Ranvier noted and described a pattern of regularly spaced gaps in the myelin sheath of an axon, which is known today as the nodes of Ranvier.

Anatomy and Physiology

An axon is a single projection of the neuron that varies in length and diameter depending on the location, function, and type of neuron. Some axons of sensory neurons located in the body can conduct action potentials from the peripheral sensory receptors, such as in the hand, toward their cell bodies located in the brain or spinal cord. In this way, the axons deliver critical information about the state of the body, such as its position and environment, to other neurons. In general, axons travel together both outside of (nerves) and within (tracts) the CNS.

The diameter of axons also affects the speed of action potential transmission. The bigger the axon diameter, the faster an action potential can travel. Numerous microtubule fibers are present within the axon and function as a set of cable systems by which vesicles containing neurotransmitters and other cellular materials are transported between the cell body and axon terminals. Neurotransmitter vesicles and other secretory products are made and packaged in the neuron cell body, which are then hooked onto the microtubule fibers and transported to the axon terminal by sliding down the microtubule fibers. Once they reach the axon terminal, neurotransmitter vesicles are stored here until the action potential arrives and triggers their release. Other cellular materials or vesicles may be transported from the axon terminal to the cell body using the microtubules as well, but in a reverse direction. In this way, the cell body and the axon terminals that may be several feet apart are still able to communicate with each other effectively.

Lisa M. J. Lee

See also: Action Potential; Nerves

Further Reading

Hodgkin, Alan L., & Andrew F. Huxley. (1939). Action potentials recorded from inside a nerve fiber. *Nature, 144*(3651), 710–711.

Poliak, Sebastian, & Elior Peles. (2003). The local differentiation of myelinated axons at nodes of Ranvier. *Nature Reviews Neuroscience, 4,* 968–980. Retrieved from http://www.nature.com/nrn/journal/v4/n12/pdf/nrn1253.pdf

B

BALANCE

Balance, or the ability to maintain body position over a center of gravity, involves many different sensory systems integrated together. The three main sources of the required sensory information are the muscles, the eyes, and the vestibular organs. Vestibular information comes from specialized organs within the inner ear and provides information about where the body is in space relative to motion. Balance is something that most people do not think about on a regular basis. However, when there are issues with balance, everyday actions become extremely difficult. Some diseases involving the balance system include benign paroxysmal positional vertigo, Meniere's disease, multiple sclerosis, and Parkinson's disease. These diseases can be related to issues arising from the vestibular system in particular or general problems involving the nervous system and brain.

Sensory Inputs

Sensory inputs originate from three main sensory systems: proprioceptive, visual, and vestibular. Information from these sensory systems is integrated in the brainstem and processed in the cerebellum. The cerebellum is responsible for sending out motor signals to help maintain balance in posture and movement.

Muscles and Joint Position

One of the biggest cues that the brain uses to determine where the body is and how it needs to move to maintain balance is the location of the joints relative to itself (proprioception). This is accomplished through joint position sense provided by receptors within the joint itself, muscle spindles (providing information about the length and motion of the muscle itself), and Golgi tendon organs (which are responsible for providing information about a sense of force on the muscle). All of these receptors help the brain determine where the body is in space and how it moves. It allows the brain to make decisions about how to move specific muscles to keep the body where it needs to be in order to maintain balance. For instance, these sensory inputs help tell you to clench your toes on your right foot if you are leaning forward too far.

Romberg Test

The ability to balance oneself is dependent on the cooperation of a minimum of two out of three subjective factors: an individual's vision, their proprioception, and the proper functioning of the vestibular organs of the inner ear. Analyzing these three factors is the basis for the Romberg test. When giving a patient a complete neurological exam, doctors will often employ the Romberg test as one of many tools designed to screen for problems with balance, particularly to determine disorders of proprioception and the vestibular apparatus.

In clinical practice, the Romberg test does not always give very precise results, and today it is used most often to monitor the progress of a patient diagnosed with a particular disease or as a general indication that the patient has difficulty with balance. The test was not designed to assess vestibular function, though it has come to be used for that purpose. There is still a lack of consistency regarding when to use the test and how to interpret the results; however, a positive Romberg's sign, meaning a loss of balance, certainly indicates a need for further testing.

One of the most common uses of the test today is by law enforcement officials to confirm positive results from standardized roadside sobriety tests. The Romberg test removes visual stimuli that a person might use to maintain balance and can therefore detect problems with proprioception or the vestibular apparatus.

Materials:

Volunteer
Enough space for two people to stand safely
Timer or watch with a second hand

Directions:

For safety, the experimenter should stand next to the volunteer with his or her arms in front of and behind the subject in all balance tests to provide support and to reduce the risk of a fall.

Test 1: Have the volunteer stand with both feet together. Ask the person to pick up one foot and balance on the other foot for 10 seconds. A normal response is that the person will not sway or need to hold on to anything for balance. Repeat this test with the other foot and compare responses.

Test 2: Have the volunteer stand with one foot in front of the other touching heel to toe. The subject can choose which foot is in front. Next, have the person fold their arms across their chest or hanging down at their sides. Have the individual stand in this position with their eyes closed for 30 seconds. Mild rotational swaying may be perceptible and is considered a normal occurrence. For a true negative test, there should be no marked swaying or loss of balance, nor should the subject have to move their feet for stability.

Erin Slocum

Visual Input

Information from the eyes comes in from light hitting the rods and cones (photo-receptors) in the retina. This information is processed in visual centers within the brain and tells the brain important information about the surrounding area. This visual input provides cues to where the body is relative to space—whether it is upright, sitting, moving in a certain direction, and so on.

Vestibular Sense

Vestibular organs reside within the inner ear and are made up of the utricle, saccule, and the three semicircular canals. The utricle and saccule are responsible for vertical and horizontal orientation within space (as relative to gravity—which way is up and which way is down), and the semicircular canals are responsible for detecting rotational motion. Typically the vestibular system works symmetrically. Ideally information from both sets of vestibular organs will match. When this sensory information does not match, it can cause a feeling of dizziness or vertigo and cause the individual to lose his or her balance.

Diseases

Diseases of the balance system typically consist of symptoms of dizziness, vertigo, and unsteadiness. One of the more common reasons for these diseases is issues involving the vestibular system. Benign paroxysmal positional vertigo (BPPV) is one of these. BPPV is due to loose vestibular crystals (otoconia). These otoconia will move when the head is tilted or jolted and will then weigh down the semicircular canals, causing them to send incorrect messages about motion to the brain. This causes a brief but intense episode of vertigo in the patient. There are multiple causes of dislodging the otoconia including head injury, age, and dehydration. Meniere's disease, another balance disorder, is still not well understood but it is believed to be related to issues with fluid filling the semicircular canals. This disease is characterized by episodes of vertigo, tinnitus (ringing in the ears), and buzzing in the ears.

Other diseases of balance are due to issues within the brain and nervous system itself. Parkinson's disease is one such disease. Parkinson's disease is a disease of the motor system characterized by tremors and muscle rigidity. Additionally, patients afflicted with Parkinson's disease may have postural instability and lose balance easily. This instability is thought to be due to problems making minute adjustments in posture to maintain a standing position.

Riannon C. Atwater

See also: Dizziness; Golgi Tendon Organs; Meniere's Disease; Tinnitus; Vestibular System

Further Reading

National Institute on Deafness and Other Communication Disorders (NIDCD). (2015). Balance disorders. Retrieved from https://www.nidcd.nih.gov/health/balance-disorders

Tassinari, Mariateresa, Daniele Mandrioli, Nadia Gaggioli, & Paola Roberti di Sarsina. (2015). Ménière's disease treatment: A patient-centered systematic review. *Audiology & Neurotology, 20*(3), 153–165.

BARORECEPTORS

Baroreceptors are unique receptors that are located within the walls of blood vessels and are part of the autonomic nervous system. These receptors are a type of mechanoreceptor that measures the amount of pressure within blood vessels. When the pressure rises, the blood vessels expand, and this expansion triggers the firing of baroreceptors within the vessels. Through the usage of baroreceptors the body regulates blood pressure. This process of regulating blood pressure is known as the baroreceptor reflex or the baroreflex.

History

In 1852, Claude Bernard (1813–1878) discovered that the sympathetic portion of the autonomic nervous system innervated blood vessels in the skin of the rabbits he was studying. This discovery was the first on the road to identifying baroreceptors and their role in regulating blood pressure. Later in 1921, Heinrich Ewald Hering (1866–1948) identified baroreceptors in the carotid artery (located in the neck) and demonstrated that stimulating them resulted in hypotension (low blood pressure) and bradycardia (very slow heart rate). Corneille Heymans (1892–1968) expanded this work and managed to successfully outline the baroreflex, leading him to win the 1939 Nobel Prize in Physiology or Medicine.

Anatomy and Physiology

Baroreceptors are primarily located in the carotid arteries and the aorta. In these locations the receptors can monitor blood pressure going to both the brain and the body. This is essential for proper blood flow to occur throughout the body. Baroreceptors are tonically active receptors. This means that they are constantly firing. Due to this, any change in blood pressure will be reflected in the rate at which the receptors fire. If blood pressure increases, then the baroreceptors fire more quickly, resulting in a physiological response that lowers arterial blood pressure.

The baroreflex is a negative feedback loop, which functions to maintain a relatively constant blood pressure. The feedback loop works in a manner similar to a thermostat that is used to regulate temperature. The baroreflex process starts when baroreceptors detect a change in blood pressure by the change in size of the vessel walls. When blood pressure is high, the vessels will expand, and as a result the baroreceptors will fire at a faster rate. This information is transmitted to the brain through the glossopharyngeal nerve to the cardiovascular control center located in the medulla oblongata of the brainstem. Here the rate of the signals will be interpreted and a response will be generated. If the blood pressure increases, the cardiovascular control center will in turn increase parasympathetic activity and decrease sympathetic activity, resulting in a decrease in heart rate and a dilation of blood vessels. This combination of actions will result in a decrease in blood pressure. The baroreceptors respond to low blood pressure in the opposite manner. Heart rate will increase and the vessels will constrict, resulting in an increase in blood pressure.

Through this process baroreceptors maintain proper blood flow when the body's position is altered rapidly, such as when a person sits up. Due to gravity, blood would naturally flow downward to the lower extremities. This lowers the amount of blood returning to the heart and in turn lowers the arterial blood pressure. The baroreceptor reflex is triggered, which then causes the heart rate to increase and vessels to constrict, which brings the blood pressure back to normal and allows blood flow to the brain to stay constant.

While the baroreflex monitors the arterial blood pressure, it is rarely attributed to long-term changes in blood pressure such as hypertension (high blood pressure). The reflex is associated with short-term changes in blood pressure. With hypertension there is a general depression of baroreflex sensitivity. Long-term changes in blood pressure are monitored primarily by the kidneys through control of blood volume. Despite this there are some cases in which baroreceptor reflex failure can result in hypertension (Heusser et al., 2005).

Disease

Baroreceptor insensitivity has been associated with various diseases and issues within the body. It has been shown that people suffering from chronic obstructive pulmonary disease (COPD) have reduced baroreceptor sensitivity. This results in a decreased response to short-term blood pressure changes as with exercise. This reduction of baroreceptor sensitivity is coupled with an increase in sympathetic activity (van Gestel & Steier, 2010).

In addition, baroreceptor insensitivity has been associated with sleep-related breathing problems (SRBP) in adolescents, which range from chronic snoring to sleep apnea. This insensitivity results in a rise in blood pressure, and researchers suggest it is likely a result of general autonomic dysfunction. Coverdale et al. (2012) have demonstrated that children with more severe SRBP had less sensitive baroreceptor reflexes. In addition to this they showed that the relationship is intensified by a higher body mass index (BMI).

Stephen Mazurkivich

See also: Autonomic Nervous System; Glossopharyngeal Nerve

Further Reading

Coverdale, Nicole S., Laura K. Fitzgibbon, Graham J. Reid, Terrance J. Wade, John Cairney, & Deborah D. O'Leary. (2012). Baroreflex sensitivity is associated with sleep-related breathing problems in adolescents. *Journal of Pediatrics, 4,* 610–614.

Heusser, Karsten, Jens Tank, Friedrich C. Luft, & Jens Jordan. (2005). Baroreflex failure. *Hypertension, 45,* 834–839.

Klabunde, Richard E. (2007). *Arterial baroreceptor.* Retrieved from http://cvphysiology.com/Blood%20Pressure/BP012.htm

van Gestel, Arnoldus J. R., & Joerg Steier. (2010). Autonomic dysfunction in patients with chronic obstructive pulmonary disease. *Journal of Thoracic Disease, 4,* 215–222.

BARTOSHUK, LINDA

American experimental psychologist Dr. Linda Bartoshuk, PhD, is the assistant director and the Bushnell Professor of Food Science and Human Nutrition at the University of Florida Center for Smell and Taste. She is an international leader in taste research and a pioneer in developing new methods of psychophysical scaling. As a Presidential Endowed Professor of Community Dentistry and Behavioral Science at the University of Florida, Bartoshuk is widely known for her work specializing in the chemical senses of taste and smell.

Born in Aberdeen, South Dakota, in 1938, Bartoshuk embraced a passion for astronomy. At Carleton College in the 1950s, Bartoshuk realized that women were not welcome in the field. On a whim, she signed up for a class in experimental psychology and discovered a new area for her scientific explorations. With a father fighting lung cancer and a brother also suffering from cancer that resulted in taste symptoms, Bartoshuk was personally motivated to research taste and discovered that nerve and tissue damage from chemotherapy caused their "taste phantoms." Bartoshuk put forth the concept that phantoms are actually caused by nerve damage.

After receiving her BA from Carleton College and her PhD from Brown University, Bartoshuk went on to explore the genetic variations in taste perception and how taste perception affects overall health. Bartoshuk was the first to discover that burning mouth syndrome, a condition that seems to be mostly experienced by post-menopausal women, is caused by damage to the taste buds at the front of the tongue and is not a psychosomatic condition as some of her contemporaries believed.

Bartoshuk was employed at Yale University prior to accepting a position at the University of Florida in 2005. She was elected a Fellow of the American Academy of Arts and Sciences in 1995. In 2003, Bartoshuk was elected to the National Academy of Sciences and is also a distinguished University of Florida William James Fellow Award winner.

Bartoshuk was the first to identify what she referred to as "supertasters," those who have an unusually high number of taste buds and experience tastes more intensely than their fellow eaters. She was responsible for contradicting the concept of the tongue map that so many of us learned about in school, making the connection between ear infections and being overweight, and creating new magnitude scales to measure subjective experiences. Her current research focuses on the connections between taste damage and obesity and on methods for comparing taste or pain experiences across people.

Corporate influence in science is something Bartoshuk has been vocal about. She is on the front lines of making inroads for women in science, and early in her career, she faced sexism from multiple sources. She encourages young people interested in science to pursue what they love, as she has—even at 70, she says, she "still can't wait to get into the lab every day."

Lin Browning

See also: Burning Mouth Syndrome; Supertaster; Taste System

Further Reading

Association for Psychological Science. (2010). *Experimental psychology, inside the psychologist's studio, taste.* Retrieved from http://www.psychologicalscience.org/index.php/video/linda-bartoshuk-itps.html

Bartoshuk, Linda. (2014). *The measurement of pleasure and pain.* Department of Food Science and Human Nutrition, University of Florida. Sage Journals. Retrieved from http://pps.sagepub.com/content/9/1/91.full

King, Camille Tessitore. (2004). On blue tongues, undergraduates, and science: An interview with Linda M. Bartoshuk. *Teaching of Psychology, 31*(3), 212–217. Retrieved from http://eric.ed.gov/?id=EJ683185

University of Florida. (n.d.). Center for Smell and Taste. UFCST Faculty. Retrieved from http://cst.ufl.edu/faculty.html

BELL'S PALSY

Bell's palsy is a peripheral nerve disorder affecting the facial nerve, or cranial nerve VII. While the exact mechanism of Bell's palsy is unknown, it is thought to be caused from edema (swelling) and inflammation of the facial nerve. It is characterized by unilateral (one side) and temporary weakness or total paralysis of the facial nerve, which originates in the brainstem and is responsible for controlling the muscles of facial expression and for the sense of taste from the anterior two-thirds of the tongue. Cranial nerve VII also provides innervation to lacrimal glands (tears), salivary glands, and the stapes (a bone in the middle ear used for hearing). Patients with Bell's palsy suffer a temporary inability to control the muscles of the face that include movements like smiling and raising eyebrows. Bell's palsy occurs in approximately 40,000 people in the United States each year and is most common among 15- to 60-year-olds (NINDS, 2012).

History

Disorders of facial nerve paralysis have been recorded in medical texts as early as the Persian physician Rhazes (865–925) who described the disorder in his text *al-Hawi.* It was later described by authors in the Greek and Roman empires and then later by European physicians in the 17th and 18th centuries. Bell's palsy is formally named after Scottish physician Sir Charles Bell (1774–1842) after he introduced the disorder to the Royal Society of London in 1829.

Diagnosis and Symptoms

Bell's palsy is diagnosed when a person suffers acute onset, unilateral, hemifacial weakness or paralysis with no other signs or symptoms and no other disorder can be attributed to the facial weakness or paralysis. It is not thought to be infectious, although some researchers are still investigating viral etiology. Bell's palsy is more common during pregnancy and in people who suffer from obesity, diabetes, hypertension, upper respiratory infections, or compromised immune systems. Patients with Bell's palsy usually recover completely, although some may never fully recover. Bell's palsy is a diagnosis of exclusion, meaning that all other disorders must be ruled out before a diagnosis of Bell's palsy can be given. Differential diagnoses for Bell's palsy that must be considered include stroke, herpes zoster virus (Ramsay Hunt syndrome type 2), Lyme disease, HIV (human immunodeficiency virus) infection, head trauma, tumors, meningitis, and inflammatory diseases of the cranial nerves such as sarcoidosis or brucellosis. Both physicians and dentists in the United States are trained in the diagnosis, treatment, and management of Bell's palsy.

There are both short-term and long-term signs and symptoms of Bell's palsy including:

- Unilateral facial weakness or paralysis
- Inability to smile and raise eyebrows on affected side
- Inability to close eye on affected side
- Alteration of taste
- Difficulty chewing food
- Numbing or tingling in cheek or mouth
- Dryness of the affected eye
- Corneal ulceration
- Vision loss
- Permanent facial disfigurement
- Ringing in the ears
- Headache
- Dizziness
- Impaired speech
- Depression
- Acute and rapid onset within 72 hours
- No other disorder, tumor, or illness can be identified

Treatment

The current treatment of choice for patients with Bell's palsy is oral corticosteroid treatment and antiviral treatment, although antiviral treatment has not been found to have a clear benefit to Bell's palsy patients. Physicians most commonly prescribe a six-month course of prednisone, and the most common antivirals prescribed are acyclovir or valacyclovir. It is recommended to begin treatment within three days of onset of symptoms for optimal results.

Physical therapy is also recommended to reduce the symptoms of Bell's palsy and may be helpful in some patients. Physical therapy stimulating the facial nerve aids in maintaining muscle tone and reeducating the muscles of facial expression so they may return to the most normal functioning upon recovery. Palliative treatment and eye care are crucial in preventing overdrying of the eye and eventual loss of vision. Frequent lubrication and protection with an eye patch of the affected eye is recommended. Heat application has been shown to reduce pain associated with Bell's palsy in some patients. Surgical decompression of the facial nerve has been done but has not been shown to be beneficial in most patients. Surgery is no longer recommended by the American Academy of Neurology. Finally, most persons will recover within three to four months after the initial signs.

Elizabeth Shick

See also: Dizziness; Facial Nerve; Ptosis

Further Reading

Baugh, Reginald F., Gregory J. Basura, Lisa E. Ishii, Seth R. Schwartz, Caitlin Murray Drumheller, Rebecca Burkholder, . . . William Vaughan. (2013). Clinical practice guidelines for Bell's palsy. *Otolaryngology–Head and Neck Surgery, 149*(3), S1–S27.
Gronseth, Gary S., & Remia Paduga. (2012). Evidenced-based guideline update: Steroids and antivirals for Bell palsy. *Neurology, 79*(22), 2209–2213.
National Institute of Neurological Disorders and Stroke (NINDS). (2012). *Bell's palsy fact sheet.* Retrieved from http://www.ninds.nih.gov/disorders/bells/detail_bells.htm
Ragupathy, Kalpana, & Eki Emovon. (2013). Bell's palsy in pregnancy. *Archives of Gynecology and Obstetrics, 287,* 177–178.

BIETTI'S CRYSTALLINE DYSTROPHY

Bietti's crystalline dystrophy (BCD) is a rare autosomal recessive eye disease that appears to be more common in people with Asian ancestry compared to any other race or ethnicity. Depending on how the disease affects a person's eyes, BCD is also known as Bietti crystalline corneoretinal dystrophy (BCCD), Bietti crystalline retinopathy (BCR), or Bietti tapetoretinal degeneration with marginal corneal dystrophy. In this disorder yellow or white crystal-like deposits of lipid (fat) accumulate in the retina. The deposit damages the retina, which leads to progressive vision loss and potentially blindness. The disease was named after Dr. G. B. Bietti, an Italian ophthalmologist who first described the symptoms in 1937.

Inheritance of Bietti's Crystalline Dystrophy

To understand how a disease is inherited, it is important to understand what a gene is and its role in metabolic and molecular cell activities. A gene is a molecular unit of an organism's heredity that codes for specific genetic traits, such as hair color and height. Each person receives one allele of the gene from his or her mother and the other from his or her father. Both alleles will determine the genetic trait. If one allele or both alleles are damaged or mutated, this can result in an abnormal trait or disease. Bietti's crystalline dystrophy is an autosomal recessive disorder, which means the offspring must inherit the defective or mutated allele from both parents. The disorder occurs in 1 of 67,000 people and is more common in people of East Asia, especially those of Chinese and Japanese descent (Okialda et al., 2012).

Cause of the Disease

Bietti's crystalline dystrophy is caused by the mutation of the *CYP4V2* gene, which is located on chromosome 4. The *CYP4V2* gene codes for members of the cytochrome P450 enzymes, which are known for breaking down various chemicals in cells. Specifically, the CYP4V2 enzyme is involved in fatty acid oxidation, which breaks down lipids (fatty acids). Even though the specific mechanism is not well understood, it is estimated that the dysfunction of the CYP4V2 enzyme in breaking down lipids affects the accumulation of lipid deposits in the retina of the eye.

Symptoms

Bietti's crystalline dystrophy is characterized by the accumulation of crystals in the cornea (which covers the eye) and yellow, shiny deposits on the retina. This leads to atrophy of the retina, choriocapillaries, and choroid, which are associated with the back layers of the eye where the optic nerve is located. Patients with BCD can have some white blood cells that can be seen with crystalline deposits when viewed under the electron microscope. The crystalline deposits seem to harm only the vision. Progressive atrophy and degeneration of the retinal pigment epithelium lead to symptoms similar to other retinal degenerations like retinitis pigmentosa. Patients suffering from BCD can have reduced visual acuity, poor night vision, visual field loss, abnormal retinal electrophysiology, and often impaired color vision. Marked asymmetry between a person's eyes is also common. Gradually, the peripheral visual field, central acuity, or both are lost, leading to blindness. The onset of the disease is usually during the second and third decades of life, but ranges can vary from early teenage years to beyond 30 years old.

Diagnosis and Treatment

The disease can be recognized by the yellow-white crystals on the retina, dysfunction of rod and cone photoreceptors on electroretinography (ERG), visual field defects, and reflective dots by spectral domain optimal coherence tomography (sdOCT). Rod and cone electroretinography tests the electrophysiology of the rod and cone cells of the retina. Persons with BCD often have reduced amplitude responses to no responses at all. Although an abnormal ERG is not required to diagnose BCD, an ERG is useful in determining the significance of the damage of the retina. To date, there is no treatment for BCD. Physicians work to reduce the damage to the retina but are not able to stop the progression of the dystrophy.

Future Work

Screening and testing can be done to detect carriers of the defective gene. However, additional research is required to better understand the gene and its defect before new treatments can be developed to slow or stop the disease.

Paul Hong

See also: Blindness; Color Blindness; Color Perception; Cones; Retina; Retinopathy; Rods; Visual System

Further Reading

National Eye Institute (NEI). (2009). *Facts about Bietti's crystalline dystrophy*. National Eye Institute (NEI). Retrieved from https://nei.nih.gov/health/biettis/bietti

Okialda, Krystle A., Niamh B. Stover, Richard G. Weleber, & Edward J. Kelly. (2012). Bietti crystalline dystrophy. In Pagon, R.A., M. P. Adam, H. H. Ardinger, et al. (Eds.). *GeneReviews*® [Internet]. Seattle, WA: University of Washington, 1993–2015. Retrieved from http://www.ncbi.nlm.nih.gov/books/NBK91457/

BITTER SENSATION

Bitter sensation, the detection of a diverse array of organic compounds, is one of the five basic tastes. Bitter is an aversive sensation in that it is regarded as unpleasant. Of the three tastes that sense organic compounds (bitter, sweet, and umami), it is the only one that is aversive, and the only taste that senses a broad range of unrelated molecules. It has likely been advantageous in human evolution by facilitating the detection and avoidance of toxic organic compounds. Most medications are considered to have a bitter taste, as well as coffee, unsweetened cacao, various leaf vegetables, and chicory. The standard substance used to compare the bitterness of compounds is quinine.

Bitterness is determined by affinity to bitter receptors, which are the taste receptor 2 family of receptors (Tas2R). There are approximately 25 functional Tas2R genes in humans. The receptor is expressed on the surface of taste receptor cells (TRCs). Only TRCs that express the Tas2R receptors sense bitterness, and TRCs that detect bitterness do not detect other tastes. Different TRCs are responsible for all five of the primary tastes. TRCs are organized into taste buds, which contain 50–150 TRCs each. Taste buds throughout the tongue contain TRCs for all five primary tastes; therefore, there is no topographic taste map. The specificity of the TRC to one taste alone is essential for the way that the different taste sensations are encoded.

Depolarization of the bitter TRCs following a signaling cascade triggered by the taste receptor transmits a signal to afferent neurons. The signal is relayed by the facial nerve (cranial nerve VII) in the anterior two-thirds of the tongue and glossopharyngeal nerve (cranial nerve IX) in the posterior third of the tongue. Sensory afferents synapse in the rostral portion of the nucleus of the solitary tract in the brainstem and are relayed to the thalamus with projections to the primary gustatory cortex.

The Tas2R receptors include receptors that detect specific compounds with high affinity, and others that detect a broad range of compounds with lower affinity. Though many different molecules may be detected, the primary bitter taste of one compound is indistinguishable from another. The affinity required for detection of bitter is much lower than those of the sweet and umami receptors. These attributes are consistent with the likely role of bitter taste to indicate the presence of potentially harmful molecules, which could be toxic at miniscule amounts and thus would need to be detected within the same range.

Bitterness is not directly correlated with toxicity. While many toxic substances are bitter, bitterness is a poor predictor of toxicity. This likely reflects a system designed to err on the side of caution—substances that are unfamiliar and do not have sufficient caloric or protein content are detected as bitter to facilitate rejection, regardless of actual toxicity. There is evidence that the full spectrum of bitter taste has lost some of its evolutionary importance in humans, as there has been some loss of function within the Tas2R receptor family. An example of loss of function is the population variation in phenylthiocarbamide (PTC) detection. PTC is sensed as bitter by the receptor T2R38, but not all humans have a functional version of this receptor, leading some people to identify the normally bitter PTC as tasteless.

Michael S. Harper

See also: Facial Nerve; Glossopharyngeal Nerve; Supertaster; Taste Aversion; Taste Bud; Taste System; Type II Taste Cells

Further Reading

Meyerhof, Wolfgang, Maik Behrens, Anne Brockhoff, Bernd Bufe, & Christina Kuhn. (2005). Human bitter taste perception. *Chemical Senses, 30* (Suppl. 1), i14–i15.

Wang, Xiaoxia, Stephanie D. Thomas, & Jianzhi Zhang. (2004). Relaxation of selective constraint and loss of function in the evolution of human bitter taste receptor genes. *Human Molecular Genetics, 13*(21), 2671–2678.

BLIND SPOT

Each vertebrate animal has a natural blind spot or scotoma in its vision. The term scotoma is derived from the Greek word meaning "darkness." Thus, a scotoma is an obstruction of the visual field surrounded by a field of normal vision. The field of vision is everything that a person sees either straight ahead or peripherally. Abnormal or pathological scotomata (plural form of scotoma) can develop from disease processes that affect the retina or the optic nerve.

History

The first documented recording of the eye's blind spot was by French physicist and priest Edme Mariotte (ca. 1620–1684). While at the French royal court, Mariotte showed this phenomenon by placing a small coin at a certain distance from a person's right eye. He asked the volunteer to close his left eye and with his right eye to look left. The coin instantly disappeared from the person's vision, which made people think it was a "magic coin." For his research in physics, particularly for acknowledging Boyle's law and its inverse relationship for gases, Mariotte was asked to join the French Academy of Sciences.

Anatomy and Physiology

In vertebrates, there is an anatomical blind spot that is caused by the lack of photosensitive receptors (rods and cones) and cells in one location of the retina. This area is called the optic disc, which can be viewed using specific tools such as an ophthalmoscope. In most humans, the optic disc is found in each eye about three to four millimeters toward the nasal side of the fovea. The fovea is the center of the macular region of the retina, which is the section responsible for precise and high-resolution vision. The optic disc is an oval shape that is thinner vertically and about 0.2 millimeter wider horizontally. The optic disc is the beginning of the optic nerve, or cranial nerve II, and it is where the optic nerve exits the eye. Anatomically, the output of the retina, called the retinal ganglion cell axons, all come together at the optic disc while blood vessels enter and exit the eye at the same spot. Thus, there are no light-sensitive receptors or neurons within the optic disc to receive and interpret signals. This makes a true anatomical blind spot.

However, the blind spot is generally not perceived during vision, especially when both eyes are open. This is because the signals of the visual fields have an overlap or are slightly different. The blind spot in one eye will not be noticed because the visual cortex of the opposite eye will take over that portion of the entire visual field. In general, the brain takes the surrounding information around the blind spot in each eye as well as information from the opposite eye to compensate for the blind spots. The blind spots are not perceived and normal vision is the result. It is only in certain circumstances, as in the "magic coin" experiment performed by Mariotte, that the blind spot can be tested. To test your own blind spot, see http://faculty.washington.edu/chudler/chvision.html.

There are some animals that do not have an anatomical blind spot, such as octopuses or other cephalopods. In their eyes, the optic nerve fibers all group together behind the retina. This is different from vertebrates whose optic nerve fibers group together in front of the retina. Not only does this anatomical orientation in vertebrates make a scotoma, but it also blocks some of the light that should "hit" the retina.

Diseases, Disorders, and Treatments

Some diseases or disorders that affect the retina or the optic nerve can result in a pathological scotoma that can be temporary or permanent depending on whether permanent damage occurs to the retina or the optic nerves. These scotomata are abnormal and can be seen in any part of the visual field, can have any shape, and can be any size. Additionally, these pathological scotomata can enlarge the normal anatomical blind spot. If the scotoma affects the macula, it can cause severe vision loss, as high-resolution vision will be compromised. On the other hand, if the scotoma affects peripheral vision, people may not even notice it because they can turn their heads to see what they are missing. This adjustment does not help with scotomata in the macular region.

The most common causes of pathological scotomata are multiple sclerosis, high blood pressure, drinking methyl alcohol, nutritional deficiencies, and tumors that block or damage the retina and/or the optic nerve. In most patients, a scotoma affects only one eye. However, in rare cases, bilateral scotomata can occur if there is a tumor of the pituitary gland. This is because the pituitary gland is inferior to the optic chiasm. When the tumor enlarges, it compresses the optic chiasm, causing a bitemporal paracentral scotoma, which can lead to bitemporal hemianopsia that extends to the periphery. If a person presents with bitemporal hemianopsia, it is usually the first sign of a pituitary tumor. Temporary pathological scotomata can occur (1) during migraines, when a bright light during the aura causes the blind spot; and (2) during pregnancy, especially if the woman is having severe hypertension (also called severe preeclampsia).

Patricia A. Bloomquist

See also: Occipital Lobe; Optic Nerve; Retina; Sensory Receptors; Tunnel Vision; Visual Fields; Visual Perception; Visual System

Further Reading

Bear, Mark F., Barry W. Connors, & Michael A. Paradiso. (2007). *Neuroscience exploring the brain* (3rd ed.). Baltimore, MD: Lippincott Williams & Wilkins.
Chudler, Eric H. (n.d.). *Neuroscience for kids: The blind spot.* Retrieved from http://faculty.washington.edu/chudler/chvision.html
Tasman, William, & Edward Jaeger. (2012). *Duane's ophthalmology* (13th ed.). Philadelphia, PA: Lippincott Williams & Wilkins.

BLINDNESS

Blindness is a condition of poor visual perception. There is a range of vision loss as defined in the *International Classification of Diseases* (ICD) of the World Health Organization (WHO). ICD-10 states the categories as: (1) normal vision, (2) moderate visual impairment, (3) severe visual impairment, and (4) blindness. Blindness can be acquired at birth or in life due to injury, genetics, and other life events. As of August 2014, according to WHO, there were an estimated 285 million people who are visually impaired worldwide, of whom 39 million are blind.

History

Blindness is a condition that has been frequently noted in history. Many cultures have viewed blindness in different aspects of mythology, social value, and legal definition. No one person can be attributed with the discovery of this condition, but many have recorded individuals in stories, official documents, and personal entries. An important figure in the history of blindness is Louis Braille (1809–1852). Braille was a French educator who became blind at age three as a result of an eye injury. He created the tactile system used by the visually impaired and blind to read and write, known simply as braille.

Types and Symptoms

The more common diseases that can cause blindness are cataracts, glaucoma, age-related macular degeneration (AMD), and pregnancy-related issues. Blindness can result from genetic defects, certain chemicals, eye injuries, and abnormalities of related tissues, such as the optic nerve.

Cataracts are the change in lens color that leads to clouding. This is associated with aging, smoking, and diseases such as diabetes. Early changes in lens color do not affect vision, but vision is impaired over time as the clouding becomes thicker.

Glaucoma is a disease in which retinal cells are damaged as a result of increased pressure within the eye. When aqueous humor, the liquid within the eyeball, is drained slower than it is produced, it can lead to increased pressure within the eye. This can also compress the optic nerve, which is responsible for transporting information about light received by the retina to the brain for processing. This disease is a major cause of irreversible blindness. Late signs of the disease include blurred vision, headaches, and reported halos around sources of light.

Age-related macular degeneration (AMD) is the progressive deterioration of the retina. It affects a specific region on the retina called the macula lutea, a pigmented region that deals with high acuity vision. There are two forms of AMD: wet and dry. In the "wet" form new blood vessels grow and cause retinal detachment by scarring, and in the "dry" form excessive accumulation of visual pigments causes many more to die off.

Treatments and Outcomes

Cataracts can be surgically corrected. The removal of the clouded lens and implantation of an artificial lens can restore effective vision. Long-term exposure to ultraviolet radiation may play a role in developing cataracts, so wearing sunglasses is recommended by many experts as a preventive measure to delay the onset.

Glaucoma can be caught early; however, it takes sight away so slowly and painlessly that many do not realize the damage until it is done. An examination for high inner eye pressure is done by administering a directed puff of air toward the cornea to measure the deformation of the sclera, the white area of the eye. The amount of deformation can detect possible glaucoma. A glaucoma exam should be performed annually after age 40 since it affects 2 percent of people over that age (Marieb et al., 2011). If caught early, glaucoma can be treated with eye drops that either increase drainage or decrease production of the aqueous humor.

AMD is mostly untreatable, but laser treatment can remove some of the growing blood vessels to slow the progression of the disease in "wet" form. To date, there are no viable treatments for the "dry" form.

Prevention and Research

The majority of these diseases have few effective preventive measures. Most are successful in the early stages of these diseases, thus most experts recommend annual eye exams, especially for persons over age 40 as many diseases seem to manifest around this age. Additionally, examinations should always be performed after any trauma to the eyes or head to ensure eye health and vision will not be affected.

A study published in the *New England Journal of Medicine* (Bainbridge et al., 2008) shows the potential of gene therapy to improve vision in subjects with an inherited blindness called LCA (Leber's congenital amaurosis). The gene therapy involved using a virus to deliver a gene into the eyes of patients with LCA, with most reporting improved vision.

In summary, several diseases that can render their victims blind may not have exact known causes or effective treatments. Ongoing research is currently exploring the effects of techniques such as gene therapy to help restore vision and reverse the effects of vision-impairing diseases. Prevention can be limited, but early signs of these sight-stealing diseases can be caught with routine eye examinations.

Eric B. Moore

See also: Optic Nerve; Optic Nerve Hypoplasia; Retina; Visual Fields; Visual Perception; Visual System

Further Reading

Bainbridge, James W., Alexander J. Smith, Susie S. Barker, Scott Robbie, Robert Henderson, . . . & Robin R. Ali. (2008). Effect of gene therapy on visual function in Leber's congenital amaurosis. *New England Journal of Medicine, 358*, 2231–2239. http://dx.doi .org/10.1056/NEJMoa0802268
International Council of Ophthalmology. (2002). *Visual standards: Aspects and ranges of vision loss with emphasis on population survey* [Report prepared for 29th International Congress of Ophthalmology]. Retrieved from http://www.icoph.org/downloads/visual standardsreport.pdf
Marieb, Elaine N., Patricia B. Wilhelm, & Jon Mallatt. (2011). *Human anatomy* (6th ed.). San Francisco, CA: Pearson Benjamin Cummings.
World Health Organization. (2014). Visual impairment and blindness. Retrieved from http://www.who.int/mediacentre/factsheets/fs282/en/

BLINK REFLEX

Blinking, or blink reflex, is the involuntary movement (opening and closing) of either one or both eyelids simultaneously. It is essential in the function of spreading tears and removing irritants from the surface of the cornea (front part of the eye) and the conjunctiva (the mucous membrane that covers the cornea and the lining of the eyelids). The rate or frequency of a blink varies between species. Each mammalian species expresses a characteristic blink rate that is constant under unchanging conditions. However, the blink rate can be affected by factors such as fatigue, eye injury, disease, or medication. In humans, the blink reflex is the first and most reliable form of the startle reflex, which is an avoidance response induced by a threatening stimulus. Further, the blink reflex can be increased by emotional stimuli.

Function and Purpose of the Blink Reflex

The blink reflex seen in animals and humans is made for the local protection of the cornea and the conjunctiva. This is because animals are highly visual and need to protect their ability to see. It enables self-preservation of the eyes, either from a threat of real danger to the animal's life (like being attacked) or from undefined fears of the surrounding conditions.

Blinking also provides moisture to the eye by irrigation. Specifically, the eyelid provides suction across the eye from the tear duct (located in the lower eyelid near the nose) to the rest of the eyeball; this prevents the eye from drying out. Thus, the tears and lubricant that the eyes secrete are essential for eye health.

Lastly, blinking protects the eye from irritants in the environment. A second line of defense against dust and other elements that could irritate the eye is eyelashes, which are hairs attached to the upper and lower eyelids. Eyelashes function to catch these irritants during a blink reflex before they reach the eyeball.

Anatomy of the Blink Reflex

Several muscles control the blink response. The main muscles in the upper eyelid are the obicularis oculi and the levator superioris muscles. These control the opening and closing of the eye. The obicularis oculi muscle closes the eye, while the levator superioris muscle contracts and opens the eye. The contraction of the obicularis oculi muscle protects important structures, like the retina (the photosensitive lining of the back of the eye), from external trauma. The smooth muscle of the upper lid, the Muller's muscle (also known as the superior palpebral muscle), also helps in widening the lid aperture, which enables the widening of the eyes.

The nerves that supply the blink reflex are cranial nerves V and VII (or trigeminal and facial nerves). Specifically, the ophthalmic branch (V_1) of the trigeminal nerve senses the stimulus on the cornea, lid, or conjunctiva. The temporal and zygomatic branches of the facial nerve initiate the motor response, or blinking action.

Vivian Vu

See also: Facial Nerve; Reflex; Trigeminal Nerve; Visual System

Further Reading

Hall, Arthur. (1945). The origin and purposes of blinking. *British Journal of Ophthalmology, 29*(9), 445–467.

Pearce, J. M. S. (2008). Observations on the blink reflex. *European Neurology, 59*(3–4), 221–223.

Shahani, Bhagwan. (1970). The human blink reflex. *Journal of Neurology, Neurosurgery, and Psychiatry, 33*(6), 792–800.

BOWMAN'S GLANDS

Bowman's glands, which are unique to the olfactory epithelium, release fluids to protect the olfactory sensory neurons from infection as well as trap odor molecules. Once an odorant is trapped, it binds to specific receptors located on olfactory sensory neurons, which begins the process of perceiving a smell.

History

Sir William Bowman (1816–1892), an English surgeon, histologist, and anatomist, is best known for his research using microscopes to study human organs. Sir William was also a successful ophthalmologist. Throughout his life, many anatomical structures were named after him including Bowman's capsule, which is a cup-like sac at the tubular portion of the nephron of the kidney and is the first step in filtering blood from urine; Bowman's membrane, which is the anterior limiting membrane in the cornea of the eye; and Bowman's glands, which are below the olfactory epithelium to secrete fluid that traps odorants.

Anatomy and Physiology

The nasal cavity is found between the ethmoid bone superiorly and the palate inferiorly. It is divided into two sections by the nasal septum. The nasal cavity is essential for conditioning the air that passes into the lungs as well as acting as a resonance chamber to enhance a person's speech. Within the nasal cavity lie the nasal and olfactory epithelia. The nasal epithelium is a pseudostratified ciliated layer with goblet cells, which secrete mucous to trap small foreign particles so that they are breathed into the lungs. The olfactory epithelium is also pseudostratified but has a columnar look to it and does not contain goblet cells. Instead it contains ciliated olfactory sensory neurons. Just beneath this epithelium are the Bowman's glands.

Also known as olfactory glands, Bowman's glands penetrate to the surface of the olfactory epithelium. The glands consist of an acinus (cluster of cells that resembles a "berry" shape) in the lamina propria (thin layer of loose connective tissue) and a secretory duct that exits through the olfactory epithelium. Bowman's glands are situated in the dorsal (roof of the nasal cavity) and caudal (toward the back) portions of the nasal cavity. Secretions from Bowman's glands, including lysozyme (a type of protein or enzyme that damages bacterial cell walls to fight and/or prevent infection), amylase (an enzyme that breaks up starches), and immunoglobulin A (an antibody that is necessary for mucosal immunity), help moisten the epithelium in the nasal passages. Additionally, these secreted enzymes are essential for maintaining the immune system of the nasal cavity, and particularly the olfactory epithelium. As a person ages, Bowman's glands are lost or disrupted in their main function. Infection can also cause Bowman's glands to be lost or damaged, particularly if the olfactory epithelium is damaged.

Research

For decades the main function of the Bowman's glands was unknown. Recent research completed at the University of Oslo (Solbu & Holen, 2011) showed that in rats and mice (1) Bowman's glands secreted mucin (a protein found in mucus), and that (2) aquaporin-5 (a water channel protein) was present at the apical face of the olfactory epithelium. Immunogold electron microscopy analysis revealed an intricate network of fine aquaporin-1-positive fibroblast processes (principal water-transporting proteins) surrounding Bowman's glands. These results show how the olfactory mucosa could be protected from infection and dehydration as well as how neuronal function is protected against ion concentration changes. This is done by the rapid replacement of water loss through aquaporin pathways.

Renee Johnson and Jennifer L. Hellier

See also: Anosmia; Dysosmia; Olfactory Mucosa; Olfactory Sensory Neurons; Olfactory System

Further Reading

Ablimit, Abduxukur, Toshiyuki Matsuzaki, Yuki Tajika, Takeo Aoki, Haruo Hagiwara, & Kuniaki Takata. (2006). Immunolocalization of water channel aquaporins in the nasal olfactory mucosa. *Archives of Histology and Cytology, 69,* 1–12.

Jayaraman, Sujatha, Nam Soo Joo, Bruce Reitz, Jeffery J. Wine, & A. S. Verkman. (2001). Submucosal gland secretions in airways from cystic fibrosis patients have normal [Na(+)] and pH but elevated viscosity. *Proceedings of the National Academy of Sciences of the United States of America, 98,* 8119–8123. Retrieved from http://www.pnas.org/content/98/14/8119.abstract?ijkey=668b36099966ef706e75d33c9b2a9c6a78668cad&keytype2=tf_ipsecsha

Solbu, Tom T., & Torgeir Holen. (2011). Aquaporin pathways and mucin secretion of Bowman's glands might protect the olfactory mucosa. *Chemical Senses, 37(1),* 35–46. Retrieved from http://chemse.oxfordjournals.org/content/37/1/35.full

BRAILLE

For persons who are blind or hard of seeing, it can be difficult or impossible to read written communication that is printed. For centuries, rudimentary forms of raised dots on paper have been developed to help the blind read as well as for military use in night activities. Since 1858, the braille system has been the official standardized reading and writing system for the blind as voted by the World Congress for the Blind.

History

Louis Braille (1809–1852) was born in France and at the age of three years he accidentally punctured his right eye with a sharp tool used by cobblers. A few months later, his left eye began to be inflamed, most likely by sympathetic ophthalmia. Medical technology at the time could not save either eye and thus, by the age of five years old Braille was completely blind. Nonetheless, Braille's parents wanted Louis to receive an education, so his father taught him the French alphabet by hammering nails into wooden blocks in the shapes of letters. Louis would run his finger over the nail heads to learn the alphabet. By 10 years old, Braille entered the Royal Institute for Blind Youth in Paris to have a formal education.

Through time, simple forms of raised-letter systems have been developed for written communication with the blind. One of the first recorded raised-letter systems was designed by Valentin Haüy (1745–1822), who was the founder of the Royal Institute for Blind Youth in Paris, France, which opened in 1784. About 20 years later, Napoleon Bonaparte's (1769–1821) army created another raised-dot system (or code) specifically for military use during night activities. Artillery captain Charles Barbier invented this system and brought it to the Royal Institute for Blind Youth as another option for blind readers. This raised-dot system was based on a six-by-six grid with each box representing a sound of the French alphabet.

Braille first learned Haüy's raised-letter system but eventually converted to Barbier's coded system as Braille felt it was a superior system. Over time, Braille improved on Barbier's original raised-dot system so that (1) each combination of dots represented an actual letter of the alphabet and not just the sound, (2) there were fewer dot combinations to memorize, and (3) the organization of the raised dots could be read by a single finger. This allowed the user to learn the system quickly, increase speed in reading, and spell words that sighted people could read. Because of his improved design, this raised-dot system was named after Louise Braille and is still used today.

Components of Braille

Braille consists of a grouping of six raised dots, which is called a cell. Each cell is organized by six dots organized in three rows and two columns, having the same organization as a number six playing card. The dot or dots that are raised determine the letter, number, or punctuation. This combination allows braille to have 64 different characters, including spaces, accent marks (required in the French language), and symbols.

Braille organized the letters of the alphabet by decades, with A–J being the first decade, K–T being the second decade, and U–Z being the third decade. This means that the first decade only has raised dots on the top and middle rows of the cell. The second decade has raised dots in each row but only in the first dot (or left dot) on the bottom row. This bottom left raised-dot denotes the second decade. Finally, the third decade has raised dots in each row but both dots are raised in the bottom row. The English-language W letter is not the same as in French and thus, it is represented by the letter J raised-dots combination along with only the right bottom dot being raised.

There are three additional decades (fourth, fifth, and sixth decades) that are used for numbers, punctuation, symbols, and spaces. These are denoted by raised dots in all rows but only the right bottom dot is raised for the fourth decade. The fifth decade only has the middle and bottom rows with raised dots, called "shift down." Finally, the sixth decade is shifted to the right with the majority of cells' first columns not having any raised dots.

Jennifer L. Hellier

See also: Blindness; Keller, Helen; Visual Motor System; Visual System; Visual Threshold

Further Reading

Braille Institute of America. (2016). About: Braille Institute. Retrieved from http://www .brailleinstitute.org/about-braille-institute.html

Bullock, John D., & Jay M. Galst. (2009). The story of Louis Braille. *Archives of Ophthalmology, 127*(11), 1532–1533.

Jiménez, Javier, Jesús Olea, Jesús Torres, Inmaculada Alonso, Dirk Harder, & Konstanze Fischer. (2008). Biography of Louis Braille and invention of the braille alphabet. *Survey of Ophthalmology, 54*(1), 142–149.

BRAIN ANATOMY

The anatomy of the brain is very complex because of its intricate structure and function in the body. The central nervous system (CNS) acts as a control system by receiving, interpreting, and directing sensory information from the body to the brain. In turn, the CNS reacts to the sensory information by initiating motor movements such as sniffing and talking.

Brain Divisions

There are three major divisions in the brain, all of which have prime responsibilities for the normal functions of the body. These divisions are called the forebrain, midbrain, and hindbrain.

The forebrain is responsible for receiving and processing sensory information as well as thinking, perceiving, producing, and understanding language. It also controls voluntary motor function. The forebrain contains structures such as the thalamus and hypothalamus, which are responsible for motor control and relaying sensory information. It also contains the cerebrum, which is the largest part of the brain where most of the processing of sensory information takes place.

The midbrain makes up part of the brainstem with the hindbrain. The midbrain is the portion of the brain that connects the hindbrain to the forebrain. This region is responsible for auditory and visual responses as well as voluntary motor function.

The hindbrain contains structures such as the pons and cerebellum. This region of the brain assists in maintaining balance and equilibrium, coordinating voluntary movement, and conducting sensory information.

Brain Building with Clay

The central nervous system (CNS) consists of the brain, brainstem, and spinal cord. The brain serves as the control center for the CNS, is responsible for coordinating responses to stimuli, and exerts control over the body. The divisions and functions of the brain are: cerebrum, higher-order functions; cerebellum, modulation of brain signals; and brainstem, regulating the cardiovascular and respiratory systems and connecting the brain to the spinal cord. The cerebrum is further divided into lobes. The frontal lobes are responsible for motor responses, reward, attention, and motivation. The temporal lobes retain visual memories, language, storage of memories, and emotions. The occipital lobes are the visual processing center, and the parietal lobes integrate sensory information and special awareness (particularly body position).

Materials:

Five colors of clay (red, green, yellow, blue, and white), waxed paper, tabletop, toothpick, and paper towels

Directions:

Place the waxed paper on the tabletop and roll a gumball-size piece of yellow clay into a worm approximately one-eighth of an inch thick. Take this worm and slowly fold it into a loose ball in your hand. This will represent the frontal lobe of the cerebrum. Set this aside and clean your hands with the paper towels. Clean them between each color.

Next, roll a gumball-size piece of green clay and roll it as done previously. This will represent the temporal lobe of the cerebrum. Fold this clay into a loosely shaped ball and set aside.

Take a gumball-size piece of blue clay and roll it into a worm approximately one-eighth of an inch thick. Fold this clay into a ball; this will represent the occipital lobe of the cerebrum.

Then take a gumball-size piece of red clay and roll it as done previously. Fold the clay into a ball; this represents the parietal lobe of the cerebrum.

Repeat the aforementioned steps to make the other half of the brain and arrange the balls of clay into a brain. The frontal lobes sit in front followed by the parietal lobes, under which the temporal lobes sit. In the back sit the occipital lobes.

Next, use a gumball-size piece of white clay and flatten one side. Using a toothpick, carve several horizontal lines across the rounded side of the ball. Add a short tail; this represents the cerebellum and brainstem. Place the cerebellum and brainstem under the occipital lobes so that the brainstem points down.

Riannon C. Atwater

Structures

The brain contains many identifiable structures. Each structure/region is responsible for different aspects of bodily function, either sensory, motor, or both. The major structures of the brain are listed here in alphabetical order.

Amygdala—an almond-shaped region just anterior to the hippocampus. Its main functions are emotional responses and memory. Damage to this region is associated with posttraumatic stress disorder (PTSD).

Basal ganglia—deep structures near the midline of the cerebrum. The basal ganglia are four distinct groups of neurons consisting of the striatum (caudate and putamen), globus pallidus, substantia nigra, and subthalamic nucleus. Together these structures are involved in cognition and voluntary movement. Generally, damage to this area is associated with both Parkinson's and Huntington's diseases.

Brainstem—a set of structures located below the cerebrum and ventral to the cerebellum. The brainstem connects the spinal cord to the cerebrum and cerebellum. It consists of the midbrain, pons, and medulla oblongata. The brainstem relays information between the peripheral nerves to the CNS as well as regulating heart rate and breathing.

Cerebellum—the "little brain" found posteriorly and below the cerebrum. It is a "quality control center" for voluntary movement coordination. It also maintains balance and equilibrium.

Cerebral cortex—the gray matter of the cerebrum. It is divided into four lobes named after the bone they lie beneath. The frontal lobe is involved with decision making, problem solving, and planning. The occipital lobe's function is vision. The parietal lobe receives and processes sensory information and language. Lastly, the temporal lobe processes emotions, memories, and speech.

Corpus callosum—a thick band of fibers connecting the left and right cerebral hemispheres.

Hippocampus—located in the temporal lobe. It is hypothesized as being the region involved with learning and long-term storage and retrieval of memories.

Hypothalamus—a structure deep in the brain and below the thalamus. It directs a multitude of important functions such as metabolism, body temperature, and hunger.

Pituitary gland—an endocrine gland located below the optic chiasm. It regulates other endocrine glands and maintains homeostasis.

Thalamus—a structure deep in the center of the cerebrum that modulates all sensory and motor responses except for olfaction.

Damage to the Brain

Although the meninges and the skull protect the brain, it still can be injured by a lack of oxygen. A stroke occurs when a blood vessel in the brain is blocked or bursts. Without the constant blood flow and oxygen required for a healthy brain, the neurons in the region of the stroke start to die. Brain damage can occur within minutes of the insult. Thus it is imperative to recognize symptoms of stroke and to act quickly. Stroke symptoms include but are not limited to sudden numbness or tingling, sudden change in vision, inability to smile on demand, or trouble speaking (slurred speech). In general, managing high blood pressure, cholesterol levels, and diabetes may prevent the probability of a stroke. Thus, it is necessary to take medication exactly as a health care provider prescribes it. A stroke is an emergency and always needs immediate emergency care.

Renee Johnson

See also: Brainstem; Cerebral Cortex; Olfactory Bulb; Visual System

Further Reading

The brain from top to bottom. (2013). http://thebrain.mcgill.ca/index.php

Hines, Tonya. (2011). Anatomy of the brain. *Mayfield Clinic for Brain & Spine.* Retrieved from http://www.mayfieldclinic.com/PE-AnatBrain.htm

WebMD. (2009). *Brain & nervous system health center.* Retrieved from http://www.webmd .com/brain/picture-of-the-brain

BRAINSTEM

The brainstem is a small yet very important component of the brain that serves a multitude of functions affecting the whole body. The structure is located on the posterior side of the brain and connects directly to the spinal cord. The brainstem is essential for regulating basic processes including breathing, heart rate, sleep, and digestion. Furthermore, it transmits information between the central and peripheral nervous systems through nerve tracts. The brainstem supplies many cranial nerves to the face and neck, allowing for sensory and motor conduction. Conversely, it also receives sensory and motor input from peripheral nerves for appropriate interpretation by the brain. Through its vast range of functions that are crucial for living, the brainstem proves to be a vital part of the central nervous system.

Anatomy and Physiology

The brainstem is positioned at the base of the cerebrum, above the spinal column, and anterior to the cerebellum. It consists of three distinct structures called the midbrain, pons, and medulla oblongata.

Midbrain

The midbrain, also called the mesencephalon, is the superior-most portion of the brainstem. Its name is derived from the Greek terms *mesos*, meaning middle, and *enkephalos*, meaning brain. The midbrain is located adjacent to the cerebral hemispheres, just below the cerebral cortex and above the pons. This structure is further organized into parts known as the corpora quadragemina, cerebral aqueduct, tegmentum, and cerebral peduncles. Within these components exist many nuclei (collection of cell bodies) and fasciculi (clusters and bundles of axons). One well-established nucleus of the midbrain is the substantia nigra, which releases the neurotransmitter dopamine that plays an important role in movement control. Other functions of the midbrain include regulation of arousal, sleep/wake cycles, and temperature. This structure also contains auditory and visual reflex centers to control proper hearing and vision.

Pons

The pons is an approximately 2.5-centimeter-long section of the brainstem, located between the midbrain and medulla oblongata. Based on its location it was given the name pons, which is derived from the Latin term meaning bridge. Functions of the pons include regulation of the sleep cycle and the development of dreams. Also, the pons contains four cranial nerves (V, VI, VII, and VIII), which it supplies to the face and neck. Through this innervation, the structure is essential for sensory functions such as taste, facial sensation, and hearing, as well as motor functions such as eye movement, facial expression, chewing, and swallowing. The pons also plays a role in bladder control, posture, and balance. Located within the pons is the pneumotaxic center, a nucleus that is responsible for regulating the switch from inspiration (breathing in) to expiration (breathing out). Therefore, the pons is also essential in proper respiratory function.

Medulla Oblongata

The medulla oblongata is the inferior-most part of the brainstem, located adjacent to the spinal column. In this position, it acts as a connector of motor tracts between the higher centers of the brain and the spinal cord. The superior sections of the medulla oblongata also form a wall of the fourth ventricle, a compartment where cerebrospinal fluid is maintained. Key functions of the medulla oblongata include regulation of basic yet fundamental autonomic processes. These include respiration, vasodilation (blood vessel relaxation), and cardiac function. Additionally, the medulla oblongata controls reflexes such as vomiting, sneezing, coughing, and swallowing.

Diseases

Due to its vast range of functions, damage to the brainstem can manifest in a variety of serious outcomes. Diseases that damage the brainstem can do so through bleeding, tumors, formation of plaques, lack of oxygen supply, or demyelination (unsheathing of neurons' axons). If a cranial nerve within the brainstem is affected, the subsequent sensory and motor stimuli will not be experienced or performed properly by the face and neck. Additionally, if a nerve tract is altered, there may be improper perception of peripheral stimuli. Based on the presentation of symptoms, whether they are visual, auditory, speech, or otherwise, the location of damage can be determined. Regardless, damage to the brainstem may be irreversible and requires immediate, invasive medical attention. Therefore, preservation of a healthy brainstem is vital, as this structure is responsible for many basic functions of life.

Vidya Pugazhenthi

See also: Auditory System; Autonomic Nervous System; Inferior Colliculus; Superior Colliculus; Taste System

Further Reading

Haines, Duane E., & M. D. Ard. (2013). *Fundamental neuroscience for basic and clinical applications*. Philadelphia, PA: Elsevier/Saunders.
Tortora, Gerard J., & Bryan H. Derrickson. (2012). *Principles of anatomy & physiology*. Hoboken, NJ: Wiley.
Urban, Peter P., & Louis R. Caplan. (2011). *Brainstem disorders*. Berlin: Springer.

BRAINSTEM AUDITORY EVOKED POTENTIALS

Brainstem auditory evoked potentials (BAEPs), also known as brainstem auditory evoked responses (BAERs), are small auditory evoked potentials that are recorded in response to an auditory stimulus from electrodes placed on the scalp. BAEPs reflect neuronal activity in areas including the inferior colliculus of the brainstem, the auditory nerve (cranial nerve VIII), and the cochlear nucleus. They all have a response latency of six milliseconds or less and have an amplitude of about one microvolt. It is possible to obtain a BAEP to a pure tone stimulus, but it is more effective when the auditory stimulus contains a range of frequencies in the form of a short, sharp click.

Test for BAEPs

When being tested for BAEPs, patients lie on their back in a reclining chair or bed and remain as still as possible. Electrodes on the scalp and each earlobe help record the response after a brief click or tone is transmitted through earphones. The person does not need to be awake for this test. The results of this test have been shown to (1) help diagnose nervous system problems including hearing loss, (2) determine the efficiency and health of a person's nervous system, and (3) test hearing ability in people who cannot have their hearing tested by other means. Abnormal BAEP responses may result from but are not limited to (1) a brain injury, (2) developmental malformation(s) of the brain, (3) a brain tumor, and (4) speech disorders. The main indication to have this test performed is when an acoustic neuroma, a nonmalignant tumor of the vestibulocochlear nerve, is suspected.

Using BAEP in Research and Case Studies

Ondine's curse—also known as congenital central hypoventilation syndrome (CCHS) or primary alveolar hypoventilation—is a respiratory disorder that is fatal if untreated. It is the failure of automatic control of ventilation (breathing) during sleep. In 1984, Long and Allen published a case report of a woman with alcoholism who was hospitalized with complications of CCHS. During her extended hospitalization, she had abnormal BAEPs in conjunction with hyperactive muscle reflexes and bilateral Babinski signs (abnormal flexion of the foot). They hypothesized that the patient's brainstem had been poisoned by her chronic alcoholism, which may have resulted in her CCHS and abnormal BAEPs.

A recent study by Akin and colleagues (2016) investigated alterations in BAEPs in children with obesity. They tested the BAEPs in just under 100 children with an average age of 12 years old. The obese cohort contained roughly 65 children while the remaining 35 children were control subjects (within normal weight ranges). The researchers performed BAEP tests and measured the latency and amplitude of BAEP from the obese and control subjects. They found that the average latency was significantly longer in children who were obese compared to the control subjects. They also tested insulin resistance (IR), which can lead to diabetes among the obese children and split them into two separate groups, those with IR and those without IR. Performing the same tests, they found that children with IR had longer latency periods than those without IR. Thus, this suggests that BAEPs can be used to determine early subclinical auditory dysfunctions of obese children with insulin resistance (Akin et al., 2016).

Finally, Zafeiriou and colleagues (2000) hypothesized that BAEPs can be utilized in children with spastic cerebral palsy to test hearing. They tested 75 patients with cerebral palsy (CP) and found that 17 patients had abnormal BAEPs while 58 had normal BAEPs. They reported no statistical significance between genders, but the mean birth weight of those with abnormal BAEPs was significantly higher than for those with normal BAEPs. Several hypotheses have been proposed to explain the abnormal BAEP findings in those with spastic CP; however, nothing has been supportive of these results as of yet.

Renee Johnson

See also: Auditory Processing Disorder; Auditory Threshold; Inferior Colliculus; Vestibulocochlear Nerve

Further Reading

Akın, Onur, Mutluay Arslan, Hakan Akgün, Süleyman Tolga Yavuz, Erkan Sarı, Mehmet Emre Taşçılar, . . . Bülent Ünay. (2016). Visual and brainstem auditory evoked potentials in children with obesity. *Brain & Development*, 38(3), 310–316. Retrieved from http://ac.els-cdn.com/S0387760415002090/1-s2.0-S0387760415002090-main.pdf?_tid=1b83719e-eeb7-11e5-bed1-00000aacb35e&acdnat=1458490771_e31b3db75c76fa1e4ee340a3708132f6

Long, Kevin J., & Neil Allen. (1984). Abnormal brain-stem auditory evoked potentials following Ondine's curse. *Archives of Neurology, 41*(10), 1109–1110. Retrieved from http://archneur.jamanetwork.com/article.aspx?articleid=583557

Zafeiriou, D. I., A. Andreou, & K. Karasavidou. (2000). Utility of brainstem auditory evoked potentials in children with spastic cerebral palsy. *Acta Paediatrica, 89*(2), 194–197.

BRODMANN AREAS

Regions of the cerebral cortex of the brain have been defined according to the structure and organization of the neurons that they contain. These regions are called Brodmann areas. It is important to note that the term—Brodmann area—is not possessive but refers to the numbering system that Brodmann used to describe the regions. Recently, it was found that Brodmann areas also contain brain regions that are now thought to share similar functions. Though there is ongoing debate about the definition and border of the regions, Brodmann areas are still useful in describing regions of the brain in terms of both function and susceptibility to pathology. Advances in imaging techniques will continue to allow for a more refined description of Brodmann areas.

History

Brodmann areas were originally described by German anatomist Korbinian Brodmann (1868–1918). He became interested in neuroscience due to the influence of Alois Alzheimer (1864–1915), a German scientist after whom Alzheimer's disease is named. Brodmann used a histological method known as the Nissl staining method to examine the structure and organization of cells in different regions of the brain. This stain was developed by the German neuropathologist Franz Nissl (1860–1919). It labels neuronal cell bodies, specifically a particular kind of RNA in the rough endoplasmic reticulum, which are also known as Nissl bodies. Brodmann applied this stain to very thin sections of brain specimens that he had acquired. This allowed him to visualize the structure and organization of cells, which is often referred to as their cytoarchitecture. Brodmann published his original cortical maps in 1909 and described the layout of the brains of humans, monkeys, and other organisms. Additionally, neuroanatomists such as Georg Koskinas (1885–1975), Constantin von Economo (1876–1931), and Alfred Walter Campbell (1868–1937) followed in his footsteps. Though Brodmann's original cortical maps labeled 52 individual areas, several of them are found only in nonhuman primates and thus there are fewer areas in the human brain. His original descriptions included 43 areas in the human cortex. Drs. von Economo and Koskinas followed up on Brodmann's original mapping of the brain in 1925, 16 years after it was published.

More than 50 years later, in the 1980s, the Brodmann area map experienced a resurgence. This was because several new imaging techniques, such as magnetic resonance imaging (MRI), had been invented and could be used to view the brain. These new modalities utilized variants of Brodmann's maps to detail structures of the brain. Specifically, the imaging could define regions of patients' brains that were undergoing some sort of pathology, such as a tumor or tissue loss following a stroke. Furthermore, as some of these new imaging techniques allowed for visualization of brain activity under various conditions, scientists and physicians could begin to correlate the cytoarchitecture of brain regions defined by Brodmann with the functions that they coordinated.

Examples of Brodmann Areas

There are several Brodmann areas that are more widely known or more often referenced. This is because they correspond to a common action, such as movement or sensory perception, or they are involved in certain pathologies.

Brodmann areas 1, 2, and 3 (often referred to in the order 3, 1, and 2) are collectively known as the primary somatosensory cortex. They are located in the parietal lobe of the brain in a region known as the postcentral gyrus. The postcentral gyrus corresponds roughly to a location starting at the top of one's ear and ending at the top of the head. There is a primary somatosensory cortex in both the right and left halves of the brain. The primary somatosensory cortex serves as the final destination of sensory inputs, such as touch or limb position, from the entire body. An interesting characteristic of the primary somatosensory cortex is that different regions along the postcentral gyrus correspond to sensory input from specific regions in the body. For instance, sensory input about touch perceived in the leg is processed by neurons closer to the top of the head, whereas input from the mouth or tongue activates neurons on the side of the head. This arrangement of inputs that maintains a regional separation according to the location of the sensory or motor input is known as somatotopy or as a homunculus. Somatotopy is Greek for "body" and "place" while homunculus is a Latin word meaning "little man."

Whereas the primary somatosensory cortex is devoted to the perception of touch, there are other regions in the brain that are responsible for detection of other senses. For example, a region designated by Brodmann areas 41 and 42 is known as the primary auditory cortex. Located in the upper part of the temporal lobe on both the right and left sides of the brain, the primary auditory cortex is responsible for processing auditory information that originates in the ears and is what dictates the perception of sound. Similar to the homunculus of the primary somatosensory and motor cortices, the primary auditory cortex is also organized in a particular manner. Different regions of the primary auditory cortex correspond to sounds of different frequencies; this has been termed a tonotopic organization.

Christopher Knoeckel

See also: Brain Anatomy; Cerebral Cortex; Homunculus; Somatosensory Cortex; Somatosensory System

Further Reading

Augustine, James R. (2008). *Human neuroanatomy: An introduction.* Burlington, MA: Elsevier Science.

Dubin, Mark. (n.d.). *Locational descriptions of human Brodmann areas,* edited from Neuro Names. Retrieved from http://spot.colorado.edu/~dubin/talks/brodmann/neuronames .html

Zilles, Karl, & Katrin Amunts. (2010). Centenary of Brodmann's map—conception and fate. *Nature Reviews Neuroscience, 11,* 139–145.

BUCK, LINDA

American biologist Linda Brown Buck, faculty member of the Fred Hutchinson Cancer Research Center in Seattle, is a 2004 Nobel Prize winner for Physiology or Medicine. Buck's work shared with the world the discovery of odorant receptors and the organization of the olfactory system.

Born in Seattle, Washington, in 1947, Linda Buck enjoyed an explorative childhood and was influenced to pursue greatness by close family members. Her childhood passion for understanding her world and a supportive environment for critical thought prepared her for a life of discovery. As an undergraduate at the University of Washington, Buck struggled to find the right career path. When studying immunology, her fascinations led her to pursue biology. Attending graduate school in the Microbiology Department at the University of Texas Medical Center in Dallas, Buck truly embraced the role of a scientist and began thinking in terms of molecules and the molecular mechanisms underlying biological systems.

Realizing she needed to grow in her understanding of the techniques of molecular biology, Buck moved to Columbia University to work with a team under the direction of Richard Axel (1946–). While working on the neuropeptide gene, Buck encountered puzzles surrounding olfaction and was intrigued. She wanted to understand how humans and other mammals are able to detect 10,000 or more odorous chemicals. She set about to find odorant receptors, a class of molecules that had been proposed to exist, but had not yet been found. Together with Richard Axel in 1991, Buck published her discovery showing how hundreds of genes in our DNA are responsible for the coding of the odorant sensors located in the olfactory sensory neurons in our noses. It was this work for which Axel and Buck were awarded the 2004 Nobel Prize in Physiology or Medicine.

In 1991, Buck joined the Neurobiology Department at Harvard Medical School in Boston as an assistant professor where she expanded her understanding of the nervous system. In 1994, Buck became an investigator at the Howard Hughes Medical Institute. Over the next decade, Buck went on to become an associate and then a full professor at Harvard Medical School and continued with her discoveries, focusing next on learning how signals from the olfactory sensory neurons are organized in the brain to generate diverse odor perceptions. Joined by a series of excellent students and postdoctoral fellows, Buck spent many years experimenting and discovering additional layers of knowledge surrounding olfactory sensation.

In 2002, Buck became a member of the Division of Basic Sciences at Fred Hutchinson Cancer Research Center in Seattle and Affiliate Professor of Physiology and Biophysics at the University of Washington. In 2015, Buck was awarded an honorary doctorate by Harvard University and elected a Foreign Member of the Royal Society (ForMemRS).

Buck continues to research odor perception in addition to pheromone and instinctive behaviors. Her work continues to help the scientific community understand the neural circuits that underlie innate behaviors and basic drives, such as fear, appetite, and reproduction.

Lin Browning

See also: Axel, Richard; Olfactory System; Society for Neuroscience

Further Reading

Howard Hughes Medical Institute. (2016). Linda B. Buck, PhD. Retrieved from http://www.hhmi.org/scientists/linda-b-buck

Nobel Media AB. (2014). Linda B. Buck—Facts. *Nobelprize.org*. Retrieved from http://www.nobelprize.org/nobel_prizes/medicine/laureates/2004/buck-facts.html

BURNING MOUTH SYNDROME

Burning mouth syndrome is a physical condition known to arise spontaneously, characterized by a burning sensation in the mucous membrane of the mouth that persists for extended periods of time; the burning usually originates with the tongue, but has been known to spread to the lips, gums, and inside of the cheeks. The most common symptoms of burning mouth syndrome, in addition to a burning sensation in the mouth, include dry mouth (xerostomia), increased thirst, taste changes, and loss of taste.

The Mouth

The inside of the mouth is lined with mucous membranes, referred to as oral mucosa, that serve to protect fat and muscle tissue from mechanical injury and bacterial infection. The oral mucosa contains a vast network of nerves, which allows for parts of the mouth to be incredibly receptive to temperature and pressure. On the tongue, soft palate, upper esophagus, and parts of the cheek, the mucosa contains taste buds that serve to recognize various aspects of taste, such as sweet, salty, sour, bitter, and umami (a Japanese word meaning "savory").

Diagnosis

There are no universally accepted diagnostic criteria, laboratory tests, or imaging studies that definitively diagnose or exclude burning mouth syndrome. Therefore, it is a clinical diagnosis that can only be made after the exclusion of all other causes. Currently, there are three classifications of burning mouth syndrome that are dependent on the apparent cause of the condition. Type 1, or "true burning mouth syndrome," arises spontaneously: upon waking, no symptoms are initially present, but as the day progresses there is a gradual escalation in the severity of the condition. While Type 1 has no clear cause, Type 2 is often associated with chronic anxiety. Patients diagnosed with Type 2 have continuous symptoms that persist throughout the day, but typically cease upon going to sleep. A Type 3 diagnosis is dependent on the consistency of symptoms; often, patients will have intermittent symptoms throughout the day and even symptom-free days (Bergdahl & Bergdahl, 1999). Since there is clear flux in the prominence of symptoms, food allergies have been suggested as a potential mechanism for the portrayal of the condition.

Epidemiology

While no definitive connections have been established, burning mouth syndrome seems to be most prevalent in women. Specifically, older women who are postmenopausal face the greatest risk for developing the condition. Burning mouth syndrome rarely presents in individuals under the age of 30 and has not been associated with any particular race. While the majority of diagnosed cases are Type 1, cases that begin spontaneously with no known triggering factor, other types are suggested to be correlated with upper respiratory tract infections, food allergies, medications, and anxiety. However, these conditions have not been consistently linked with the syndrome. Additionally, treatment of suspected correlated conditions has done little to consistently reduce the prevalence of the syndrome. Currently, there is no definitive cure for the condition.

Future Research

There is no consensus regarding a definitive cause for burning mouth syndrome. Understanding the cause for the condition could provide insight into how the oral mucosa is connected to other aspects of the body. Specifically, a better understanding of how the taste buds and sensory nerves relay information about temperature to the brain could reveal possible ways to treat the syndrome. The broad definition of the condition and variability in the way the condition presents have prevented homogeneous research from being established. For instance, Type 1 burning mouth syndrome is, by definition, not known to be linked to other factors, whereas Type 2 is suspected of being connected to the endocrine system, nutritional habits, bacterial infection, pharmaceutical drugs, and possibly even neuropsychiatric factors. Currently, the broad definition serves to fill an absence of knowledge in the medical community. Research should be directed at developing methodologies to test for the presence or absence of the condition, and at the ways in which burning mouth syndrome is connected to other aspects of the body.

James Danahey

See also: Bartoshuk, Linda; Nociception; Taste Aversion; Taste Bud; Taste System

Further Reading
Bergdahl, Maud, & Jan Bergdahl. (1999). Burning mouth syndrome: Prevalence and associated factors. *Journal of Oral Pathology & Medicine, 28*(8), 350–354. http://dx.doi.org/10.1111/j.1600-0714.1999.tb02052.x

Gruska, Miriam, Joel B. Epstein, & Meir Gorsky. (2002). Burning mouth syndrome. *American Family Physician, 65*(4), 615–620. Retrieved from http://www.aafp.org/afp/2002/0215/p615.html

Nelson, Linda P. (2013). Consumer version: Biology of the mouth—Mouth and dental disorders. *Merck Manuals.* Retrieved from http://www.merckmanuals.com/home/mouth-and-dental-disorders/biology-of-the-mouth-and-teeth/biology-of-the-mouth

C

CAROTID BODY

An animal's body must balance and control the amount of oxygen and carbon dioxide within its cardiovascular system (heart and lungs) to maintain good health. In mammals, this process is controlled by a feedback system between the cardiovascular system and the central nervous system. This is done by specialized chemoreceptors (proteins that sense changes in chemical concentrations) called the carotid body (also known as the carotid glomus or glomus caroticum). These chemoreceptors and other support cells form a small cluster located within the left and right carotid arteries just before they branch (bifurcate) into the internal and external carotid arteries. These four arteries are found on both sides of the throat and bring blood to the brain. The function of the carotid body is to sense the amount of oxygen within the blood. Specifically, it detects the partial pressure of oxygen by the glomus type I (chief) cells. This triggers a nerve impulse via the glossopharyngeal nerve (also called cranial nerve IX). The glossopharyngeal nerve is a paired cranial nerve that serves sensory and motor function to the head and neck. In turn, cranial nerve IX relays the partial pressure of oxygen within the blood to the medulla oblongata of the brainstem. In addition to measuring the partial pressure of oxygen, the carotid body detects changes in the amount of carbon dioxide, subtle changes in pH (the measurement of acidity or basicity of the blood), and temperature. Because of the location of the carotid body, it is suggested that persons who are working out and who want to take their pulse do so on their wrist. If they take their pulse on their neck, they may press too hard, altering their blood chemistry, and thus causing them to become lightheaded and possibly pass out.

Anatomy and Physiology

Two types of cells make up the carotid body, the glomus type I (chief) cells and glomus type II (sustentacular) cells. The glomus type I cells are similar to neurons in the central nervous system as they have the ability to release neurotransmitters, which are chemicals that transmit nerve signals. Specifically, glomus type I cells release acetylcholine, adenosine triphosphate (ATP), and dopamine to neurons located in the respiratory center of the brainstem. Glomus type II cells are support cells and have similar functions as glia (non-neuronal cells that maintain homeostasis) in the central nervous system. Because the carotid body is essential for maintaining homeostasis (balance) within the cardiovascular system, they are continually sensing the ratio of oxygen to carbon dioxide in the blood and constantly sending this information to the brain. For example, if the oxygen partial pressure is normal (about 100 mm Hg) and the pH is normal (around 7.2), then the glomus type I cells send out a relatively low output of action potentials to the brainstem. However, if the oxygen partial pressure is low (less than 60 mm Hg), then the glomus type I cells significantly increase their output, which causes the brainstem to significantly increase the person's breathing.

Pathology

In rare cases, carotid bodies can become tumorous and alter a person's blood pH and oxygen to carbon dioxide ratios. There are three types of carotid body tumors: familial, hyperplastic, and sporadic. Although rare, familial tumors are most common in younger patients while sporadic is the most common form overall, representing about 85 percent of all carotid body tumors. Sporadic tumors are generally seen in adults over the age of 45. People who live at a high elevation, such as in Denver, Colorado (a mile high), are more prone to hyperplastic carotid body tumors. Hyperplastic tumors have been associated with chronic hypoxia, as seen in patients with chronic obstructive pulmonary disease (COPD). Nonetheless, carotid body tumors are generally slow growing and persons may be asymptomatic for years. The tumors can be palpated in the neck near the carotid bifurcation. If the tumor is large enough, it may press on the nerves that supply the muscles of speech and swallowing, leading to other symptoms, such as pain, dysphagia, and hoarseness. The best treatment for carotid body tumors is surgical removal.

Jennifer L. Hellier

See also: Cranial Nerves; Sensory Receptors

Further Reading

Chaaban, Mohamad. (2014). *Carotid body tumors.* Medscape. Retrieved from http://emedicine .medscape.com/article/1575155-overview
Schultz, Harold D., Noah J. Marcus, & Rodrigo Del Rio. (2013). Role of the carotid body in the pathophysiology of heart failure. *Current Hypertension Reports, 15*(4), 356–362.

CATARACTS

The term "cataract" is used to describe a condition when the lens of the eye becomes opaque over time, often resulting in decreased visual acuity and overall visual function, which commonly results in increased falls, difficulty reading, difficulty driving, or decreased night vision. In most cases, the cataract (lens of the eye) can be removed using minimally invasive surgery and replaced with a new artificial lens that is inserted below the cornea of the eye, providing increased visual acuity postoperatively.

Types of Cataracts

There are two primary categories of cataracts. They are defined by (1) their location and (2) their point of origin.

Cataracts Defined by Location

Nuclear sclerotic cataracts are the most common type and are based on age. They often develop very gradually, resulting in the lens becoming more yellow in color and much more rigid in consistency. What is unique about nuclear sclerotic cataracts is that a patient's near vision may actually improve for a period of time before all vision becomes more difficult. Cortical cataracts usually present as a cloudiness or opaqueness in the cortical region (outer ring) of the lens. They tend to have a "wheel" appearance with spokes that project from the outer portion of the lens to the center, causing light to refract or scatter as it enters the eye and resulting in impaired vision. Posterior subcapsular cataracts occur when the opacity or cloudiness of the lens develops on the back side of the lens, which results in increased sensitivity to light, decreased near vision, and haloing of light.

Cataracts Defined by Their Point of Origin

These types of cataracts include (1) age-related cataracts, which start to develop as a function of aging, often beginning at age 40, but not really becoming significant until after age 70; (2) secondary cataracts, which are frequently a secondary effect of surgery for some other type of eye pathology, most commonly after surgery to release intraocular pressure associated with glaucoma or in patients who are on steroids for an extended period of time; and (3) traumatic cataracts, which can develop as a result of direct trauma to the eye. These types of cataracts can develop either very shortly after an injury or, more often, develop many years after an injury, probably in association with aging. In addition to direct trauma, exposure to chemicals or other caustic agents can also cause rather immediate cataracts.

Risk Factors

There are a number of health and environmental factors that often result in the development and onset of cataracts or that can increase the severity of cataracts. Individuals with long-term diabetes mellitus are thought to have an increased risk of developing cataracts due to the buildup of sorbitol, a sugar that is a breakdown product of glucose. The exact mechanism of how this might work is not well understood. Smoking and the long-term use of alcohol have also been shown to increase a person's risk for cataracts. In fact, both males and females who are heavy smokers double their risk of developing cataracts. This is thought to be due to the increased number of free radicals that can be found in the circulating blood of smokers. Smokers also experience a decrease in oxygen flow to the cornea and lens of the eye, resulting in a decrease in the turnover of nutrients necessary for proper function of the eye. Third, long-term use of corticosteroids is also being looked at closely now as a potential cause of cataracts. In fact, a recent study showed that individuals with asthma who have a history of long-term use of inhaled corticosteroids have a 90 percent greater risk for developing cataracts than nonasthmatics. Lastly and probably the most common cause of cataracts is overexposure or prolonged exposure to bright sunlight, which exposes the lens of the eye to high doses of ultraviolet light.

Treatment

Treatment for cataracts can be either nonsurgical or surgical in nature. Nonsurgical treatment is an option with the very early onset of cataracts. These treatments include using various types of corrective lenses to decrease light intensity, or the use of high-intensity reading lamps and other behavioral activities. It also includes trying to decrease or eliminate the factors that might be contributing to the onset of cataracts.

There are two primary surgical treatments. The first and most common procedure used today is called phacoemulsification, in which sound waves (ultrasound) are used to break up the lens of the eye, and then the debris is simply removed from the eye capsule. The removed lens is then replaced with an artificial lens, which often gives a patient nearly normal vision. The second surgical procedure uses an extracapsular approach: the lens is removed from the eye as a single entity. It is not broken up by chemical or ultrasound procedures. This procedure has more risk involved due to the larger incision that needs to be made to remove the lens.

Charles A. Ferguson

See also: Blindness; Visual Fields; Visual System

Further Reading

Christen, W. G., J. E. Manson, J. M. Seddon, R. J. Glynn, J. E. Buring, B. Rosner, & C. H. Hennekens. (1992). A prospective study of cigarette smoking and risk of cataract in men. *Journal of the American Medical Association, 268*(8), 989–993.

Mathew, Milan C., Ann-Margaret Ervin, Jeremiah Tao, & Richard M. Davis. (2012). Antioxidant vitamin supplementation for preventing and slowing the progression of age-related cataract. *Cochrane Database of Systematic Review, 6*, CD004567.

Neale, Rachel E., Jennifer L. Purdie, Lawrence W. Hirst, & Adele C. Green. (2003). Sun exposure as a risk factor for nuclear cataract. *Epidemiology, 14*(6), 707–712.

CENTRAL NERVOUS SYSTEM

The central nervous system (CNS) is composed of the brain, brainstem, and spinal cord. It is responsible for receiving and interpreting signals from the peripheral nervous system (PNS). The brain integrates sensory information and coordinates body function, both consciously and unconsciously. Complex functions including thinking, feeling, and regulation of homeostasis take place in various parts of the brain. The spinal cord enables communication between the brain and the rest of the body and controls musculoskeletal reflexes.

Anatomy and Physiology

The basic unit of the CNS is the neuron, which is specialized for rapid nerve impulse conduction and for exchanging signals with other neurons. Billions of neurons allow different parts of the body to communicate with one another via the brain, brainstem, and the spinal cord. Glia (plural), which is a Greek word for "glue," are supportive non-neuronal cells that surround the cell bodies, dendrites, and axons of neurons. Glial cells of the CNS include astrocytes, oligodendrocytes, microglia, and ependymal cells. Their main functions are to ensure neurons are "glued" together; nutrients and oxygen reach the neurons; neurons are insulated from one another; and pathogens are destroyed while removing dead neurons.

Brain

The cerebral cortex is the outermost part of the brain and consists of gyri and sulci, which give it a wormy appearance. It is the largest part of the brain and controls higher thought, language, consciousness, and memory. The cerebrum is divided into two hemispheres that are connected by the corpus callosum. Each hemisphere is responsible for controlled, voluntary limb movement of the contralateral side of the body.

The brain is divided into four lobes: frontal, parietal, temporal, and occipital. The frontal lobe contains dopamine-sensitive neurons that are associated with reward, attention, short-term memory, planning, and motivation. Executive functions of the frontal lobe include choosing between good and bad and recognition of consequences. In humans, the frontal lobe is not fully developed until the early 20s. The motor cortex is located in the frontal cortex and receives information from various parts of the brain to control movement.

The parietal lobe processes sensory information including pressure, touch, and pain via the somatosensory cortex. It integrates this sensory information and determines spatial sense and navigation. Attentiveness to the position of one's body and one's relationship to space is organized in this lobe. Additionally, language processing also takes place here.

The temporal lobe allows for interpretation of sounds and language and is the primary location of the auditory cortex. The hippocampus is also located in the temporal lobe and is important in the formation of memories. Damage to this area of the brain may lead to problems with memory, speech perception, and language skills.

The occipital lobe is associated with interpreting visual stimuli and information. The primary visual cortex is located in the occipital lobe and is responsible for receiving and interpreting information from the retina of the eye. These lobes are the smallest of the four.

The cerebellum, "little brain," is a complex motor coordination structure and has gyri and sulci similar to the cerebral cortex. It is connected to the brainstem by motor fiber tracts called peduncles. Its function is to produce changes in muscle tone in relation to equilibrium, locomotion, and posture and to coordinate the timing of contraction of muscles being used for skilled movements. In general, the cerebellum can be thought of as the quality control center of the CNS.

The diencephalon contains two structures: the thalamus and hypothalamus. The thalamus serves as a relay station, taking in sensory information and passing it to the cerebral cortex. The hypothalamus regulates autonomic, endocrine, and visceral functions including hunger, thirst, emotion, body temperature, and circadian rhythm.

Brainstem

The brainstem consists of the medulla oblongata, pons, and midbrain. The midbrain is located at the most anterior portion of the brainstem and contains ascending and descending pathways, which play roles in the visual and auditory systems. Located below the midbrain, the pons contains nuclei that mediate several auditory and balance functions. The pons receives input from the vestibular system within the inner ear and communicates with the cerebellum for balance. Below the pons, the medulla oblongata consists of neural fiber tracts, called pyramids, which are large and pyramidal-shaped. The pyramids travel toward the CNS with sensory information from the skin, muscles, and tendons and travel away from the CNS with motor information to control the body's muscles in the periphery.

Spinal Cord

The spinal cord is the central processing and relay station that transmits both sensory and motor information. It receives and projects information via peripheral nerves and ascending and descending tracts. Afferent sensory fibers enter the spinal cord through the dorsal roots of spinal nerves, and efferent motor fibers leave by way of ventral roots. Sensory signals travel via ascending tracts to the brain, while motor signals travel to the PNS via descending tracts. Vertebrae, three layers of meninges, and cerebrospinal fluid protect the spinal cord. The spinal column is divided into four sections: cervical, thoracic, lumbar, and sacral.

Danielle Stutzman

See also: Afferent Tracts; Brain Anatomy; Brainstem; Cerebral Cortex; Cranial Nerves; Peripheral Nervous System; Somatosensory Cortex; Somatosensory System

Further Reading

Kiernan, John A. (2009). *Barr's the human nervous system: An anatomical viewpoint* (9th ed.). Baltimore, MD: Lippincott Williams & Wilkins.
Noback, Charles R., N. L. Strominger, R. J. Demarest, & D. A. Ruggiero. (2005). *The human nervous system structure and function* (6th ed.). Totowa, NJ: Humana Press.

CEREBRAL CORTEX

The cerebral cortex is the thin, outermost layer of the brain of any animal with a cerebrum. It is approximately two to three millimeters thick and includes only the outer layer of the brain proper. In humans, it is where approximately 19 percent of all neurons' cell bodies exist in the brain.

The cerebral cortex is also known as "gray matter." This is based on how it looks to the naked eye, as the cell bodies are not myelinated. Thus the cerebral cortex does not include the underlying "white matter" through which the neurons' axons project. The cerebral cortex is the most easily visible part of the brain and has a highly characteristic folded appearance, particularly in humans. Its folded nature accommodates a tremendous amount of surface area. In fact, the human cerebral cortex contains three times the amount of surface area compared to that of the chimpanzee, the nearest primate relative of humans. If unfolded completely, this part of the brain would cover three sheets of notebook paper.

The cerebral cortex appears to have discrete, functional units. Several research experiments have identified distinct regions of the cerebral cortex that handle their own discrete tasks, such as visual processing, understanding verbal communication, and so on. In some cases, however, if one of these areas becomes damaged, studies have shown that other regions of the cortex may be able to learn new tasks and help the person compensate for the loss of that ability. This action indicates that the cerebral cortex might be somewhat modular and plastic, meaning it has the ability to adapt.

In the human brain, most of the cell-to-cell communication that exists in the cerebral cortex occurs between different regions of the cortex itself, but there is also communication with other structures buried deep underneath, including those that regulate emotion. This may help to explain why emotions can impinge strongly on thoughts and actions.

Histology and Function

The cerebral cortex is made up of three regions: archicortex—meaning the "ancient outer layer," paleocortex—which translates to the "old outer layer," and lastly, neocortex—which is the "new outer layer." These layers are named according to their phylogeny. Specifically, the archicortex is the most phylogenetically conserved across all animals with a cerebrum while the neocortex is the most recently developed portion of the cerebral cortex and is only conserved through mammals. The paleocortex shows intermediate conservation between the other two cortical regions.

The cellular organization is different within each region. The archicortex, which forms the hippocampal formation, has three layers, and the paleocortex has a variable number of cell layers. The neocortex is a six-layered structure with each layer being numbered with the corresponding Roman numeral: I–VI. As the neocortex is common in all mammals, this entry will focus on its distinct characteristics.

The neocortex's outermost layer is the "molecular layer" and is also called layer I. Alternating layers of neurons that have either a granular or pyramidal shape follow the molecular layer, thus these layers are called granular and pyramidal layers. Layer VI is polymorphic, meaning it consists of several cell types and is the deepest layer. In mammalian brain development, these layers develop in an "inside out" migration, meaning higher numbered layers are formed first, and then lower numbered layers migrate past them. For example, layer V forms, then layer IV forms and moves past layer V into position, followed by the formation of layer III that moves past both of these layers into position. The exception is layer I, which forms first and demarcates the boundary of the cortex. Within layers II–V, the granular cells act as the principal interneurons, and their projections do not leave the local cortex. The pyramidal cells act as the primary output neurons, and typically do send projections out of the cortex. These projections frequently contact other cortical areas of the brain or subcortical areas. Sometimes, the inputs and outputs are fairly consistent by layer. For example, the afferent inputs into layer IV frequently come from thalamic nuclei, while efferent output from layer III is predominantly corticocortical fibers, meaning fibers from one part of the cortex to another. Although this layered architecture is the general layout for the neocortex, it is not always clearly visible. The motor cortex, for example, is so dominated by large pyramidal cells that individual layers are difficult to identify.

The neocortex is profoundly enlarged in humans compared to all nearby species. In human fetal development, the neopallium gives rise to the neocortex, and this is initially a smooth structure. As development continues, however, the neopallium becomes the largest and fastest growing cortical area, eventually covering more than 90 percent of the total cortical area. By six months in development, the cortex begins to invaginate to accommodate the profound cortical growth and to increase its surface area. These folds are called gyri while the grooves are named sulci.

The cerebral cortex can be further subdivided into regions based on function or by cellular organization. In 1909, the German neurologist Korbinian Brodmann

(1868–1918) established a map of the human brain based on cytoarchitectonics, which is defining how cells are organized in a tissue. Since then, this map has been closely correlated to functional areas of the brain. This means that experiments investigating regional function, such as brain imaging, have found close overlap of Brodmann areas with discrete, functional units. For instance, Brodmann area 17 has axons from the retina ending in the occipital cortex, which is considered the visual cortex. From brain imaging experiments, Brodmann area 17 does appear to be the primary visual cortex, although these are approximations because it is currently not possible to obtain cellular-level resolution with current imaging techniques.

Jonathon Keeney

See also: Brain Anatomy; Entorhinal Cortex; Occipital Lobe; Parietal Lobe; Somatosensory Cortex; Somatosensory System

Further Reading

Creutzfeldt, O. D. (1995). *Cortex cerebri: Performance, structural and functional organisation of the cortex.* Oxford Scholarship Online. Retrieved from http://www.oxfordscholarship.com/view/10.1093/acprof:oso/9780198523246.001.0001/acprof-9780198523246
Herculano-Houzel, Suzana. (2009). The human brain in numbers: A linearly scaled-up primate brain. *Frontiers in Human Neuroscience, 3*(31), 1–11.

CHEMORECEPTION

The term *chemoreception* refers to an organism's ability to perceive and react to different chemicals. It is comprised of a sensory system that is activated by exposure to chemicals. Special sensory receptors called chemoreceptors are stimulated by chemicals and relay signals to the nervous system. The nervous system will then respond accordingly. This mechanism is important for survival because these receptors enhance the organism's perceptions of its surrounding.

Olfaction and gustation are the systems most often discussed when referring to chemoreception. Both sensory systems utilize chemoreceptors. Olfaction refers to the ability to smell, and gustation refers to the ability to taste. Both systems utilize chemical interaction to create signals for the organism to process. Chemoreceptors are made up of specialized cells called neurons, which enable them to convert chemical signals into action potential. These signals are then relayed to the central nervous system.

Anatomy and Physiology

Different organisms have varying chemoreception systems. The scientific community believes that all organisms have some level of chemoreception, and many vertebrates have different classes of chemoreception (Starenchak & Bissonnette,

2014). Chemoreception is controlled by the autonomic nervous system. In vertebrates, chemoreceptors function as pH balance sensors to maintain homeostasis (respiratory chemoreceptors), detect vapors (olfactory chemoreceptors), and taste potential food (gustatory chemoreceptors). The respiratory chemoreceptors are made up of the central and peripheral chemoreceptors. In vertebrates, the central chemoreceptors are located on the medulla oblongata of the brain. Periphery chemoreceptors, also known as arterial receptors, are located on the carotid and aortic bodies. The carotid body can be found on the bifurcation of the carotid artery of the heart and the aortic body by the aortic arch. Olfactory chemoreceptors are found at the top of the nasal passages. The synapses of these nerves are ultimately connected to the olfactory cortex of the brain. Gustatory chemoreceptors are found in the mouth and are commonly called taste buds. However, these chemoreceptors are found on taste cells that are located within taste buds.

Classes of Chemoreceptors

Chemoreceptors are divided into two classes: indirect chemoreceptors and direct chemoreceptors (Starenchak & Bissonnette, 2014). Indirect chemoreceptors work from a distance. Only a low concentration of chemical is necessary for these chemoreceptors to convert the stimulus into an action potential. The olfactory system is an example of a sensory system that utilizes indirect chemoreceptors. The olfaction system can detect odors and associate them to a source that may be located quite far away. Direct chemoreceptors involve many of the chemical compounds making actual contact with the neurons. There needs to be a high enough concentration of the chemical to trigger a cascade of action potentials all the way to the central nervous system. More stimuli will result in more frequent and rapid action potentials. An example of a direct chemoreceptor is the gustation system. Chemicals must physically touch the taste cells within the taste buds in order for the brain to interpret taste. The more flavor something has, the stronger the taste. Respiratory chemoreceptors also fall under the class of direct chemoreceptors because these receptors maintain homeostatic pH levels by directly detecting hydrogen ions in the blood.

Diseases and Defects

A defect in chemoreceptors can impair an organism's ability to sense its environment. This may leave the organism vulnerable to predators, especially those who rely heavily on their olfactory senses. Impaired olfactory chemoreceptors are also known to affect appetite. Defects in gustatory chemoreceptors are presented in many forms including reduced ability to taste (hypogeusia), phantom taste perception (parageusia), and even complete loss of tasting ability (ageusia). The respiratory chemoreceptors are arguably the most vital for survival. Diseases such as coronary heart disease and chronic obstructive pulmonary disorder (COPD) have been shown to affect these receptors (van Gestel & Steier, 2010). COPD may develop following chronic inhalation of toxic smoke, which impairs the body's ability to expel carbon dioxide. Aortic bodies are thought to provide a compensatory mechanism in these patients, but research in this field is currently in its infancy.

Melissa Tjandra

See also: Ageusia; Hypogeusia; Taste Bud; Taste System

Further Reading

Starenchak, Holly, & Nicole Bissonnette. (2014). Developmental and comparative aspects of chemoreception in the vertebrates. *Anatomy, Phylogeny, and Ontogeny of Chemoreceptors.* Retrieved from https://sites.google.com/a/ncsu.edu/anatomy-phylogeny-and-ontogeny-of-chemoreceptors/

Sundin, Lena, Mark L. Burleson, Adriana P. Sanchez, Jalile Amin-Naves, Richard Kinkead, Luciane H. Gargaglioni, . . . Mogens L. Glass. (2007). Respiratory chemoreceptor function in vertebrates: Comparative and evolutionary aspects. *Integrative and Comparative Biology, 47*(4), 592–600. Retrieved from http://icb.oxfordjournals.org/content/47/4/592.full

van Gestel, Arnoldus J. R., & Joerg Steier. (2010). Autonomic dysfunction in patients with chronic obstructive pulmonary disease (COPD). *Journal of Thoracic Disease, 2*(4), 215–222. Retrieved from http://www.ncbi.nlm.nih.gov/pmc/articles/PMC3256465/

CHORDA TYMPANI NERVE

The chorda tympani is a nerve that relays information between portions of the tongue and the brain. There are two types of fibers contained within the chorda tympani—sensory fibers and autonomic fibers, which are motor fibers that control involuntary actions. The sensory fibers innervate taste buds on the front part of the tongue and the autonomic fibers provide stimulation to the salivary glands, which in turn produce saliva. Hence, the chorda tympani is involved in transmitting taste sensations to the brain as well as producing the saliva needed to eat and begin digesting food.

The chorda tympani is one of two nerves that transmit taste information to the brain from the taste buds on the tongue. The glossopharyngeal nerve, or cranial nerve IX, is the nerve that innervates taste buds on the back of the tongue while the chorda tympani innervates taste buds on the front of the tongue. In addition, different nerves innervate taste buds located in other structures throughout the oral cavity such as the palate on the roof of the mouth and the epiglottis in the throat. All of these taste nerves connect to the base of the brain in the brainstem. Here the taste nerves form a complicated circuit where each taste nerve inhibits the signals from other taste nerves. The chorda tympani in particular strongly inhibits the other taste nerves as well as the pain nerve fibers from the tongue. Damage to the chorda tympani nerve can cause a disruption of this inhibitory function, resulting in making the sensation of taste irregular and unpredictable.

Anatomy and Physiology

The chorda tympani nerve originates from cranial nerve VII, also called the facial nerve. As the facial nerve travels along the facial canal, the chorda tympani branches off and travels through the middle ear along the eardrum. The chorda tympani takes a winding path from the ear down into the neck and eventually emerges into the mouth near the base of the tongue. At this point, the autonomic fibers continue toward the salivary glands located under the tongue and the sensory fibers extend to the taste buds on the front of the tongue.

The taste information that the sensory fibers transmit to the brain begins when taste molecules stimulate the taste cells. Once taste cells are stimulated, they communicate this information by releasing chemicals onto the taste nerve fibers. This causes an action potential to travel along the nerve, which is ultimately transmitted to the brain. As the brain processes the incoming taste signals, several outgoing neural pathways are activated in order to digest the food. One of the beginning steps of the digestive process is the increased production of saliva.

Saliva is produced and secreted by the salivary glands. Most animals have three major pairs of salivary glands. The autonomic fibers of the chorda tympani stimulate two pairs of these glands—the sublingual glands located underneath the front of the tongue and the submaxillary glands located beneath the lower jaw. Together these glands are responsible for about 75 percent of saliva production. Under normal conditions, the human salivary glands in adults produce up to one and a half quarts, or six cups, of saliva per day.

Saliva is a clear liquid consisting largely of water but also containing small amounts of electrolytes, mucus, and enzymes. Saliva serves to moisten and break down food so that it can be swallowed easily. Because chemicals in food must first be dissolved in order to bind to the taste cells, saliva also assists in mammals being able to taste food. You can appreciate the fact that taste molecules need to be in solution and the role of saliva by using a clean paper towel to thoroughly dry your tongue and then eat dry food, such as pretzels or crackers. In general, the taste of food is decreased or even absent without saliva or other aqueous liquids.

In addition to direct injury to the nerves or salivary glands, certain diseases and medicines can affect how much saliva is produced. Without enough saliva, the mouth can become very dry. This condition is called dry mouth or xerostomia. Patients who suffer from this condition often have difficulty chewing, swallowing, and tasting food. A dry mouth also causes the gums and tongue to become swollen and uncomfortable, making it difficult to talk. Further, the risk of gum disease, tooth decay, and infections of the mouth increases as saliva normally clears food particles and cavity-causing bacteria from the teeth. While the benefits of saliva often go unnoticed, it plays important roles in oral health, the digestive process, and the enjoyment of food.

Dianna Bartel

See also: Cranial Nerves; Glossopharyngeal Nerve; Nerves; Taste System

Further Reading

Bowen, Richard A. (2002). *Salivary glands and saliva*. Retrieved from http://www.vivo.colostate
    .edu/hbooks/pathphys/digestion/pregastric/salivary.html
National Institute on Deafness and Other Communication Disorders. (2009). *NIDCD fact
    sheet taste disorders*. Retrieved from http://www.nidcd.nih.gov/staticresources/health
    /smelltaste/TasteDisorders.pdf
Yale School of Medicine. (1998). *Course of the chorda tympani*. Retrieved from http://www
    .yale.edu/cnerves/cn7/cn7_18.html

CHROMESTHESIA

Imagine if every time you listened to music in high octaves, you immediately saw pale lavender. Or while listening to lower octaves, you saw deep blue, and rapid major chord sequences elicited rapid flashes of colors. These are symptoms of one specific form of synesthesia—chromesthesia. Synesthesia is a neurological condition in which stimulation of one sense triggers another. In chromesthesia, sounds heard automatically and involuntarily evoke color experiences. Chromesthesia occurs in only about 1 in 3,000 people, including a remarkable number of famous painters and musicians, such as Pharrell Williams (1973–), Leonard Bernstein (1918–1990), Duke Ellington (1899–1974), Vincent Van Gogh (1853–1890), and Wassily Kandinsky (1866–1944), who used Wagner's *Lohengrin* to help create wild, crazy lines of color. Pharrell Williams views his chromesthesia as an indispensable gift and the secret behind his music, fundamental to his creative processes.

The same categories of synesthetes who see alphanumerical figures in color exist for those who hear in color: projectors are people who perceive color in the external space and associators are persons who perceive color in their minds. Some individuals with chromesthesia find it to be much more than just perceptual. Some have chromesthesia with any kind of sound; others have it with specific types of sound only. Musicians and those with musical training have more distinct colors for specific notes if they are chromesthetes. And each individual experiences his or her own unique color connection, which explains why we all do not have Pharrell Williams's talent. People with chromesthesia have higher creativity and sound memory but at the same time are more likely to have difficulty with numbers. Levels of concentration, fatigue, emotions, sleep habits, fever, and consumption of caffeine, alcohol, or hallucinogens can contribute to the perception of sound as color. They can also alter how chromesthetes experience colors in response to sound.

When synesthesia was first discovered in the 19th century, it was traced back to the eyes until it was discovered that the same phenomenon could be experienced with the eyes closed, confirming a neurological basis. Signals from the five senses originate in different anatomical regions of the brain. Why then do auditory and visual experiences interact with each other? The main reason is that these interactions enable the human brain to make sense of sensory information that corresponds to the same event; for example, the ears register the sound of a lightbulb shattering as it hits the floor at the same time as the eyes register the sight of it hitting the floor. Sensory cross-modal connections help the brain integrate and make sense of the constant complex multisensory inputs we experience. Synesthesia is a part of this cross-modal connections, often the result of unusual connections.

Many nonsynesthetes have music-to-color associations similar to those of chromesthetes. Music with lively tempos in a major key elicit dominate yellow hues that are bright and vivid. Slower melodic music in a minor key elicits more dark blues to grays. High-energy rock music with prominent drums and fast, loud guitar riffs elicit colors that are predominantly reds, blacks, and other dark colors, as opposed to laid-back, easy-listening music and simple piano melodies that bring out blues, purples, and cool, muted colors. Distortion, volume, keys, tempo, pitch, energy, complexity, and harmonic and melodic content all play a part in determining the colors chosen by chromesthetes and nonchromesthetes. In addition, the emotional qualities of the music correlate to the colors elicited. Lively music in a major key sounds strong and happy; slower melodic music or music in a minor key sounds weak and sad; rock music can sound angry and aggressive; and easy-listening music can sound calm and introspective.

Colors and music have very few sensory similarities in common. Color is visual, music is auditory; color has the properties of hue, lightness, and vividness; music has the properties of pitch, timber, tempo, and rhythm—but both share aspects of emotion. Happy emotion is correlated with bright yellows (sunshine), anger with red (red faces and bloodshed from violence), and depression with grays and darker colors (under a cloud or a rainy day). For most people, whether they are chromesthetes or not, music tends to elicit an emotional response.

Carolyn Johnson Atwater

See also: Auditory System; Grapheme-Color Synesthesia; Synesthesia

Further Reading

Dutton, Jack. (2015). The surprising world of synaesthesia. *British Psychological Society, 28*, 106–109. Retrieved from https://thepsychologist.bps.org.uk/volume-28/february-2015/surprising-world-synaesthesia

Palmer, Stephen E. (2015). What color is this song? Retrieved from http://nautil.us/issue/26/color/what-color-is-this-song

CHRONOCEPTION

Chronoception refers to the sense of time that almost everyone experiences. This can refer to the lapse of time between events or the duration of the event. Chronoception is largely related to consciousness and memory. Because of this, many of the brain regions associated with chronoception also play a role in consciousness and memory. Additionally, chronoception plays a role in maintaining circadian rhythms in mammals. Some research suggests a connection between many psychological diseases (for example, schizophrenia or bipolar disorder) and a malfunction in the natural chronoception of the afflicted individual.

Associated Brain Regions

Widely spread throughout the brain, chronoception is linked to regions of the cerebral cortex, cerebellum, and basal ganglia. Chronoception is not specifically linked to one sensory system, but rather has nuclei spread throughout the brain. Moreover, this sense has nuclei located in almost all the other sensory systems. Research has shown that estimating the time it would take for something to happen in one of your senses activates that region. For example, if you are attempting to determine the duration of an auditory stimulus, regions of the auditory cortex are more activated. Similarly for visual stimuli, visual cortex regions are more active, and estimating the time it would take to complete an action stimulates regions in the primary motor cortex. This breadth of association is important as it takes the brain longer to process some stimuli over others. By having a larger associated region within the brain, chronoception is able to help combine the senses into a cohesive temporal experience. It is capable of integrating the time it will take you to respond to a stimulus that combines two or more of the senses, such as the approach of a fire engine with its siren on simultaneously providing a unified estimation of time.

Associated Rhythms

Chronoception has been shown to play a very large role in the maintenance of circadian rhythms. One specific region chronoception has been closely associated with is the suprachiasmatic nucleus (SCN), which is located in the hypothalamus above the optic chiasm (crossing of the optic nerves into the brain). The SCN plays a large role in maintaining the body's circadian rhythm, or sleep-wake cycles. Reduction of the light entering the eyes triggers the release of melatonin in the brain, which helps to signal that it is time to sleep. However, the circadian rhythm is not completely controlled by this, and a large part of it is due to the body's natural sense of time. This has been demonstrated in the fact that most mammals, including humans, maintain their circadian rhythm during 24 hours of darkness.

It is likely that chronoception also plays a role in many other natural rhythms such as sleep patterns and circalunal rhythms (such as the human menstrual cycle). The brain cycles through sleep patterns during slumber. The two main patterns are REM (rapid eye movement) and non-REM sleep. These cycles are repeated throughout the duration of sleep at approximately 90-minute intervals. Chronoception likely plays a role in the maintenance of these cycles. Additionally, menstruation is timed by the body. While a large portion of this is controlled by hormones, chronoception does help with the timing of the cycle. However, a large number of inputs also play a role in the human menstruation cycle, including but not limited to stress, hormonal fluxes, pheromones, medications, and sex.

Associated Diseases

Time perception issues have been associated with a large number of neurological diseases and disorders. These include depression, Parkinson's disease, attention deficit hyperactivity disorder (ADHD), and schizophrenia. Chronoceptive hallucinations are considered symptoms of these diseases. In these hallucinations the individual perceives time as moving much differently than it is. For example, something that happened an hour ago might appear to the person as having happened months ago or vice versa. Part of the reason for the association is that these diseases include an abnormality in dopamine levels within the brain. Some research has demonstrated that dopamine plays a large role in the integration of chronoception within the basal ganglia.

Riannon C. Atwater

See also: Circadian Rhythm

Further Resources
Lacquaniti, Francesco, Gianfranco Bosco, Silvio Gravano, Iole Indovina, Barbara La Scaleia, Vincenzo Maffei, & Myrka Zago. (2015). Gravity in the brain as a reference for space and time perception. *Multisensory Research, 28*(5–6), 397–426.

CIRCADIAN RHYTHM

In synchrony with the rotation of the earth, all biological organisms have an internally controlled or endogenous cycle referred to as a circadian rhythm. During this approximately 24-hour period, organisms undergo a cyclical regulation of physiological events and behaviors. In mammals, this internal clock is driven by a nerve bundle in the hypothalamus called the suprachiasmatic nucleus (SCN). To synchronize the body with the local environment, the SCN uses external cues, such as light and temperature. An adaptive mechanism called temperature compensation prevents variation in external temperature from disrupting the body's daily cycle. Using information from the eyes about the length of day and night, the SCN regulates the sleep-wake cycle. Additionally, the SCN acts as a pacemaker for daily rhythms in peripheral cells and tissues, resulting in the regulation of many other physiological processes including release of hormones at specific times, changes in body temperature, peak times for cell regeneration, and digestion.

In humans, the circadian rhythm forms during the first few months of life and starts to deteriorate in advanced age. Without changes in influencing external cues or disease to disrupt the rhythm, it should remain unchanged.

Physiology

In the late 1960s, scientists discovered that vision and its pathways had a substantial role in the metabolic processes of the hypothalamus, a region in the brain that regulates metabolism through the autonomic nervous system. These scientists discovered that in rodents, the retinohypothalmic tract (RHT) projected from the eye directly to the SCN. Upon further research, lesions performed in mice to this part of the hypothalamus resulted in arrhythmia of the circadian clock. With this function established, follow-up research focused on understanding the function of the SCN in circadian rhythm.

In one critical set of experiments, neuroscientists found that with a total lesion of the SCN, the endogenous clock ceases to function. However, when new SCN tissue from another animal species with a shorter circadian period was grafted to the animal with the lesion, the rhythm was restored. Additionally, the period exhibited was that of the donor animal and not of the receiving animal. These experiments confirmed that the SCN acts to synchronize all biorhythms of the organism and that the period of the daily cycle is determined by this group of cells.

One of the defining factors of circadian rhythms is the ability to be entrained, or adapt to the local environment, particularly light. As light enters the eye, several types of photoreceptive cells in the retina are activated, including rods, cones, and photosensitive retinal ganglion cells that contain the light-sensitive pigment melopsin. Activation of these cells sends information about the amount of environmental light along the RHT, which directly synapses to the SCN via the optic nerve. The SCN passes this information to other parts of the hypothalamus and the pineal gland, which modulates the secretion of a hormone called melatonin throughout the day. Increased amounts of melatonin are released during the nighttime hours. Melatonin inhibits activation of cells in the SCN, ultimately resulting in the modulation of the sleep-wake cycle.

Circadian Rhythms and the Sleep-Wake Cycle

The sleep-wake cycle includes approximately 8 hours of nocturnal sleep and 16 hours of daytime wakefulness. The circadian system works with the homeostatic system to maintain this cycle via mutually inhibited groups of neurons in the hypothalamus and brainstem. From the moment a person wakes, adenosine levels rise in the blood. As adenosine blood levels continue to increase throughout the day, the need for sleep significantly increases. This occurs regardless of the time of day when that person wakes up. The secretion of melatonin from the pineal gland keeps the circadian system synchronized with external light cues and promotes wakefulness during the daylight hours. However, both photic (light) and nonphotic (food availability and temperature) cues can promote a sleep-wake schedule most adaptive for the organism. A normal circadian rhythm is characterized with increased desire for sleep between midnight and dawn, but this can be artificially affected with indoor lighting and blackout conditions. Artificial changes to light conditions can change the circadian rhythm but seem most disruptive to the sleep-wake cycle when they occur in the morning hours.

B. Dnate' Baxter

See also: Chronoception; Cones; Optic Nerve; Retina; Rods; Sensory Receptors; Visual System

Further Reading

National Institute of Neurological Disorders and Stroke (NINDS). (2007). *Brain basics: Understanding sleep.* Retrieved from http://www.ninds.nih.gov/disorders/brain_basics/understanding_sleep.htm

Williams, Ruth. (2006). Circadian rhythms: SCN synchronicity . . . hup, two, three, four. *Nature Reviews Neuroscience, 7,* 328. http://dx.doi.org/10.1038/nrn1913. Retrieved from http://www.nature.com/nrn/journal/v7/n5/full/nrn1913.html

Zivkovic, Bora. (2011). Circadian clock without DNA—History and the power of metaphor. *Scientific American.* Retrieved from http://blogs.scientificamerican.com/observations/2011/02/11/circadian-clock-without-dna-history-and-the-power-of-metaphor/

CIRCUMVALLATE PAPILLAE

Papillae (from the Latin word meaning "nipple") are present as hair-like, bulb-shaped, or domed structures on the tongue. The majority of papillae contain taste buds, which are essential for mediating the sense of taste. Four types of papillae are found in specific regions of the human tongue: circumvallate (or simply vallate), filiform, foliate, and fungiform. Circumvallate papillae are located the deepest in the mouth and look like large domes. This type of papillae is the biggest and may vary in number depending on the individual. Most people have 8 to 14 circumvallate papillae oriented in two rows, which are V-shaped and pointing toward the throat.

Structure and Function

To the naked eye, circumvallate papillae appear as large domed formations on the posterior one-third of the tongue. The structure of circumvallate papillae resembles an upside down "U" with the opened end serving as the attachment point to the body of the tongue. A microscopic view of these structures will show that the flat apical (top) surface is actually covered in tiny secondary papillae; the taste buds are housed in these smaller papillae. It is important to note that the sides of the circumvallate papillae "U" shapes are not attached to one another. They are instead surrounded by mucosa tissue, which forms slick walls called the vallum (Latin for "wall"). The trench that is created between the papillae is called the fossa, and it provides a channel for saliva flow.

Circumvallate papillae are most commonly known in association with von Ebner's glands, specialized saliva glands located under the body of the tongue. These glands are named after the Austrian histologist Victor von Ebner (1842–1945) who discovered them. When we eat, von Ebner's glands proceed to fill the empty fossa with saliva; when the saliva is swallowed, it washes away any taste molecules that were previously attached to the taste buds and prepares the papillae to detect new food molecules. This process allows circumvallate papillae to detect small changes in taste almost immediately. In order to handle this volume of taste information, the circumvallate papillae are connected to different cranial nerves than papillae on the anterior portion of the tongue. The saliva produced by von Ebner's glands provides an important additional function: the enzyme lingual lipase is produced and secreted by these glands in order to begin lipid hydrolysis (the process of fat digestion) in the mouth.

Medical Conditions

There are few diseases that directly affect the structure or function of the circumvallate papillae. The most common form of loss of function is due to aging, which has been studied in both mouse and human models. This loss of taste buds seems to increase with age, but aging does not seem to affect some of the other papillae types.

Circumvallate papillae commonly become swollen or enlarged. Sometimes these swollen papillae are mistaken for something more serious (such as tumors), but for the most part it is not a serious issue and swelling will disappear after several days. This enlargement is suspected to be a result of viral infection, exposure to irritants, burning of the taste buds by hot food or drink, or by excessive smoking. Cigarette smoking may also affect the function of taste buds. A recent study by Jacob and colleagues (2014) has shown that current smokers and even former smokers are not able to distinguish between or identify bitter and nonbitter foods. Bitter foods can be easily identified at low concentrations by nonsmokers, yet as a result of toxicity produced by cigarette smoking on the tongue's taste receptors, smokers and former smokers have a significantly decreased ability to identify this taste.

Kendra DeHay

See also: Fungiform Papillae; Supertaster; Taste Aversion; Taste Bud; Taste System

Further Reading

Jacob, Nelly, Jean-Louis Golmard, & Ivan Berlin. (2014). Differential perception of caffeine bitter taste depending on smoking status. *Chemosensory Perception, 7*(2), 47–55.

Mistretta, Charlotte M., & Bruce J. Baum. (1984). Quantitative study of taste buds in fungiform and circumvallate papillae of young and aged rats. *Journal of Anatomy, 138*(2), 323–332. Retrieved from http://www.ncbi.nlm.nih.gov/pmc/articles/PMC1164072/pdf/janat00202-0126.pdf

Owen, David. (2015). Beyond taste buds: The science of delicious. *National Geographic*. Retrieved from http://ngm.nationalgeographic.com/2015/12/food-science-of-taste-text

Sbarbati, A., C. Crescimanno, & F. Osculati. (1991). The anatomy and functional role of the circumvallate papilla/von Ebner gland complex. *Medical Hypotheses, 53*(1), 40–44.

COCHLEA

The cochlea is an organ within the auditory system that is responsible for the sensation of sound. It is located within the last part of the auditory canal called the inner ear. This organ gets its name from the Latin word for snail since its hollowed tube structure coils in on itself like a snail's shell. The cochlea is a long tube that is open to the middle ear at one end and closed and tapered at the opposite end. The tube is composed of three fluid-filled sections separated by thin membranes. This particular organ has one main function: the transformation of physical waves from sound into electrical signals that can be sent to the brain. The cochlea is also attached to three separate half circle–shaped tubes that help maintain balance as a part of the vestibular system.

Anatomy and Physiology

The cochlea is the final organ of the auditory canal and is located in the inner ear. The inner ear is found within the bony structure just behind the outer ear called the temporal bone. There are two noticeable landmarks on the external surface of the cochlea, the oval and round windows. These structures are adjacent to each other, the oval window on top and the round window on the bottom. An extremely thin membrane covers each of these windows in order to contain the fluid within the cochlea. The oval window is attached to one of the ossicles located within the middle ear called the stapes. The round window is left open to the environment external to the cochlea and helps to reduce pressure within the cochlea.

The coiled snail shell–like structure is best pictured as an uncoiled stretched-out tube. Within this tube there are three compartments: (1) the scala vestibuli can be found at the top of the tube and has the oval window at one end, (2) the scala tympani is found at the bottom of the tube and contains the round window on the same end as the oval window, and (3) the scala media lies between the scala vestibuli and the scala tympani and contains the organ of Corti. The scala media is separated from the top compartment by Reissner's membrane and from the bottom compartment by the basilar membrane. The organ of Corti rests on top of the basilar membrane and contains millions of hair cells, which respond to physical movement and produce a neural signal.

The transduction of sound into a neural signal occurs when a sound wave travels down the auditory canal and reaches the stapes. As the stapes vibrates from the sound wave, it acts like a piston on the oval window and produces a wave within the fluid of the topmost chamber. The membrane between the top and bottom chambers is thin enough that the wave can continue past it. The wave travels down the length of the top chamber and returns down the bottom chamber until it reaches the round window, which releases the pressure wave. As the sound wave disrupts the fluid within the top and bottom chambers of the cochlea, the fluid within the middle chamber moves as well, which in turn moves the basilar membrane. The basilar membrane is thin and stiff at one end and the other end is wide and floppy. This property allows high-frequency noises and low-frequency noises to be converted into a neural signal at different places along the membrane. High-frequency noises are perceived at the thin stiff region of the basilar membrane and low-frequency noises are perceived at the wide floppy region.

Hair cells have tiny hair-like projections on their top surface called cilia that are embedded into a nonmoving shelf-like membrane called the tectorial membrane. Once a sound wave causes the basilar membrane to move, the hair cells move as well. Since the cilia are stuck in place, the base of the cilia attached to the cell will bend back and forth as the sound wave hits it. It is this bending motion that produces an action potential within the hair cells. The action potentials produced in the hair cells are then transmitted down small individual nerves to join the auditory or cochlear nerve.

Diseases

A normal functioning human cochlea is able to perceive sounds ranging from 20 to 20,000 hertz. The most common disease of the cochlea is deafness or loss of the ability to hear. Hearing loss specific to the cochlea and neural pathways is referred to as sensorineural hearing loss. Hearing acuity within the cochlea generally decreases with age, but it also can be due to prolonged exposure to loud noises. High-frequency sounds are typically lost first. Other causes of sensorineural hearing loss are illness, genetic disorders, head trauma, or tumors.

Lynelle Smith

See also: Action Potential; Auditory System; Cochlear Implants; Deafness; Vestibulocochlear Nerve

Further Reading

Bear, Mark F., Barry W. Connors, & Michael A. Paradiso. (2007). *Neuroscience exploring the brain* (3rd ed.). Baltimore, MD: Lippincott Williams & Wilkins.

COCHLEAR IMPLANTS

Cochlear implants are used in patients who are extremely hard of hearing or deaf as a treatment for deafness caused by damage to the sensory hair cells within the cochlea, which transmit vibrations to the brain via the auditory nerve. Rather than amplifying the sound as hearing aids do, cochlear implants perform the same function as the sensory hair cells within the cochlea: they both amplify vibrations and transmit them to the auditory nerve, which makes up part of the vestibulocochlear nerve (cranial nerve VIII). Cochlear implants are electronic devices with both an external portion and an internal portion. Cochlear implants do not transmit the same sound that would be heard by someone with normal hearing; rather, they offer a close enough facsimile that the patient can interact with his or her environment and participate in conversations. Surgery is required to install the implant.

How the Implants Work

Cochlear implants bypass the damaged portions of the patient's ear to directly stimulate the auditory nerve. To do this, the cochlear implant uses four major parts: (1) a microphone—responsible for catching any noises from the external environment; (2) a speech processor—determines which sounds are to be amplified and how; (3) a transmitter—converts those noises allowed through the microphone and speech processor into electrical impulses the brain will recognize; and (4) an electrode array—a group of electrodes that collects the impulses from the transmitter and sends them to the auditory nerve to travel to the brain. The auditory nerve then conducts this electrical signal primarily to the temporal nerve where the sound is converted into something the patient perceives as sound. Cochlear implants only work if the patient's brain is capable of taking this electrical signal and converting it into what the patient hears as a sound. The sounds heard by the patient's brain are not the same as normal hearing, but they still allow the patient to hear and react to noises in the environment, including carrying on a normal conversation.

Implantation and Treatment

The only way for cochlear implants to be installed is through expensive surgery—in 2010 the average cost of the cochlear implant, surgery, and postoperative aural rehabilitation was well over US$40,000. If the surgery is successful, patients still have to undergo extensive therapy to learn how to interpret the sound that they hear. Results are often the best for patients who fairly recently lost their hearing, as they can learn to associate certain sounds that they hear with sounds from before. Children who undergo early implantation also experience pretty good results with intensive postimplantation therapy. The U.S. Food and Drug Administration (FDA) has reported that approximately 324,200 people in the world have received a cochlear implant and approximately 58,000 U.S. adults and 38,000 U.S. children have received cochlear implants (NIDCD, 2013). The National Institute on Deafness and Other Communication Disorders (NIDCD) supports further research in the field of treatments for deafness, including the cochlear implant to improve its function. One group of studies is looking at ways to make the sound heard through the implant sound more like normal hearing and to convey speech in an easier to understand way. Additional research is also looking into ways to use the cochlear implant to treat a variety of other hearing losses.

Famous People with Cochlear Implants

There are a few famous persons who lost their hearing as a young child and have decided to undergo cochlear implant surgery. In 1999, *Guiding Light* actress Amy Ecklund received her cochlear implant (Ecklund, 1999). Ecklund lost her hearing at age six and was enrolled in drama classes to maintain her speaking ability. In 1995, she was hired to play deaf hospital administrator Abigail Bauer. After Ecklund received her cochlear implant, her character also underwent cochlear implant surgery. Former Miss America Heather Whitestone recovered her hearing with a cochlear implant in 2003. She was the first deaf woman to be crowned Miss America (1995) and is now the first Miss America alum to receive a cochlear implant. She decided to have the surgery after her son hurt himself in the backyard and was crying. Whitestone was inside and did not know that he was injured. This incident made her want to better connect with the hearing world.

Riannon C. Atwater

See also: Auditory System; Cochlea; Cranial Nerves; Deafness; Sensory Receptors; Vestibulocochlear Nerve

Further Reading

Ecklund, Amy. (1999). Now hear this! *People, 52,* 1. Retrieved from http://www.people.com/people/archive/article/0,,20128697,00.html

National Institute on Deafness and Other Communication Disorders (NIDCD). (2013). *Cochlear implants.* Retrieved from https://www.nidcd.nih.gov/health/hearing/pages/coch.aspx

COLOR BLINDNESS

A person who is unable to see or distinguish colors has a dysfunction called color blindness. However, this term is a misnomer. It is rare to be totally color-blind, meaning a person can only see shades of gray. Most persons who have difficulty in discriminating colors or shades of colors, such as reds and greens, are more correctly diagnosed with poor color vision. The majority of persons with decreased color vision inherit this disorder. Men inherit poor color vision more often than women.

Causes

In poor color vision, patients have deficits in the neural receptors (specialized proteins) that sense color. These receptors are found on the retina, the photosensitive portion of the eye that lines the posterior (back) part of the globe. The retina has photoreceptors called rods, which are activated in dim light and produce black and white vision, and cones, which are activated in bright light and produce color vision. There are three types of cones that are activated by specific wavelengths of light: red retinal photoreceptors, green retinal photoreceptors, and blue retinal photoreceptors. Therefore, poor color vision is due to a deficit in the cones, particularly in missing only one pigment retinal photoreceptor.

Poor color vision is a genetic disorder that is linked to the X chromosome (the genetic material that helps determine the sex of the organism). This means that the part of the X chromosome that codes for cones has a mutation. Men are more likely to have poor color vision because they only have one X chromosome, while women have two. For a woman to be affected with poor color vision, both of her X chromosomes would have a mutation. In rare cases, a person may not see any color and can only see in shades of gray. This condition is called achromatopsia. Persons with achromatopsia generally have other vision problems including lazy eye, light sensitivity, nystagmus (abnormal, erratic movements of the eye), and poor vision.

Signs, Symptoms, Diagnosis, and Treatment

The most common form of poor color vision is having difficulty in distinguishing between shades of red and green. However, some persons may have difficulty in determining between shades of blue and yellow. Persons with blue-yellow poor color vision may also have difficulty with red-green color vision. If the color vision deficit is mild, people may not realize that they have poor color vision.

Poor color vision is normally detected when a child is learning colors. In general, the child will not be able to tell the difference between reds and greens. A health care professional can test color vision during a routine eye exam and determine the type of poor color vision. Specifically, patients are given a card that has various sized spots or splotches of several shades of red and green or blue and yellow on the paper. One of the colors is used to make the background spots and the other color is in the form of a shape, number, or letter. Patients are then asked what they see. If patients have normal color vision, they will easily be able to see the shape, number, or letter. If they have poor color vision, they will not be able to see a difference between the two colors and see "nothing." Some persons with a mild form of poor color vision may only have difficulty if the shades of both colors are very similar, meaning both colors are fairly light, instead of one being light in color and the other bright in color. To determine mild poor color vision, the test may only use several shades of reds/oranges/yellows for both the background and shape colors. Readers can test their own color vision at the following link: http://www.colour-blindness.com/colour-blindness-tests/ishihara-colour-test-plates/

There is no known treatment for poor color vision or for achromatopsia as both are genetic disorders. Persons with poor color vision can live normal lives, but may not be able to have certain jobs that depend upon color vision, such as painting, electrical work (to determine the color of the wires), and cooking (to determine the color of cooked meats).

Jennifer L. Hellier

See also: Color Perception; Cones; Nystagmus; Rods; Visual Perception; Visual System

Further Reading

Color Matters. (n.d.). *What is color-blindness?* Retrieved from http://www.colormatters.com /color-and-vision/what-is-color-blindness. There is a short color blindness test that the reader can use.

Mayo Clinic. (2011). *Poor color vision.* Retrieved from http://www.mayoclinic.com/health /poor-color-vision/DS00233

COLOR PERCEPTION

Color is an integral part of life. It tells us if a piece of fruit is ripe, if the sky is about to rain, or if the grass and trees are healthy. However, since we all have unique life experiences, it begs the question, "can one person perceive color differently than someone else?" For the most part, we all have the same anatomical and physiological means to see color, but do our brains interpret it differently? For decades, color perception was thought to be based on the amount of light available to illuminate an object. More recently, however, research has shown that color perception is controlled more by the brain than by how many cones in the retina are activated by light.

Anatomy and Physiology

There are two types of light-sensing cells in the retina of vertebrates: cones and rods. The main function of cones and rods is to convert light into impulses to the optic nerve. Three types of cones process color vision—a spectrum of colors based on the primary colors of red, blue, and yellow—as well as details of an object. Rods, however, are used for night and peripheral vision. Cones are named by their size and shape, and they are more prominent in humans and other diurnal animals compared to nocturnal animals.

Research studies have measured the spatial density of cones and rods in the adult human eye. Specifically, it has been estimated that there are 4.6 million cones and roughly 92 million rods (Curcio et al., 1990). The location of cones and rods in the retina differs as well. Specifically, cones are concentrated in the central portion of the retina, called the macula, while rods are found on the elliptical ring of the optic disc, mainly on the lateral and superior portions. The three types of cones are named by the length of light waves that activate them. Thus, there are the short wavelengths (S-cones) that perceive blue colors; medium wavelengths

(M-cones) that perceive yellow; and, long wavelengths (L-cones) that perceive red colors.

Perception

As light hits an object, the color an individual perceives is actually the color of light being reflected by the object's surface. Ratios of S-, M-, and L-cones will be activated based on the amount and wavelengths of light that enter the eye. As more cones are activated, the eye is able to differentiate more hues and vibrancy of a color. Additionally, color perception requires visual experience so that the brain can interpret what the person is seeing. This is called visual-experience-dependent neural plasticity, which was originally thought to occur only in preadult brains. For example, when a child is learning colors, the brain is wired so that the color yellow is associated with the word "yellow." Thus, plasticity allows the color sensory experience to act as a guide so that the brain does not need to hard-wire all the necessary connections for a single hue and brightness of the color yellow. Since light is a spectrum, there are hundreds of ways yellow can be seen. This plasticity allows the brain to remodel the neural connections and produce adaptive adjustments as the person's experiences change.

Within the past decade, neuroscientists have shown that between individuals the ratio of L- to M-cones in the retina is highly variable, meaning that some people have more M-cones than L-cones and vice versa. For our previous example of perceiving the color yellow, we would expect that a person with fewer M-cones would not be able to perceive yellow or not as many hues of yellow because there simply is not enough M-cone activation. On the other hand, a person with more M-cones would be able to perceive all hues of yellow. But Roorda and Williams (1999) showed that there was no difference in individuals perceiving or seeing the same color and hue of yellow. Thus, it is hypothesized that the visual cortex is able to use a plastic normalization mechanism along with previous experience to compensate for individual differences in cone ratios, which ultimately allows color perception to be uniform.

Jennifer L. Hellier

See also: Color Blindness; Cone Dystrophy; Cones; Fovea Centralis; Retina; Rods; Visual System

Further Reading

Curcio, Christine A., Kenneth R. Sloan, Robert E. Kalina, & Anita E. Hendrickson. (1990). Human photoreceptor topography. *Journal of Comparative Neurology, 292*(4), 497–523.

Neitz, Jay, Joseph Carroll, Yasuki Yamauchi, Maureen Neitz, & David R. Williams. (2002). Color perception is mediated by a plastic neural mechanism that is adjustable in adults. *Neuron, 35,* 783–792.

Roorda, Austin, & David R. Williams. (1999). The arrangement of the three cone classes in the living human eye. *Nature, 397*(6719), 520–522. http://dx.doi.org/10.1038/17383

CONE DYSTROPHY

In rare cases, cone cells in the eye can be damaged, resulting in a type of cone dystrophy, which is a general term to describe rare disorders that affect cone cells.

Types of Cone Dystrophies

To date, cone dystrophies have been classified into two groups: stationary and progressive disorders. Stationary cone dystrophies are usually present at birth (congenital disorder) or in early childhood and continue to be stable over the lifetime of the patient. The opposite is true for progressive cone dystrophies in which symptoms worsen over time. Progressive dystrophies tend to occur in late adolescence to early adulthood. Health care professionals, however, have differed in how to use the term cone dystrophy. Some use the term only for progressive disorders, while others will use the term for both stable and progressive disorders.

Cone dystrophies can be inherited or occur spontaneously without a specific cause for the disease. Some health care providers also call spontaneous cone dystrophies sporadic dystrophies. Types of cone dystrophies include complete and incomplete achromatopsia—a stationary and inherited disorder in which a person has the inability to see color as well as having a sensitivity to light (photophobia) and decreased vision; blue cone monochromatism—a rare X-linked disorder in which persons have poor or no color discrimination, increased sensitivity to light, and decreased central vision; and X-linked progressive cone dystrophy—an uncommon disorder that may also cause degeneration in rod cells.

Inherited dystrophies are caused by a mutation in one or several genes that are associated with cone proteins and can be inherited as an autosomal dominant (only a single copy of the gene, either from the mother or father, is mutated) or recessive (both copies of the gene are mutated) trait or as an X-linked recessive trait (the abnormal gene is located on the X chromosome). If a cone dystrophy is X-linked, then males are affected more often than females as they only have one X chromosome. Females can either be a carrier—having one mutated X chromosome—or have the disorder if both X chromosomes are affected. In sporadic, autosomal dominant and recessive cone dystrophies, males and females are affected at the same rate.

Signs and Symptoms

Symptoms in persons with cone dystrophies can vary between patients as does the progression and severity of the degeneration. In cone dystrophies, cone cells can degenerate, resulting in loss of color vision (not color blindness as this is generally caused by a different mechanism) and loss of vision acuity particularly in central vision—when looking straight ahead. Often, this also causes an increased sensitivity to light that can be painful. In sporadic dystrophies, the age of onset can vary, as does the amount of visual deficits. In some cases, patients may become legally blind, meaning their vision is 20/200 or worse and cannot be corrected with glasses or contact lenses.

Other symptoms may include patients developing a nystagmus (rapid, involuntary movements of the eyes) associated with their disorder. Generally, persons do not become completely blind as the rod cells are often spared. In cases where the onset of the dystrophy began later in life, rod cells may be affected, reducing peripheral and low-light vision in these patients.

Treatments

To date, there are no known cures for cone dystrophies. Treatments are provided to alleviate specific symptoms, such as wearing dark sunglasses in brightly lit areas and using magnifying devices to help improve clarity when reading.

Jennifer L. Hellier

See also: Color Blindness; Color Perception; Fovea Centralis; National Organization for Rare Disorders; Retina; Visual System

Further Reading

Hamel, Christian P. (2007). Cone rod dystrophies. *Orphanet Journal of Rare Diseases, 2*, 7. http://dx.doi.org/10.1186/1750-1172-2-7

Kohl, Susanne. (2009). Genetic causes of hereditary cone and cone-rod dystrophies. *Der Ophthalmologe: Zeitschrift der Deutschen Ophthalmologischen Gesellschaft, 106*, 109–115.

Michaelides, M., David M. Hunt, & Anthony T. Moore. (2004). The cone dysfunction syndromes. *British Journal of Ophthalmology, 88*, 291–297.

CONES

There are two types of light-sensing cells in the retina of vertebrates: cones and rods. The main function of cones and rods is to convert light into impulses to the optic nerve. Cones process color perception and details of an object, while rods are used for night and peripheral vision. Cones are named by their size and shape, and they are more prominent in humans and other diurnal animals compared to nocturnal animals. Because cones identify details of an object, they need plenty of light to be activated. This is called photopic vision, while rods mediate scotopic (dark) vision.

Anatomy and Physiology

Research studies have measured the spatial density of cones and rods in the adult human eye. Specifically, it has been estimated that there are 4.6 million cones and roughly 92 million rods (Curcio et al., 1990). The location of cones and rods differs as well. Cones are concentrated in the central portion of the retina, called the macula, while rods are found on the elliptical ring of the optic disc mainly on the lateral and superior portions. The macula also contains a depression called the fovea (or fovea centralis), which is a rod-free zone. This densely cone-packed region is roughly about 0.3 millimeters in diameter and contains the majority of cone cells. The number of cones drastically decreases in number as you move away from the fovea centralis and toward the periphery of the retina.

As light enters the eye, it is bent and refracted via the cornea and lens of the eye. This allows an image to be focused onto the retina where the cones are located. Light then activates the cones, which starts a chemical reaction that propagates an electrical impulse from the cone cells to the axons of the optic nerve. This signal continues through the brain until it ends at the primary visual cortex of the occipital lobe. Cones have a faster response time to light stimuli compared to rods, thus allowing details of objects to be viewed and/or perceived.

There are three types of cone cells in humans: S-cone, M-cone, and L-cone cells, with each containing a protein called photopsin. Slight conformational changes in photopsin will determine how light is absorbed in each of the three cone types. As light enters the eye, all three types of cones will be stimulated and absorb the light. However, only at specific wavelength ranges will the peak absorption take place, best activating the cone cells. For instance, each cone type responds best to a specific color range of visible white light, which ranges from 400 to 700 nanometers (nm). S-cone cells are activated by short wavelengths with peak stimulation from 420 to 440 nm, detecting violet to blue colors. M-cone cells are called medium-wavelength sensitive cells and have peak activation from 534 to 545 nm. Finally, L-cone cells are called long-wavelength sensitive cells and have peak stimulation from 564 to 580 nm. However, medium to long wavelengths of light will activate both M-cone and L-cone cells at the same time. The cone type that has more cells stimulated at a time will determine the color that is perceived by the person. For instance, if more M-cones are activated compared to L-cones, then the color yellow is perceived. However, if significantly more L-cones are stimulated than M-cone cells, then the color red is perceived. The more cone cells that are activated at one time will allow a continuous range of colors to be perceived by the human eye.

Diseases of the Cones

In rare cases, cone cells can degenerate, resulting in loss of color vision (not color blindness, as this is generally caused by a different mechanism) and loss of vision acuity, particularly in central vision. Often, this also causes an increase in sensitivity to light that is painful. Degeneration of the cones is a type of cone dystrophy, which is a general term used to describe a group of rare disorders that affect cone cells. Cone dystrophies have been classified into two groups: stationary and progressive disorders. Stationary cone dystrophies are usually present at birth (congenital disorder) or in early childhood and continue to be stable over the lifetime of the patient. The opposite is true for progressive cone dystrophies in which symptoms worsen over time. Cone dystrophies can be inherited or occur spontaneously without a specific cause for the disease. Symptoms in persons with cone dystrophies can vary between patients as does the progression and severity of the degeneration. To date, there are no known cures for cone dystrophies and treatments are provided to alleviate specific symptoms, such as wearing dark sunglasses in brightly lit areas and using magnifying devices to help improve clarity when reading.

Patricia A. Bloomquist and Jennifer L. Hellier

See also: Color Blindness; Color Perception; Cone Dystrophy; Fovea Centralis; Retina; Rods; Visual System

Further Reading

Curcio, Christine A., Kenneth R. Sloan, Robert E. Kalina, & Anita E. Hendrickson. (1990). Human photoreceptor topography. *Journal of Comparative Neurology, 292*(4), 497–523.
Kostic, Corinne, & Yvan Arsenijevic. (2016). Animal modeling for inherited central vision loss. *Journal of Pathology, 238*(2), 300–310. http://dx.doi.org/10.1002/path.4641
Roorda, Austin, & David R. Williams. (1999). The arrangement of the three cone classes in the living human eye. *Nature, 397*(6719), 520–522. http://dx.doi.org/10.1038/17383

CONGENITAL INSENSITIVITY TO PAIN

A person with congenital insensitivity to pain never feels any physical pain from the start of his or her life. This is a very dangerous disease as these people may not be able to determine if a bone is broken or if they have bitten off the tip of their tongue unless they see the swelling of the surrounding tissue or taste blood in their mouth. Because of this inability to sense pain, it is common for patients with congenital insensitivity to pain to have unseen infections as well as have a multitude of bruises, wounds, and broken bones over their lifetime. It is important to note, however, that persons with congenital insensitivity to pain do not have cognitive defects and they have normal light and crude touch sensations. This means they can sense sharp and dull pressures on their skin. Temperature sensation may be normal. People with congenital insensitivity to pain can tell if something is hot or cold to the touch, but they are not able to sense pain caused by extremely hot temperatures, which is abnormal. For example, they may not realize that by touching a hot stove, they are burning their skin.

In general, persons with congenital insensitivity to pain have a shortened life expectancy, as they have repeated burn injuries. Most of these burns are severe (third-degree burns) and may become a life-threatening injury. Additionally, children with congenital insensitivity to pain tend to have mouth wounds because they do not know that they are biting their tongue or cheek, and tend to have finger and hand injuries.

Other disorders that have difficulty with pain and touch sensitivity are autism and its related autistic-spectrum disorders like Asperger's syndrome. These disorders are associated with an overall dysfunction of the sensory system, and pain or touch insensitivity can be one of the symptoms of the syndrome.

Anatomy and Physiology

Congenital insensitivity to pain is considered to be a neuropathy of the peripheral nervous system as it is a sensory system dysfunction. Recent studies have identified a mutation in the *SCN9A* (sodium channel, voltage gated, type IX alpha subunit) gene that causes congenital insensitivity to pain. The *SCN9A* gene codes for part of a sodium channel, specifically the NaV1.7 channel. These sodium channels are found in pain fibers (nociceptors) and are essential in transmitting pain from the periphery to the central nervous system. Defects in the *SCN9A* gene cause the NaV1.7 channel to not be formed or made, thus sodium is not able to enter the channel and transmit the pain signal. NaV1.7 channels are also found in olfactory sensory neurons. This means that many persons with congenital insensitivity to pain will also have anosmia, or the inability to smell.

Congenital insensitivity to pain is a very rare disease with less than 50 cases found in scientific literature. It is an autosomal recessive gene dysfunction, which means that both copies of the *SCN9A* gene must have a defect. Thus, a person with congenital insensitivity to pain must receive a mutated *SCN9A* gene from both his or her mother and father. The parents of children with congenital insensitivity to pain are considered to be carriers as they have at least one mutated gene. The parents generally do not have any signs or symptoms of abnormal perception of pain nor do they have congenital insensitivity to pain.

Jennifer L. Hellier

See also: Anosmia; National Organization for Rare Disorders; Nociception; Sensory Receptors; Somatosensory Cortex; Somatosensory System

Further Reading

Capsoni, Simona, Sonia Covaceuszach, Sara Marinelli, Marcello Ceci, Antonietta Bernardo, Luisa Minghetti, . . . Antonino Cattaneo. (2011). Taking pain out of NGF: A "painless" NGF mutant, linked to hereditary sensory autonomic neuropathy Type V, with full neurotrophic activity. *PLoS One, 6*(2), e17321.

Genetics Home Reference: Your Guide to Understanding Genetic Conditions. (2010). Congenital insensitivity to pain. *U.S. National Library of Medicine.* Retrieved from http://ghr.nlm.nih.gov/condition/congenital-insensitivity-to-pain

Golshani, Ashkahn E., Ankur A. Kamdar, Susanna C. Spence, & Nicholas M. Beckmann. (2014). Congenital indifference to pain: An illustrated case report and literature review. *Journal of Radiology Case Reports, 8*(8), 16–23. Retrieved from http://www.ncbi.nlm.nih.gov/pmc/articles/PMC4242143/

CONSENSUAL PUPILLARY LIGHT REFLEX

The pupillary light reflex is a reflex that constricts or dilates in response to increased or decreased illumination of the retina (the photosensitive lining of the posterior part of the eye). Most mammals experience consensual pupillary light reflex in which light directed at one eye causes increased illumination of the retina not only of the same eye, but also that of the other eye. Therefore, light directed at one eye causes the stimulated eye to constrict as well as the opposite pupil. Among vertebrates, there is a wide range in the size of consensual pupillary light reflex compared to direct pupillary light reflex. In humans, 100 percent of pupillary light reflex is consensual, while there is 0 percent in rabbits (Trejo et al., 1989). This variation may be related to the proportion of uncrossed fibers in the optic tract and the extent of binocularity in the mammal. However, some animals exhibit inconsistent observations and therefore further research must be conducted in order to solidify this theory.

Clinical Significance

The pupillary light reflex provides a useful diagnostic tool in testing the integrity of the sensory and motor functions of the eye. A lack of a consensual pupillary light reflex is often taken as a sign of serious neurological disorder involving the brainstem. In general, cranial nerve reflexes fall into the polysynaptic category due to interneurons that take sensory signals and transmit motor signals to bilateral sides. For instance, a bright penlight in one eye causes both pupils to constrict. If the light causes only the eye with the light to constrict, there is a problem with the motor neuron (oculomotor nerve) on the contralateral side. If there is no pupillary constriction when a penlight is shone, the problem likely exists with that ipsilateral (same side) optic nerve. This understanding can help identify problems with the nerves (such as inflammation or tumors) or with the brain itself (such as tumors or strokes).

Vivian Vu and Jennifer L. Hellier

See also: Blink Reflex; Brainstem; Central Nervous System; Cranial Nerves; Neurological Examination; Visual System

Further Reading

Bear, Mark F., Barry W. Connors, & Michael A. Paradiso. (2007). *Neuroscience exploring the brain* (3rd ed.). Baltimore, MD: Lippincott Williams & Wilkins.

Kandel, Eric R., James H. Schwartz, Thomas M. Jessell, Steven A. Siegelbaum, & A. J. Hudspeth (Eds.). (2012). *Principles of neural science* (5th ed.). New York, NY: McGraw-Hill.

Trejo, L. J., M. N. Rand, & C. M. Cicerone. (1989). Consensual pupillary light reflex in the pigmented rat. *Vision Research*, 29(3), 303–307.

CRANIAL NERVES

The cranial nerves are a series of 12 paired nerves that originate from the cranium, as opposed to the spinal nerves that originate from the spinal cord. These nerves are responsible for conducting both motor and sensory information to and from the head, face, and neck. Additionally, some of these nerves are responsible for conducting the information of the special senses such as olfaction, vision, gustatory, auditory, and equilibrium to the brain. Most cranial nerves carry only sensory or motor information. However, one-third of the cranial nerves are "mixed" because they carry both sensory and motor information. In animals, sensory information is the input from the outside world; motor information causes a reaction in response to the outside world. In most bilaterally symmetrical animals, including humans, many of the specialized senses are found in the cranium.

Consider the example of a person eating a strawberry. The perception of the strawberry includes its appearance, taste, smell, and texture. Each of these sensory modalities is mediated by a different cranial nerve. Additionally, the physical action of eating the strawberry requires specific movements of the tongue and jaw, which are caused by other cranial nerves. All these nerves and organs that allow for these sensations and movements are present in the head.

Naming Technique

Cranial nerves are named by the special sense they serve or for the muscles they innervate. In addition to their names, cranial nerves are numbered by Roman numerals starting with the most rostral—the olfactory nerve or cranial nerve I—to the most caudal—the hypoglossal nerve or cranial nerve XII. A popular way to remember the names and the order of the 12 cranial nerves is by using mnemonic devices, which is a learning technique to help retain information. The most famous mnemonic device used to remember the cranial nerves is "On old Olympus's towering tops, a Finn and German viewed some hops." For this saying, the first letter of each word represents the first letter of each cranial nerve in order. Students use this device to remember the order of the 12 cranial nerves, which is olfactory, optic, oculomotor, trochlear, trigeminal, abducens, facial, auditory (or vestibulocochlear), glossopharyngeal, vagus, spinal (or accessory), and hypoglossal.

There are also mnemonic devices for remembering which cranial nerves are sensory, motor, or both. The most common of these phrases is "Some say marry money, but my brother says big brains matter most." For this saying, the first letter of each word indicates if the nerve is sensory, motor, or both.

Anatomy and Physiology

Cranial nerves are bundles of axons that exit or enter the cranium. For sensory cranial nerves, the cell bodies are usually found in specialized structures called ganglia. These ganglia are generally located between their peripheral target (somewhere on the head and/or neck) and the central nervous system. This is not particularly true for motor cranial nerves. Motor nerves generally have their cell bodies located in the brainstem in structures called nuclei and their axons travel toward their target. Most of these nerves do not cross the midline and synapse on the same side of the face, head, or neck.

The simplest cranial nerves—meaning that only motor information is carried to skeletal muscles—are the oculomotor (III), trochlear (IV), abducens (VI), and hypoglossal (XII). All four of these nerves arise from nuclei located near the midline of the brainstem. Cranial nerves III, IV, and VI are used in concert to control eye movement, particularly during complex actions like tracking moving objects. The oculomotor nerve is also responsible for the shape of the lens and pupil size of the eye, which is evident in the consensual pupillary reflex. This is a normal reflex that is caused when one pupil is stimulated with light, causing both the stimulated and nonstimulated pupils to constrict. This is a fast, easy, and noninvasive cranial nerve test that is used to help diagnose concussions.

More complex cranial nerves are the trigeminal (V), facial (VII), glossopharyngeal (IX), vagus (X), and accessory (XI). In vertebrates, these nerves innervate skeletal muscles that originate from the brachial arches. Of these more complex cranial nerves, all but XI are mixed nerves, meaning that they carry both sensory and motor axons. The accessory nerve consists of purely motor axons that assist in moving shoulder and neck muscles.

The trigeminal nerve receives its name because it has three distinct branches—V_1, V_2, and V_3. Both V_1 (ophthalmic) and V_2 (maxillary) branches carry only sensory information, specifically somatosensation from the top third of the face and the upper jaw, respectively. The mandibular branch (V_3) is mixed and carries somatosensation from the lower jaw as well as movement of the muscles involved in chewing.

The facial nerve (VII) is mixed and brings taste information from the anterior tongue, somatosensation from the ear, and controls tear and saliva secretion. The motor axons of nerve VII are essential for controlling the muscles used for facial expression in the ipsilateral half of the face as well as the stapedius muscle of the middle ear. Damage to cranial nerve VII will cause the ipsilateral half of the face to have weakness and the decreased ability to have facial expressions such that the person cannot smile or frown. Furthermore, tear and saliva secretion may be altered on the same side of the face. This type of damage is generally called Bell's palsy.

The glossopharyngeal is also a mixed nerve. It carries the sense of taste and somatosensation from the posterior tongue. Along with the facial nerve, it helps control saliva secretion. Portions of the glossopharyngeal nerve called the carotid bodies sense chemical changes in the blood, which are visceral sensations. For the motor component of the glossopharyngeal nerve, it controls the muscles of the larynx and pharynx along with the motor portion of the vagus nerve (X). These muscles are used in the action of swallowing and speech.

The vagus nerve is very thick and large in humans compared to other cranial nerves. This is because the vagus nerve, which means wandering in Latin, exits the medulla from the brainstem down to the abdomen. It is here that cranial nerve X serves autonomic functions for the gut, heart, and lungs. These are the primary preganglionic parasympathetic neurons used in the autonomic nervous system. The sensory portion of the vagus nerve innervates the external ear and carries somatosensory information.

Lastly, there are three pure sensory cranial nerve pairs, which are the olfactory (I), optic (II), and auditory (or vestibulocochlear, VIII) nerves. The axons of olfactory sensory neurons (OSN) make up cranial nerve I and pass through the ethmoid bone between the eye sockets and terminate in the olfactory bulb. OSNs are unique in that they are in direct contact with the outside world in the nasal cavity and synapse directly into the brain. These neurons are also exceptional because they are continually replaced throughout the life of the animal. Thus, newborn OSNs must guide their axons through the ethmoid bone and synapse in the correct location in the olfactory bulb to maintain the sense of smell.

The optic nerve (II) is relatively thick compared to most cranial nerves. It consists of axons from ganglion cells that leave the retina of the eye, cross at the optic chiasm, and terminate in the occipital lobe. Through the optic nerve, vision is conveyed from the eye to the brain. Most mammals are highly visual and in these animals the majority of the brain is wired to understand the outside world through vision, such as location in space, shape and color of an object, and determining brightness.

Finally, the auditory (vestibulocochlear, VIII) nerve is used for both hearing and balance (equilibrium). It travels from the inner ear to the brainstem. Together with the optic nerve, the vestibulocochlear portion provides the perception of orientation and head movement in space. For example, people who become "seasick" may be able to alleviate/overcome that sensation by looking at the horizon where visually it is more stable.

C. J. Saunders and Jennifer L. Hellier

See also: Bell's Palsy; Facial Nerve; Glossopharyngeal Nerve; Nerves; Olfactory Nerve; Optic Nerve; Trigeminal Nerve; Vagus Nerve; Vestibulocochlear Nerve

Further Reading

Appendix A: The brainstem and cranial nerves. (2004). In D. Purves, G. J. Augustine, D. Fitzpatrick, W. C. Hall, A. LaMantia, J. O. McNamara, & S. M. Williams (Eds.), *Neuroscience* (3rd ed., pp. 755–761). Sunderland, MA: Sinauer Associates.

Herlevich, N. E. (1990). *Reflecting on old Olympus' towering tops.* Retrieved from www.ncbi.nlm.nih.gov/pubmed/2254946

CROSSED EYES: *See* Strabismus

D

DEAFNESS

Deafness is a functional loss in the ability to hear. It varies along a spectrum from mild hearing impairment to profound deafness and total deafness where little to no sound can be heard, even with amplification. There are two categories of deafness—conductive and sensorineural. Conductive hearing loss is the result of a disruption in sound wave conduction within the outer and middle ear. Sensorineural deafness is the result of damage or injury to the cochlea or the auditory nerve that prevents the transduction of the electrical impulse created by sound waves. A combination of both conductive and sensorineural hearing loss is called mixed deafness. Deafness can be unilateral, affecting one ear, or bilateral, affecting both ears. Tuning fork tests, such as the Weber test and the Rinne test, are used to distinguish between the type of hearing loss, the extent of the loss, as well as the differentiation between unilateral and bilateral. It is estimated that in the United States about 13 percent of the population have some form of hearing loss ranging from total deafness to hearing impairment. Deafness affects all age groups and all races equally. Typically, hearing assistive devices, including hearing aids and cochlear implants, are used for sensorineural loss, while local medical treatments are used when the hearing loss is conductive.

Conductive deafness is caused by decreased conductivity of sound waves at any point between the outer ear and the middle ear. The majority of pathologies that cause conductive hearing loss can be treated with standard medical interventions, generally with the full recovery of hearing. Causes of conductive hearing loss can include normal processes that go into overproduction. Earwax secretion is an example of a normal and beneficial process that can cause conductive deafness. When earwax buildup becomes excessive, it can collect and block the auditory canal, which thereby inhibits the passage of sound waves to the middle ear. The buildup usually causes sudden hearing loss accompanied by localized pain and irritation. To treat this issue, the wax buildup must be removed. Health care providers can either scoop the wax out of the ear with a special instrument or syringe the wax out with a warm saline lavage.

Other common causes of conductive hearing loss are otitis media and otitis externa, which are ear infections of the middle ear and outer ear, respectively. Bacteria such as *Streptococcus pneumonidae* as well as *Haemophilus influenzae* introduced to the middle ear via the auditory tubes typically cause ear infections of the middle ear and the subsequent inflammation in the outer ear. Hearing loss with ear infections is most commonly triggered by excess fluid within the middle ear, which inhibits movement of the ossicles and tympanic membrane. Ear infections are typically treated with a medicated eardrop that is combination of antibiotics and steroids.

Tympanic membrane injury is another common cause of conductive hearing loss. It can range from perforations to ruptures in the membrane. If the eardrum is injured, the conduction of sound waves to the middle ear can be decreased because the tympanic membrane is less responsive to sound waves. Eardrum trauma can be caused by direct injury to the membrane via a foreign body, significant air compression within the outer ear, or by middle ear infections when fluid buildup causes a rupture. Treatment of eardrum injury depends on the severity and cause. If the injury is mild, the eardrum should heal without direct treatment; if the injury is severe, it may have to be repaired surgically. Any injury to the eardrum accompanied by an infection should be treated with antibiotic and steroid eardrops.

Sensorineural hearing loss is caused by a decrease or complete inability to transduce sound waves into electrical impulses in the cochlea or cochlear nerve. This type of deafness is sometimes referred to as nerve deafness because the location of the deficit is at the level of the cochlear nerve or hair cells. There are various causes of sensorineural deafness including old age, loud noise, congenital defects, and infection. The pathologies that cause sensorineural hearing loss typically damage the hair cell cilia directly, or they damage the cochlear nerve in such a manner that neural impulses cannot be sent to the brain. In instances such as old age and prolonged exposure to loud noises, the damage occurs at the level of the cilia. Hearing loss caused by old age or prolonged exposure to loud noises is the result of cilia that are no longer attached to the hair cells. Without the cilia on hair cells, action potentials cannot be generated and sent to the cochlear nerve. This form of sensorineural hearing loss typically affects only some frequencies, so individuals affected can still hear other frequencies of sound. The use of a standard hearing aid can help compensate for the hearing loss caused by old age or loud noise exposure.

Congenital hearing loss occurs while a baby is still in the womb and is caused by a variety of factors. Some common causes of congenital sensorineural hearing loss are maternal infections such as rubella (German measles) or toxoplasmosis (a parasite that is often found in cat feces). In other cases, congenital hearing loss can be caused by a hereditary disease that is passed from the parents to the child genetically. Another cause of sensorineural hearing loss is infection that leads to inflammation of the inner ear. Infection-induced hearing loss occurs when an infection such as the mumps causes inflammation and swelling around the cochlea, which causes damage to the hair cell cilia. Treatment for any type of sensorineural deafness requires the use of hearing assistive devices such as hearing aids or cochlear implants.

Lynelle Smith

See also: Americans with Disabilities Act; Assistive Technology; Auditory System; Cochlea; Cochlear Implants; Vestibulocochlear Nerve

Further Reading

Gallaudet University Library LibGuides. (2012). *Deaf population in the U.S. (data file).* Retrieved from http://libguides.gallaudet.edu/content.php?pid=119476&sid=1029111

Leighton, S., A. Robson, & J. Russell. (2000). *Hall & Colman's diseases of the ear, nose and throat* (15th ed., M. Burton, Ed.). London: Harcourt Brace.

DESENSITIZATION

Desensitization can have different meanings in medicine and science. For instance, desensitization is a process to reduce or alleviate a person's or animal's adverse reaction to a stimulus. In rare cases, certain stimuli may actually cause a phobia in a person, such as seeing spiders (arachnophobia). Desensitization techniques can be used to reduce a person's phobia. In neuroscience, desensitization generally refers to receptor desensitization, where the receptor cannot be activated or opened for a specific length of time even if the neurotransmitter is present. Finally, in the field of psychology desensitization is defined as the diminished emotional responsiveness to a negative or aversive stimulus after repeated exposure. When an action tendency associated with an emotion proves irrelevant or unnecessary, an emotional response is repeatedly evoked. Developed by psychologist Mary Cover Jones (1897–1987), desensitization is a process primarily used to assist individuals to unlearn phobias and anxieties. In 1958, Joseph Wolpe (1915–1997) developed a method of a hierarchical list of anxiety-evoking stimuli in order of intensity. This allowed individuals to undergo adaption. While medication is available for individuals, evidence supports desensitization with high rates of cure, especially in those who suffer from depression or schizophrenia.

Steps to Desensitization

First, the hierarchical list developed by Wolpe ranks an ordered series of steps from the least to the most disturbing fears or phobias. This is constructed between a client and therapist. The client is taught techniques in order to produce deep relaxation. While it is impossible to feel both anxiety and relaxation at the same time, it is important to ease the client into deep relaxation. This helps inhibit any feelings of anxiety. A guided reduction in fear, anxiety, or aversion, known as systematic desensitization, can be achieved by gradually approaching a feared stimulus as well as maintaining relaxation. When individuals are directly exposed to the stimuli and situations they fear, desensitization works best as anxiety-evoking stimuli are paired with inhibitory responses. This can be carried out with in vivo desensitization (performing in real-life situations) or as vicarious desensitization (acting out steps of the hierarchy so clients can observe modules of the feared behavior). The patient and therapist will slowly move up the hierarchy until the last item on the list is performed without any fear or anxiety.

Effects on Animals

Animals can be desensitized to their fears as well as humans can. A race horse, for example, who is afraid of the starting gate can be desensitized to fearful elements. These fearful elements may include but are not limited to the creak of the gate, the starting bell, and the enclosed space. Horses can be desensitized to these one at a time, in small doses.

Effects on Violence

One topic debated in science is whether violence is caused by the exposure to violence in the media including television, video games, and movies. Desensitization can also refer to the potential for reduced responsiveness to this actual violence. It has been suggested that violence may prime thoughts of hostility with the possibility of affecting the way humans perceive others and interpret their actions. Aversive responses including but not limited to increased heart rate, fear, discomfort, perspiration, and disgust have been associated with the initial exposure to violence in the media. Prolonged and repeated exposure to violence may reduce or habituate the initial psychological impact until violent images do not elicit these negative responses. Over time, an observer could become desensitized to media violence, both emotionally and cognitively. An experiment was completed with participants who played violent video games. This showed that gaming participants had lower heart rates and electrical skin response readings. This was interpreted as the individuals displaying a physiological desensitization to violence. However, these findings have not been replicated, and it has been questioned whether becoming desensitized to media violence specifically transfers to becoming desensitized to real-life violence.

Renee Johnson

See also: Carotid Body; Excitation; Free Nerve Endings; Perception

Further Reading

Engelhardt, Christopher R., Bruce D. Bartholow, Geoffrey T. Kerr, & Brad J. Bushman. (2011). This is your brain on violent video games: Neural desensitization to violence predicts increased aggression following violent video game exposure. *Journal of Experimental Social Psychology, 47*(5), 1033–1036.

Krahe, Barbara, Ingrid Moller, L. Rowell Huesmann, Lucyna Kirwil, Juliane Felber, & Anja Berger. (2011). Desensitization to media violence: Links with habitual media violence exposure, aggressive cognitions, and aggressive behavior. *Journal of Personality and Social Psychology, 100*(4), 630–646.

Mrug, Sylvie, Anjana Madan, & Michael Windle. (2016). Emotional desensitization to violence contributes to adolescents' violent behavior. *Journal of Abnormal Child Psychology, 44*(1), 75–86.

DIPLOPIA

Diplopia is the medical term for double vision. This is when a person sees two images of the same object. The images can be side by side (horizontally), one above the other (vertically), or both, making the images diagonally across from each other. Diplopia occurs when the six extraocular muscles that surround each eye begin to weaken and have difficulty in converging the eyes. These muscles are controlled by three cranial nerves: oculomotor (cranial nerve III), trochlear (cranial nerve IV), and abducens (cranial nerve VI).

Causes

In general, diplopia is the result of an underlying systemic disease and can cause the person to have difficulty with balance, reading, and walking. Some diseases resulting in diplopia include but are not limited to brain tumors; damage to cranial nerves III, IV, or VI; diabetes; Lyme disease; migraine; multiple sclerosis; and stroke.

Types

There are four classifications of diplopia: binocular, monocular, temporary, and voluntary. Binocular diplopia is generally associated with strabismus where the six extraocular muscles do not align the eyes properly so that convergence cannot occur. For instance, one eye focuses on an object and the other eye turns inward or outward and focuses on a completely different object. Thus, two different images are sent to the brain, which can be confusing for visual perception. In young children, their brains may learn to ignore the image from the weaker eye—usually the turned eye. If the turned eye is only slightly askew, then both eyes may focus on the same object but the images are focused on different regions of the two retinas. The brain will try to determine where the object is in space based on the two images sent to the visual cortex, which can also be confusing.

Monocular diplopia or monocular polyopia is when one eye perceives more than one image. This can occur if the surface of the eye—the cornea—thins and changes shape to be more cone-like (keratoconus). Keratoconus is a degenerative disorder of the eye and is usually diagnosed in a person's teenage years. If the keratoconus is severe, surgery may be necessary to correct the shape of the cornea. However, in some cases the cornea may need to be replaced (corneal transplant). Other causes of monocular diplopia include structural defects of the eye, such as a displaced or misaligned lens, and astigmatism. Astigmatism is a common vision condition and is caused by a misshaped cornea, resulting in light not focusing properly on the retina.

Being tired, trauma to the head, or overindulgence in alcohol generally causes temporary diplopia. Temporary diplopia should resolve on its own with rest. However, if a person has trauma to the head, he or she should see a health care provider immediately for evaluation.

Finally, voluntary diplopia occurs when a person purposely crosses the eyes (such as focusing on the tip of the nose), unfocuses the eyes (which can help in viewing stereo images), or focuses on an object that is behind another object. The object closest to the person will be doubled. It is an urban legend that if you cross your eyes, it will become permanent. In reality, voluntary diplopia is not dangerous but if it is prolonged, it may cause headaches.

Treatment

Treatment for diplopia depends on the cause of the double vision. The underlying cause must be treated first for best results. If diplopia is acute, it may be resolved by restful sleep; if it is chronic diplopia, an optometrist may prescribe eye exercises, wearing an eye patch, or wearing eyeglasses with a prism correction. For severe cases and where other treatments have not been effective, eye surgery may be necessary to correct the diplopia.

Jennifer L. Hellier

See also: Astigmatism; Cranial Nerves; Myopia; Presbyopia; Strabismus; Visual System

Further Reading

American Optometric Association. (2015). Astigmatism. Retrieved from http://www.aoa.org/patients-and-public/eye-and-vision-problems/glossary-of-eye-and-vision-conditions/astigmatism?sso=y

Blumenfeld, Hal. (2010). *Neuroanatomy through clinical cases*. Sunderland, MA: Sinauer.

Graf, M., & B. Lorenz. (2012). How to deal with diplopia. *Revue Neurologique* (Paris), *168*(10), 720–728. http://dx.doi.org/10.1016/j.neurol.2012.08.001

DISCRIMINATIVE TOUCH

Distinguishing fine details—feeling the numbers on a debit card or knowing how hard to press on the screen of a smartphone—are examples of activities aided by discriminative touch. "Discriminative" in this context refers to the ability to distinguish between different shapes, textures, vibration, and other fine points of touch. A specific set of neurons and pathways into the brain is dedicated to this fine-tuned sense. Interestingly, the sensations of pain and temperature involve entirely different neurons and spinal cord pathways.

Discriminative Touch Experiment

Touch is the most basic sense for animals and discriminative touch (two-point discrimination) is essential for survival. It is used by animals to identify objects that can be tools to access or pick up food. Discriminative touch employs small receptor fields to increase the intensity of the touch sense. If a body region has an extensive number of small receptor fields, it will be more sensitive to external stimuli.

Materials:

Metric ruler
Two toothpicks or similar items
Calculator
Paper
Pencil
At least three people willing to be subjects

Directions:

One person will measure distance in millimeters and record the results, one person (tester) will test the two-point discrimination of the different body parts, and the remaining people will be the subjects. If there are only three people, rotate positions so that each person takes a turn as a subject.

1. To test two-point discrimination, the tester will take two toothpicks and simultaneously place them about eight inches (roughly 200 millimeters) apart on the upper back of the subject. The tester **does not** need to push hard to cause pain, just enough pressure so that the subject can feel the two points. Ask the subject, "How many points do you feel?" If the answer is "one," then measure and record the distance in millimeters between the two points. If it is "two," then move the toothpicks closer together about one inch (25 millimeters) and simultaneously place them on the subject's back.
2. Repeat step 1 until the subject feels only one point; measure and record the distance.
3. Repeat steps 1 and 2 on the back of the hand (starting distance will be about three inches—about 75 millimeters—apart) and ask the subject to close their eyes and turn their head. This is to ensure that the subject is only using the discriminative touch sense and not visual sense to determine the number of points. Move the toothpicks closer together about 10 millimeters at a time.
4. Repeat steps 1 and 2 on the fingertip (starting distance will be about half an inch—about 13 millimeters—apart) and ask the subject to close their eyes and turn their head. The finger is the most sensitive body part and if the points are too large, the tester will have a difficult time getting to "one point." Move the toothpicks closer together about 1–2 millimeters at a time.
5. Average the distances for each body part and graph the results.

Jennifer L. Hellier

These special nerves generally fall under the category of "mechanoreceptors." Physical stimulation depresses the neuron's plasma membrane and ions rush into the cytoplasm, creating an action potential. This signal is relayed to the spinal cord and eventually to the contralateral parietal cortex in the brain. Here the signal is interpreted. With the addition of many individual mechanoreceptors, the brain is able to create a complete picture of a coin's edge or the sticky side of a stamp.

Anatomy and Physiology

The first step in initiating a "touch" sensation is an action potential from one of the mechanoreceptors in the skin. The neuron's membrane is depressed/stretched and ions rush in, creating an action potential. While this concept can be applied broadly to discriminative touch neurons, each behaves slightly differently, creating a more detailed ability to distinguish touch. An understanding of the characteristics of each of the corpuscles helps inform the entire process of touch.

Meissner's corpuscles and Pacinian corpuscles are more similar than different. Both detect pressure, vibration, and the initiation/termination of touch. Once an initial series of action potentials are generated, these nerves slow the frequency of signaling so as not to overwhelm our sensory pathways. Take the example of putting on a shirt. Initially, the weight and texture of the material are sensed. This initial sensation is quickly ignored until there is a change such as tugging on the shirt, adding a coat, and so on. This characteristic explains why both corpuscles are described as "phasic" or "rapidly adapting."

These two neuron types differ in location within the skin and specific stimulation characteristics. Meissner's corpuscles exist on the most superficial aspect of the dermis directly below the epidermis. This allows detection of light touch and minimal vibration (approximately 10–50 hertz). They are found in highest concentration in the fingertips and the lips. Slightly deeper in the skin is where Pacinian corpuscles can be found. These neurons detect slightly greater pressure and are more sensitive to vibration (200 hertz). Interestingly, slicing a Pacinian corpuscle in two reveals an onion-like appearance of the nerve ending. This feature allows for the determination of specific surface textures like smooth or rough.

In contrast with the rapidly adapting mechanoreceptor, Ruffini corpuscles and Merkel nerve endings offer examples of slowly adapting mechanoreceptors. Existing deeper in the dermis, these receptors are sensitive to pressure and stretch. The need for a slowly adapting tactile nerve—where the action potential continues to provide information—is exemplified with a cup of water. Once the cup is initially grabbed, the rapidly adapting mechanoreceptors relay the amount of pressure needed to hold the cup as well as the surface texture. This initial signal decreases as long as the cup is held. If the cup began to slide, a signal generated at the Ruffini corpuscle would be relayed to the brain and adjustments could be made to the grip.

Adding another component to the slowly adjusting mechanoreceptors, Merkel nerve endings provide slightly different information than Ruffini corpuscles. The receptive field—or area of skin dedicated to one neuron—is smaller for Merkel nerve endings. These cells are also found in higher density in areas dedicated to discriminative touch such as fingertips. Additionally, these cells are extremely sensitive to skin stretch (only one micrometer needed, i.e., 10^{-6} meters). This allows for a fine-tuned, slowly adapting mechanoreceptor signal.

Once a signal is generated in either a rapidly or slowly adjusting mechanoreceptor, it then makes a rapid journey through the dorsal column–medial lemniscal system. The corpuscles previously mentioned make up the first-order neurons with cell bodies outside of the spinal cord. These first-order neurons are covered in insulation known as myelin and are known as fast-conducting fibers. The first-order neurons enter the posterior spinal cord and ascend toward a component in the brainstem known as the medulla.

At this point, the first-order and second-order neurons synapse at either the nucleus gracilis (sensation from the legs) or the nucleus cuneatus (sensation from the arms). The second-order neurons then cross to the contralateral medulla via the medial lemniscus pathway. These neurons continue to the thalamus where a synapse is made with third-order neurons. A signal from an initial touch sensation finally climbs to the postcentral gyrus or primary somatosensory cortex of the parietal lobe via the internal capsule.

Tactile stimulation from the skin is precisely ordered in the brain. This pattern or map of the human body within the postcentral gyrus is known as the homunculus. Imagine a small human image applied to the lateral aspect of the brain, with legs dangling into the sagittal fissure and the remainder of the body along the outside of the parietal lobe. A tactile stimulation from the hands is processed in a unique order and then compared to a similar stimulation from the feet. Though the journey is complicated—from corpuscle to postcentral gyrus—the total time elapsed is milliseconds, which is 10^{-3} seconds.

Disease and Disability

Taking a deeper look at the homunculus in the primary sensory cortex shows that not all parts are created equal. A larger portion of space is reserved for areas with more discriminative touch sensors. This dedicated space, however, is not stationary. If there is constantly more or less information from a certain peripheral location, the homunculus will restructure. Plasticity is the formal name for this restructuring.

Reading braille is an example of an increase in the amount of discriminative touch information relayed to the cortex. Persons with visual impairment have benefited from this form of written communication since the mid-1800s. Braille was initially a French military invention, a way to read without light. The series of small, palpable bumps are interpreted when fingertips gently pass over them. Utilizing the Meissner's corpuscles, Merkel nerve endings, and the dorsal column–medial lemniscal system, a signal is interpreted in the primary sensory cortex.

Over time, a greater area in the homunculus is dedicated to the processing of tactile stimulation. The primary sensory cortex remodels, allowing for physically more space and numerically more neuronal connections to be made. This neurological plasticity explains why a person with visual impairments becomes advanced in "seeing" the world through physical touch.

An extremity amputation is the converse example to visual impairment in the primary visual cortex. The space devoted to a hand, for example, in the homunculus is enormous. If there is no tactile stimulation, this area eventually diminishes in size and other sensory areas will increase in size. An ipsilateral forearm might become more receptive to discriminative touch, taking over a larger area in the primary sensory cortex.

When considering the process of neurologic plasticity, however, a simplified explanation can be given. If the area of the homunculus slowly expands with more tactile stimulation such as reading braille, so too should the primary cortex area slowly shrink if tactile stimulation is absent. Unfortunately, the process of rearranging neurons can be imprecise. The new connections in the sensory cortex might confuse a person into thinking he or she is experiencing sensation—ranging from mild tingling to intense pain—in the missing limb.

A clinical application of discriminative touch relates to the disease of diabetes. Every six months to a year, persons with this affliction are asked to visit a physician's office to have the sensation in their feet evaluated. This task is accomplished by gently touching the foot with a thin, flexible piece of plastic called a "monofilament." The longer people live with diabetes, the more likely they are to lose discriminative sensation in their extremities. This process typically starts with the toes and slowly works up the foot.

The process of diminished sensation is known as "diabetic neuropathy." How this takes place is a story of sugar. Diabetic people tend to have difficulty reducing the level of sugar in their circulation. If not well controlled, these sugar levels remain elevated and work into tissues such as the kidney, retina, and eventually small neurons. The excess sugar inside the neuron slowly builds up. Water molecules follow these additional sugar molecules and steadily cause damage to the neurons. Smallest, weakest-walled neurons are the first to be damaged. The various corpuscles and nerve endings dedicated to discriminative touch happen to be some of the smaller nerves in the extremities.

Why is this process of slow sensory loss important? Two concepts must be considered. First, damage to the tactile nerves in areas such as the foot can lead to wounds. Imagine a rock inside a shoe. A person without diabetic neuropathy would immediately sense the uncomfortable feeling and remove the offending agent. If this small irritant were not removed, it could slowly cause a blister or open wound on the foot. This becomes a problem with diabetics because of the second important concept: diabetes slows the speed and effectiveness of wound healing.

Nicholas Breitnauer

See also: Homunculus; Meissner's Corpuscles; Phantom Pain; Sensory Receptors; Somatosensory Cortex; Somatosensory System; Touch

Further Reading

McGlone, Francis, Ake B. Vallbo, Hakan Olausson, Line Loken, & Johan Wessberg. (2007). Discriminative touch and emotional touch. *Canadian Journal of Experimental Psychology, 61*(3), 173–183.

DIZZINESS

In mammals, dizziness is a symptom that causes a disruption in determining the body's location in space and physical stability. Dizziness is often classified as vertigo, disequilibrium, and presynchopy—defined as being lightheaded or faint. Conditions that cause dizziness are often wide and varied because there are many body systems that are responsible for balance, such as the inner ear, the central nervous system, and the muscular system. The most common form of dizziness is vertigo; it causes more than 50 percent of all clinical cases of dizziness (Hornibrook, 2011). Vertigo is a disease process that is defined as a type of dizziness that produces the sensation of rotational or spinning movement despite the body remaining still. In addition to the sensation of movement, affected individuals often suffer from nausea and balance issues that make it difficult to stand or walk straight. Vertigo can be classified into two categories: peripheral or central. Peripheral vertigo is the result of vestibular system dysfunction within the semicircular canals or the otolith organs. Central vertigo generally causes balance issues and not the perception of movement, as in peripheral vertigo. Causes of central vertigo are often stroke, brain tumor, hemorrhage, or epilepsy.

Dizziness and vertigo are commonly reported in the general population; it can be a primary disease or symptom that is secondary to another disorder. Individuals of all age groups can show signs and symptoms of vertigo. Individuals experiencing vertigo can have acute attacks lasting a few seconds to a few minutes, or they can have chronic symptoms with the experience lasting for hours and recurring over an extended time frame. Vertigo is caused either by a dysfunction in the peripheral nervous system or by disorders of the central nervous system. Peripheral vertigo originates in the vestibular system and common causes of peripheral vertigo are benign paroxysmal positional vertigo (BPPV), vestibular neuritis, and Meniere's disease. Central vertigo originates from issues within the central nervous system including brain hemorrhage, vestibular nerve lesions, and multiple sclerosis.

BPPV is the most common type of peripheral vertigo and is accompanied by the sudden sensation of spinning. The episode of dizziness associated with BPPV ranges from mild episodic cases to prolonged intense dizziness. In a normal functioning vestibular system, small calcium carbonate particles called otoconia are located within the otolith organs (saccule and utricle), which are part of the vestibular labyrinth of the inner ear. In BPPV, the otoconia are inappropriately displaced into the semicircular canals of the vestibular labyrinth within the inner ear. Normally, these stones are attached to a gelatinous membrane within the utricle and saccule. When the otoconia are free to move within the semicircular canal, a head tilt allows the stones to shift the endolymph, resulting in neural impulses. This creates the false sense of motion that causes the dizziness experienced in BPPV. Any head motion that would normally stimulate the semicircular canals such as head tilting, turning suddenly, looking up or down, and rolling over in bed can trigger BPPV. Unilateral BPPV is the most common form of this disease; however, BPPV can be bilateral and affect the vestibular organs on both sides of the head.

Common signs and symptoms of BPPV include (1) dizziness—the sensation that the surroundings are moving although the person is still, (2) lightheadedness, (3) loss of balance, (4) blurred vision, (5) nystagmus, (6) nausea, and (7) vomiting. In general, these signs and symptoms are recurrent and short in duration. Nystagmus is a common symptom of vertigo that is triggered by the vestibulo-ocular reflex (VOR). The VOR reflex loop connects the movements of the eye to the motions of the head sensed by the vestibular system. When an individual is dizzy, the VOR tries to compensate for the perceived movement with a rapid side-to-side eye "twitching" movement.

Specific causes of BPPV are generally linked to head injuries such as concussions or even migraine headaches. Other causes of BPPV include damage to the inner ear by some unknown cause or by damage to the inner ear during ear surgery. Doctors may use a diagnostic test called electronystamography (ENG) or videonystagmography (VNG) to determine if a patient has the nystagmus associated with inner ear BPPV. These tests measure the rapid eye movements associated with BPPV while the patient moves his or her head in different directions. However, to determine central nervous system vertigo, health care providers may use magnetic resonance imaging (MRI). The main treatment of BPPV is a simple technique called the canalith-repositioning procedure, which must be performed by a health care provider or a trained professional. This practice uses several slow, purposeful head movements, which force the loose otoconia to move back to the utricle and saccule and become reembedded into the gelatinous membrane. In general, the patient will need to have one or two treatments for this procedure to be effective. In rare cases, if the canalith-repositioning procedure is not successful, then surgical interventions must be used to alleviate BPPV.

Lynelle Smith

See also: Central Nervous System; Peripheral Nervous System; Vestibular System

Further Reading

Hornibrook, Jeremy. (2011). Benign paroxysmal positional vertigo (BPPV): History, pathophysiology, office treatment and future directions. *International Journal of Otolaryngology*, Article ID 835671. http://dx.doi.org/10.1155/2011/835671.

Vestibular Disorder Association. (2013). *Labyrinthitis and vestibular neuritis.* Retrieved from
    http://vestibular.org/labyrinthitis-and-vestibular-neuritis

DOPPLER EFFECT

The Doppler effect, also known as the Doppler shift, is the change in frequency of
a wave for an observer moving relative to its source. The Austrian physicist Christian Doppler (1803–1853) proposed this effect in 1842 in Prague. This effect is
very commonly heard in the sounding siren of an emergency vehicle as it approaches, passes, and then gets farther away from another vehicle or observer. The
received frequency is always higher than the emitted frequency during the approach of the observer, while the frequency is identical at the direct instant of passing the observer. As the source gets farther away from the observer, the received
frequency becomes lower than the emitted frequency.

Development

While the concept was first proposed by Christian Doppler in 1842, Christophorus Henricus Diedericus Buys Ballot (1817–1890), a Dutch chemist and meteorologist, tested the Doppler effect hypothesis for sound waves in 1845. His test
confirmed that the sound's pitch was higher than the emitted frequency when the
sound approached him, and lower than the emitted frequency when the sound
receded away from him. French physicist Hippolyte Fizeau (1819–1896) independently discovered the same phenomenon in 1842 with electromagnetic waves; and
in 1848, Scottish civil engineer John Scott Russell (1808–1882) made an experimental study of the Doppler effect in Britain.

Where Do We See the Doppler Effect?

The Doppler effect is seen almost everywhere we see waves. As already mentioned, humans can hear the Doppler effect in sirens or other loud passing sounds
such as airplanes flying overhead. It can also be observed within electromagnetic
waves and light waves.

In astronomy, the Doppler effect is observed in electromagnetic waves. Light is
of great use in astronomy and can result in what is called redshift or blueshift depending on the motion of the object creating the light. The Doppler effect in astronomy is used to measure the speed at which stars and galaxies are approaching
or receding from Earth (radial velocity). The spectra of stars exhibits absorption
lines at well-defined frequencies that are correlated with the energies required to
excite electrons in various elements from one level to another. These absorption
lines are not always observed at the frequencies that are expected from the spectrum of a stationary light source. Blue light has a higher frequency than red light,
and therefore the spectral lines that are an approaching astronomical light source

exhibit a blueshift and those of a receding astronomical light source exhibit a redshift.

Radar uses the Doppler effect to measure the velocity of various detected objects. A radar beam is fired at a moving target and is continually fired as the target moves farther away or closer to the source. The radar beam determines if the gap is getting bigger or smaller between firing, and the wavelength increases or decreases to compensate. If the beam travels a shorter distance, a smaller wavelength is used, and vice versa. This allows the location and velocity of various objects to be measured from a still location. Today, the weather is predicted using the Doppler effect to track storms and changes in air patterns.

In medicine, the Doppler effect is used in medical imaging and in measuring blood flow using tools such as ultrasound or echocardiogram (ECG). An ECG can produce an accurate assessment of the direction of blood flow and the velocity of blood and cardiac tissue at any arbitrary point using the Doppler effect. Although an ultrasound beam functions similarly, it unfortunately must be parallel to the blood flow in order to provide an accurate reading of the velocity. Through calculations using the Doppler effect, cardiac output can be determined.

Research

A group at Microsoft as well as a group at the University of Washington have performed research on using the Doppler effect to sense gestures while interacting with a computer. They used sonic techniques (Doppler effect) to test for gesturing (motion sensing). Some gestures they tested for include but are not limited to scrolling, single tap or double tap, and the two-handed seesaw. They used software called SoundWave to build a computer that is only capable of motion sensing via the Doppler effect. While this research is still in process, they believe that this software could be implemented among many different devices including cellphones and tablets. If this is the case, it might provide the opportunity for cheaper tools to be used in the medical world. This could have huge implications in developing countries and underserved areas where the finances for equipment are limited.

Renee Johnson

See also: Auditory System; Visual System

Further Reading

Gupta, Sidhant, Dan Morris, Shwetak N. Patel, & Desney Tan. (2012). SoundWave: Using the Doppler effect to sense gestures. *ACM SIGCHI Conference on Human Factors In Computing Systems,* May 5–10, Austin, Texas.
National Aeronautics and Space Administration (NASA). (2015). *Doppler effect.* Edited by Nancy Hall. Retrieved from https://www.grc.nasa.gov/www/k-12/airplane/doppler.html

DOUBLE VISION: *See* Diplopia

DYSGEUSIA

The medical term *dysgeusia* is derived from the Greek root words *dys* (abnormal) and *geusia* (taste). Symptoms can range from a mild distortion of taste, dysgeusia, to a complete absence of taste, ageusia. Taste is a special sense conveyed from the taste buds to the brain over several pathways. There are five basic tastes: sweet, sour, salty, bitter, and umami (savory or delicious taste).

Anatomy and Physiology

The human tongue and mouth have areas of special epithelium containing taste receptors. Roughly 50–100 taste receptor cells are gathered inside onion-shaped structures called taste buds. Taste receptors are found on the tongue, palate, epiglottis, pharynx, larynx, and upper esophagus (Simon et al., 2006). The tongue is coated with rough tufts of epithelium that help to protect taste buds and aid in food handling. Taste is sensed when food dissolves in saliva and bathes taste buds. This stimulates the receptor cells through different channels, signaling pathways, and cranial nerves to the gustatory (taste) area of the brain where basic taste is sensed.

The receptor cells from the front of the tongue and palate connect to branches of the facial nerve (7th cranial nerve), and the back of the tongue is supplied by the glossopharyngeal nerve (9th cranial nerve). The vagus nerve, or the 10th cranial nerve, brings taste information from the throat, epiglottis, and esophagus and can mediate the reflex of swallowing or gagging (Simon et al., 2006). Different tastes are appreciated by differing chemical reactions within the receptor cells. Dysgeusia results from a disruption in this process.

History

Taste is important in distinguishing safe from harmful foods and can trigger an acceptance reflex, swallowing, or an avoidance reflex, gagging. In ancient days important people had personal tasters to try their food first to avoid being poisoned. It is reported that current world leaders may have food tasters as part of their staff for similar reasons. In recent years, scientists have debunked the "taste map" myth that there are very specific areas of the tongue dedicated to each taste.

Tests

In order to test taste, the tongue should be moist. The nerves that convey taste should be tested on each side of the front and back of the tongue with the tongue protruded. The taste can be applied with a moistened cotton-tip applicator. Using a taste questionnaire can be helpful as those who state easily tasting saltiness, bitterness, sourness, and sweetness almost certainly do not have dysgeusia (Malaty & Malaty, 2013).

The majority of those complaining of taste problems are found to have smell loss instead (Cowart, 2011). Because the sense of smell is strongly linked with the perception of taste, the olfactory (smell) system should be investigated by examining smell sensation in each nostril of the person with dysgeusia. Viewing the nasal system through a special scope can help diagnose some conditions. The physician may need computerized tomography scanning of the nose and sinuses for diagnosis.

Significance

The sense of taste helps us to avoid harmful or spoiled food. Loss of taste may lead to decreased appetite, weight loss, and failure to thrive. Normally, women have better taste perception than men, and taste lessens with aging.

Dysgeusia is almost always due to loss of smell sensation resulting from diseases of the nose or sinuses, head injury, or certain neurological diseases. Dysgeusia may be caused by poor mouth hygiene or inflammation, surgery of the middle ear or dental surgery, radiation therapy to head and neck, vitamin deficiencies (copper, zinc, B_{12}, or niacin) or malnutrition, medications, head trauma, toxins, and chronic medical conditions (Malaty & Malaty, 2013).

Treatment

The treatment is to carefully examine and identify the cause of distorted taste and eliminate or treat it. Determine whether distorted taste is due to nasal or mouth disease and address the underlying problem. If applicable, limit exposures to smoke or chemicals that may affect olfaction. If dysgeusia is from a new medication, stopping medication should result in gradual return of taste. This is true for chemotherapy exposure as well since taste receptors renew themselves about every 10 days.

The prognosis of dysgeusia depends on the severity of the loss and other factors. It is reported that one-third to one-half of individuals report a returning sense of smell over time (Malaty & Malaty, 2013). If dysgeusia persists, the person should be referred to a specialist, specifically an ear, nose, and throat doctor.

Lauren C. Seeberger

See also: Ageusia; Bitter Sensation; Salty Sensation; Sour Sensation; Sweet Sensation; Taste Aversion; Taste System; Umami

Further Reading

Cowart, Beverly J. (2011). Taste dysfunction: A practical guide for oral medicine. *Oral Diseases, 17,* 2–6.

Malaty, John, & Irene A. C. Malaty. (2013). Smell and taste disorders in primary care. *American Family Physician, 88*(12), 852–859.

Simon, Sidney A., Ivan E. de Araujo, Ranier Gutierrez, & Miguel A. L. Nicolelis. (2006). The neural mechanisms of gustation: A distributed processing code. *Nature Reviews Neuroscience, 7,* 890–901.

DYSOSMIA

Dysosmia is a distortion or alteration of the perception of smell. It is considered a qualitative olfactory disorder because there is no measurable change in the ability to smell, but rather a change in how smells are perceived. Dysosmia can affect both nostrils at the same time or either nostril on its own (Kühn et al., 2013). Dysosmia can be characterized as either parosmia or phantosmia. Parosmia is when the brain misinterprets the natural smell of an odorant, and the smell is different from what a person remembers. This is considered an olfactory illusion and is more specifically characterized as cacosmia when natural odors are perceived as unpleasant aromas. Phantosmia is the perception of smell in the absence of any physical odorant and is considered to be an olfactory hallucination when the smell lasts only a few seconds.

Causes and Associations

Dysosmia is often considered to be a neurological disorder and other clinical associations have been made. Many cases have been associated with upper respiratory tract infections (URTIs) and nasal and paranasal sinus disease, like chronic rhinosinusitis. Dysosmia is also commonly associated with head trauma following an accident. Other clinical associations of dysosmia include toxic chemical exposure, nasal surgery, epilepsy, tumors on the frontal lobe or olfactory bulb, and neurological abnormalities (Nordin et al., 2011). Dysosmia has also been utilized to indicate the onset of neurodegenerative disorders such as Alzheimer's and Parkinson's diseases. Dysosmia in cases of neurodegenerative disorders presents itself about 20 years before other classic symptoms appear (Nordin et al., 2011). Smell disturbance with dysosmia is often associated with taste disturbance. People who suffer from smell and taste disturbance often have decreased food enjoyment, which results in significant weight loss and an impaired quality of life often leading to depression. Adverse effects of impaired life quality include deterioration of work life, sexual life, and social interactions (Nordin et al., 2011).

Etiology

The causes of dysosmia are unclear but there are both peripheral and central theories behind the etiology of dysosmia (Leopold, 2002). In parosmia, the peripheral theory explains that the distortion is likely due to a number of olfactory primary neurons not functioning to create a complete characterization of an odorant. The central theory describes parosmia as a result of interpretive centers of the brain forming a distorted odor. Peripherally, phantosmia is theorized to be caused by primary olfactory neurons emitting abnormal signals to the brain, or due to the loss of inhibitory cells that are typically present in normal functioning. Phantosmia is explained centrally as hyperfunctioning cells in the brain generating the perception of odor.

Diagnosis and Tests

Diagnosing dysosmia requires taking an extensive medical history. A history will reveal past respiratory infection or head trauma, which is usually precedent to parosmia. On the other hand, cases of phantosmia typically occur spontaneously without a history of such events and are then considered idiopathic. Patients often have a difficult time distinguishing whether they have a taste or smell problem (Leopold, 2002). Physicians must identify whether the smell distortion is present when patients inhale an odorant (parosmia) or if an odor is present in the absence of a stimulus (phantosmia). A complete ear, nose, and throat (ENT) examination is important in observing nerves, nasal mucosa, and airways for obstructions and infections. Also, brain imaging should be used to rule out tumors.

Treatment

Dysosmia is typically found in elderly people and symptoms tend to go away on their own. Waiting and watching is an appropriate treatment plan for dysosmia. However, if an individual is unwilling or unable to tolerate the olfactory distortions, there are medical and surgical treatments. Medical treatments include various types of nasal drops such as saline, Oxymetazoline HCl, and topical cocaine HCl, each with various advantages and side effects to consider (Leopold, 2002). There are surgical procedures to remove or excise olfactory bulbs, neurons, and olfactory epithelium in an attempt to eliminate phantosmia with the possibility of removing olfactory ability completely.

Darin T. Sisneros

See also: Anosmia; Odor Threshold; Olfactory Bulb; Olfactory Mucosa; Olfactory Nerve; Olfactory Sensory Neurons; Olfactory System; Phantosmia

Further Reading

Kühn, M., N. Abolmaali, M. Smitka, D. Podlesek, & T. Hummel. (2013). Dysosmia: Current aspects of diagnostics and therapy. *HNO, 61*(11), 975–984.

Leopold, Donald. (2002). Distortion of olfactory perception: Diagnosis and treatment. *Chemical Senses*, 27, 611–615.

Nordin, Steven, Ebba H. Blomqvist, Petter Olsson, Päär Stjäärne, & Anders Ehnhage. (2011). Effects of smell loss on daily life and adopted coping strategies in patients with nasal polyposis with asthma. *Acta Oto-Laryngologica, 131*(8), 826–832.

EAR PROTECTION

People participating in a variety of activities need ear protection. The NIDCD (National Institute on Deafness and Other Communication Disorders) estimates that 15 percent of Americans between ages 20 and 69 have hearing loss caused by loud noises (NIDCD, 2014). Ear protection prevents this hearing loss. Additionally, ear protection keeps water out of the ear canal during water sports. Ear protection is important because ear damage is preventable, and once damage occurs it may be irreversible.

Loud Noise Damages Hearing

Sound waves enter the outer ear and travel to the eardrum, causing the eardrum to vibrate. Small bones transfer vibrations to the cochlea. The vibrations in the cochlea are detected by specialized hair cells. The hair cells transmit information via the auditory nerve to the brain. Hair cells are fragile and can be damaged by loud noise. Hair cells in humans cannot regenerate, making hearing loss irreparable and irreversible.

The process of hair cell damage from noise exposure can be slow and progressive, or it can happen quickly after exposure to a loud noise. Understanding which noises pose a risk to hearing helps individuals select appropriate ear protection.

Sound is measured in units called decibels (dB). Sounds measuring less than 75 dB do not pose a risk to hearing, whereas sounds at or above 85 dB cause hearing loss. Normal conversations measure 60 dB, whereas a power mower measures 90 dB. A sound at 100 dB damages hearing within 15 minutes. Concert speakers generate sounds as high as 110 dB, damaging hearing within one minute. Similarly, stereo headphones can be as loud as 105 dB, damaging hearing within minutes. Discharges from firearms and explosions from firecrackers near 150 dB; thus ear protection is required.

Types of Ear Protection for Noise Reduction

In the United States, ear protection carries a noise reduction rating (NRR), indicating the decibel reduction provided. Wearing two types of hearing protection, such as earplugs and earmuffs, does not offer an additive advantage and only provides a few more decibels reduction than the higher NRR value.

Earplugs are available in foam, silicone, flanged, and custom molded styles. Foam earplugs are compressed and placed in the ear canal. These earplugs are used in manufacturing and construction, providing NRR values from 20 to 35 dB. Silicone earplugs are moldable, covering the external ear canal, providing NRR values from 20 to 25 dB. Flanged earplugs provide less sound distortion and have variable NRR, often around 20 dB. Some flanged earplugs offer a cap, allowing the user to hear without removing the earplugs. Custom molded earplugs may be vented for communication, may have filters allowing less sound distortion, or may contain electronics to block loud sounds and amplify soft sounds.

Earmuffs, which fit over the external ear, are used for a variety of activities including shooting and construction. Earmuffs are available with a range of NRR. Advantages of earmuffs include comfort and the ability to wear hearing aids. Disadvantages of earmuffs include bulk and difficulty getting a proper seal around hair and eyeglasses. Earmuffs passively block damaging sound waves. Electronic earmuffs have circuits that allow amplification of sound in addition to protection against loud sounds. Earmuffs can also be purchased with built-in speakers to play music.

Although some forms of hearing protection play music, headphones available with music players are not ear protection. Frequent exposure to sounds exceeding 85 dB causes long-term hearing loss. Many people listen to music players at higher levels.

Water Sports Damage Ears

Water sports pose risks for different types of ear damage; all types of ear damage can cause hearing loss. Surfer's ear, caused by repeated exposure to cold water and wind, causes bony growths in the ear canal. Swimmer's ear is an outer ear infection resulting from water exposure. Water can cause infection in people with exposed middle ears due to eardrum perforation or tube placement.

Different types of ear protection are available for water sports. Surfers need protection to keep the ear warm and dry. Swimmers who have had ear infections use earplugs to keep water out, as do people with exposed middle ears. Chisholm, Kuchai, and McPartlin (2004) found that petroleum jelly and a cotton ball kept the ear as dry as commercially available earplugs.

Effectiveness of Ear Protection

Some hearing loss caused by damage from water sports is irreversible and all hearing noise–induced hearing loss is irreversible, highlighting the importance of ear protection. With proper ear protection, hearing loss is preventable.

Lisa A. Rabe

See also: Age-Related Hearing Loss; Cochlea; Deafness; Sensory Receptors; Tinnitus

Further Reading

Chisholm, Edward J., R. Kuchai, & D. McPartlin. (2004). An objective evaluation of the waterproofing qualities, ease of insertion and comfort of commonly available earplugs. *Clinical Otolaryngology and Allied Sciences, 29*(2), 128–132. http://dx.doi.org/10.1111 /j.1365-2273.2004.00795.x. PMID 15113295

National Institute on Deafness and Other Communication Disorders. (2014). *NIDCD fact sheet: Noise-induced hearing loss* (NIH Pub. No. 14-4233). Retrieved from http:// www.nidcd.nih.gov/staticresources/health/hearing/NIDCD-Noise-Induced-Hearing -Loss.pdf

EMESIS

Emesis is the medical term for vomiting, the forceful expulsion of the contents of the stomach and upper intestinal tract through the mouth. Nausea, increased sweating, increased heart rate, and increased salivation usually precede emesis. Vomiting is a complex reflex coordinated by a region within the medulla oblongata, a portion of the brainstem. Neural input from receptors around various regions of the body can initiate vomiting (Marieb et al., 2011).

Pathophysiology

Contraction of the abdominal wall causes the lower esophageal sphincter to relax. In turn, this allows the increasing abdominal pressure to push the contents of the stomach up into the esophagus. This is called retching, commonly termed "dry-heaving." Vomiting occurs when the pressure inside the thoracic cavity, or chest cavity, is high enough to push the stomach contents up the esophagus to the mouth (Widmaier et al., 2011). Vomiting is also accompanied by strong contractions of the upper intestinal tract, which can push the intestinal contents up into the stomach to be expelled with the contents of the stomach. When this occurs bile from the upper intestinal tract can sometimes be seen, discoloring the vomit a greenish hue.

Causes of Emesis

There are a variety of causes of emesis and their frequency ranges from occasional to prolonged, repetitive events that can lead to detrimental health effects. These can involve many different regions of the body as a response to receptors encountering a stimulus that makes them initiate the vomiting reflex. The following are common initiators of the vomiting reflex:

- Distension of the stomach due to overeating, for example, is tracked by mechanoreceptors that measure the stretching of the stomach. This falls into a category of many gastrointestinal causes. Some others are inflammation of related organs, such as the pancreas and appendix.

- Chemoreceptors in the brain and digestive tract react to certain substances, such as poisons and vomit-stimulating chemicals (called emetics), to initiate vomiting in an effort to expel possibly harmful substances from the body.
- Sensory stimuli such as intense pain, rotating movement of the head that affects the sense equilibrium (motion sickness), or pressure increased in the skull or applied to the back of the throat, initiate the so-called "gag reflex" (Widmaier et al., 2011). There are conditions involving the brain that can stimulate emesis. These include concussions, brain tumors, and even migraines.
- Reactions to food allergens or drugs such as alcohol, opioids, and those used in chemotherapy can cause emesis.
- Diseases or pathogens that cause inflammation of organs related to the gastrointestinal tract as mentioned above can usually cause illnesses, such as the "stomach flu."
- Pregnancy can also stimulate emesis. The common form of nausea and vomiting is morning sickness, but there is a rare complication related to pregnancy called hyperemesis, which is a more persistent state of nausea, vomiting, and dehydration. This has an unknown cause, but it is speculated that the hormonal changes related to pregnancy are a possible factor in developing this condition (Cole, 2010).

Complications

There are many complications that arise from vomiting, usually after prolonged or excessive occurrences. Dehydration and electrolyte imbalance is one of the more common complications. This is the excess loss of water and salts that can produce circulatory and metabolic problems.

Aspiration of vomit occurs when the stomach contents enter the respiratory tract. This can lead to choking and possible asphyxiation (low levels of oxygen due to inability to breathe properly) or infection and inflammation of the lungs and bronchioles (known broadly as bronchopneumonia).

Oral health may be affected due to the high acidity of stomach contents coming into contact with the gums and teeth. Tooth enamel can be broken down over time if vomiting is excessive, which is commonly seen in those with bulimia, a condition in which a person is compelled to vomit regularly due to poor self-body image.

Prevention and Treatment

In the prevention and treatment of vomiting, substances known as anti-emetics are effective against vomiting and nausea. They are often prescribed for those who experience motion sickness, morning sickness, and the vomiting/nausea side effects to chemotherapy drugs as well as opioid general pain relievers.

Eric B. Moore

See also: Bitter Sensation; Nociception; Olfactory System; Pregnancy and Sense of Smell; Taste System

Further Reading

Cole, Laurence A. (2010). Biological functions of hCG and hCG-related molecules. *Reproductive Biology and Endocrinology, 8,* 102. http://dx.doi.org/10.1186/1477-7827 -8-102

Marieb, Elaine N., Patricia B. Wilhelm, & Jon Mallatt. (2011). *Human anatomy* (6th ed.). San Francisco, CA: Pearson Benjamin Cummings.

Widmaier, Eric P., Hershel Raff, & Kevin T. Strang. (2011). *Vander's Human Physiology: The Mechanisms of Body Function* (12th ed.). New York, NY: McGraw-Hill.

ENTORHINAL CORTEX

The entorhinal cortex (EC), where "ento" means interior and "rhino" means nose, is an area of the brain that is located in the medial temporal lobe and functions as a hub in a widespread network for memory and navigation (the sense of direction). This is the main interface between the hippocampus and neocortex. The EC-hippocampus system plays a role in declarative memories including but not limited to memory formation, memory consolidation, and memory optimization during sleep. The EC stretches dorsolaterally and is located at the rostral (closer to the nose) end of the temporal lobe. Divided into medial and lateral regions, there are three bands that each have their own distinct properties and connectivity that run perpendicular across the whole area.

History

Brodmann areas were originally described by German anatomist Korbinian Brodmann (1868–1918). He became interested in neuroscience due to the influence of Alois Alzheimer (1864–1915), another German scientist after whom Alzheimer's disease is named. Brodmann used a histological method known as the Nissl staining method to examine the structure and organization of cells in different regions of the brain. Brodmann applied this stain to very thin sections of brain specimens that he had acquired. This allowed him to visualize the structure and organization of cells, which is often referred to as their cytoarchitecture. Brodmann published his original cortical maps in 1909 and described the layout of the brains of humans, monkeys, and other organisms. Though Brodmann's original cortical maps labeled 52 individual areas, several of them are found only in nonhuman primates and thus there are fewer areas in the human brain.

The EC is also named Brodmann area 28. Interest in this area arose around the turn of the 19th century when Santiago Ramón y Cajal (1852–1934) described a peculiar part of the posterior temporal cortex, which was strongly connected to the hippocampal formation. Ramon y Cajal suggested that the physiological significance of the latter structure would relate to that of the EC. He assumed that the EC was part of the olfactory system; however, in the late 1950s, Scoville and Milner speculated that the hippocampus was a main player in conscious memory processes in humans. Now, it is well accepted that the EC is part of a strongly interconnected set of cortical areas that together form the parahippocampal region, which is closely related to the hippocampal formation.

Diseases

The EC is normally the first area affected by Alzheimer's disease, which accounts for 60–70 percent of all cases of dementia. Alzheimer's is a chronic neurodegenerative disease that typically starts slowly and worsens over time. A recent study by López and colleagues (2014) showed there are differences in the volume of the left EC between patients with progressing and stable mild cognitive impairment. They also found the volume inversely correlates with the level of alpha band phase synchronization between the right anterior cingulate and temporo-occipital regions.

The EC is also associated with temporal lobe epilepsy and schizophrenia. In epilepsy, layer III of the EC shows degeneration, while in schizophrenia the EC has a general miswiring and decreased volume. In 2012, Suthana and collaborators implanted intracranial depth electrodes in seven epileptic patients to identify seizure-onset zones for subsequent epilepsy surgery. All subjects completed a spatial learning task during which they learned destinations within virtual environments. The researchers found that when entorhinal stimulation was applied while the subjects learned locations of landmarks, their subsequent memory of these locations was enhanced and they reached these landmarks more quickly and by shorter routes. They also found that direct hippocampal stimulation was not effective. Suthana et al. (2012) concluded that stimulation of the EC enhanced memory of spatial information when applied during learning.

Renee Johnson

See also: Cerebral Cortex; Limbic System; Seizures

Further Reading

Hafting, Torkel, Marianne Fyhn, Sturla Molden, May-Britt Moser, & Edvard I. Moser. (2005). Microstructure of a spatial map in the entorhinal cortex. *Nature, 436,* 801–806.

López, María Eugenía, Ricardo Bruña, Sara Aurtenetxe, José Ángel Pineda-Pardo, Alberto Marcos, Juan Arrazola, . . . Fernando Maestú. (2014). Alpha-band hypersynchronization in progressive mild cognitive impairment: A magnetoencephalography study *Journal of Neuroscience, 34*(44), 14551–14559. Retrieved from http://www.jneurosci.org/content/34/44/14551

Suthana, Nanthia, Zulfi Haneef, John Stern, Roy Mukamel, Eric Behnke, Barbara Knowlton, & Itzhak Fried. (2012). Memory enhancement and deep-brain stimulation of the entorhinal area. *New England Journal of Medicine, 366,* 502–510. Retrieved from http ://www.nejm.org/doi/full/10.1056/NEJMoa1107212

EPINEPHRINE: *See* Adrenaline

EXCITATION

In the nervous system, neurons communicate with one another by nerve impulses or action potentials. The result is an excitatory or inhibitory response in the receiving neuron. This process is generally called excitation (excitatory circuits) or inhibition (inhibitory circuits). The normal brain is constantly balancing between excitation and inhibition as too much of one state can cause abnormal neurological activity. For instance, too much excitation can cause seizure-like activity while too much inhibition can make a person feel "hung-over" or lethargic.

For most adult neurons, excitation "turns on" a cell and inhibition "turns off" a cell. Both are very important for normal brain function. Excitation is like gasoline for a car, which allows it to turn on and move. On the other hand, inhibition is like the brakes for a vehicle. For example, a person driving a car who needs to turn must apply the brakes to navigate safely through the turn. However, if the brakes fail prior to the turn, the driver is unable to slow down to the proper speed, which results in a car accident. The case within a brain is similar. If inhibition is compromised, it can result in neurons or circuits not being turned off, which may result in seizures or seizure-like activity.

Anatomy and Physiology

Neurons consist of a cell body, several dendrites, and a single axon. The axon terminates at its target and may have collateral branches to reach additional targets. The target is usually another neuron, muscle cell, or organ. In general, action potentials are discrete electrical signals that are transmitted along the length of axons and propagate information within the nervous system. Specifically, these signals are generated as a result of a transient change in membrane permeability: from a state where it is more permeable to potassium (K^+) than sodium (Na^+), to a reversal of these permeability properties. During the action potential, a flow of Na^+ into the neuron is responsible for rapid depolarization and a flow of K^+ out of the neuron causes repolarization or hyperpolarization. These changes in membrane permeability are due to the opening and closing of voltage-gated ion channels. The speed at which the action potentials are conducted is based on the radius of the axon, the presence of a myelin sheath, and the number of ion channels.

As the action potential propagates to the terminal end of the axon, it reaches the synaptic cleft, a small space between the two neurons. The presynaptic neuron releases a neurotransmitter into this space and the postsynaptic neuron receives the chemical. This action results in a voltage change across the postsynaptic neuron's membrane. Specifically, postsynaptic potentials (PSPs) represent graded voltage changes in the electrical membrane potential of the postsynaptic neuron in a chemical synapse. If the neurotransmitter is an excitatory chemical, like glutamate, NMDA (N-methyl-D-aspartate), or AMPA (α-Amino-3-hydroxy-5-methyl-4-isoxazolepropionic acid), it results in an excitatory postsynaptic potential (EPSP). This is the opposite response of an inhibitory postsynaptic potential (IPSP), which is induced by inhibitory chemicals such as GABA (gamma-amino butyric acid) and glycine. When multiple EPSPs arrive at a postsynaptic membrane relatively closely together, they will summate their amplitudes and produce a larger EPSP. If the newly combined EPSP is large enough, it may increase the membrane's potential to produce an action potential.

In neurophysiology experiments where the circuitry of the brain is being tested, neuroscientists often refer to the PSP of the "field" or an fPSP. In general, this is an extracellular recording of all neurons within a local circuit that are firing nearly at the same time. Since a single neuron's action potential is too small to be recorded by an extracellular electrode, the population of the neurons within a small distance of the electrode's tip can be measured. Thus, an fPSP is the aggregate of all regional neurons firing action potentials near the extracellular electrode. This is recorded as excitation in the brain.

Jennifer L. Hellier

See also: Axon; Inhibition; Membrane Potential: Depolarization and Hyperpolarization

Further Reading

Baylor, Stephen M., & Stephen Hollingworth. (2012). Intracellular calcium movements during excitation-contraction coupling in mammalian slow-twitch and fast-twitch muscle fibers. *Journal of General Physiology, 139*(4), 261–272.

Fry, Chris H., & Rita I. Jabr. (2010). The action potential and nervous conduction. *Surgery (Oxford), 28*(2), 49–54.

Hellier, Jennifer L., & F. Edward Dudek. (2005). Chemoconvulsant model of chronic spontaneous seizures. *Current Protocols in Neuroscience,* Chapter 9: Unit 9.19.

Purves, Dale, George J. Augustine, David Fitzpatrick, William C. Hall, Anthony-Samuel LaMantia, James O. McNamara, & Leonard E. White. (2008). *Neuroscience* (4th ed.). Sunderland, MA: Sinauer Associates.

EXTEROCEPTION

Exteroception is the awareness of the body relative to the external environment. This includes information about its position in space (proprioception), the five main senses (auditory, visual, gustatory, olfactory, and somatosensory), pain (nociception), temperature (thermoception), and balance (equilibrioception). Counter to exteroception is interoception, which is responsible for visceral sensory information. Exteroception is incredibly important to survival as it is what allows humans to interact with their environment.

Audition

The auditory system is responsible for hearing and translates vibrations into sound. This occurs when vibrations hit the hair-like cilia within the ear and is amplified as it travels from the outer ear to the inner ear. Once there it interacts with the eardrum and is translated into an electrochemical signal and carried by the auditory nerve to the primary auditory cortex in the cerebral cortex. Errors in the auditory system result in partial or complete deafness.

Vision

Vision is created when light hits the rods and cones that reside within the retina in the eye. These rods and cones pick up different frequencies of light and send the information to the brain via the optic nerve. This information is processed as color and patterns in the thalamus. Once there it is integrated into a comprehensive image. Visual system errors can result in partial or complete blindness as well as poor vision either close or far.

Gustation

Taste is conveyed by the gustatory system to the brain. Taste cell receptors on the tongue reside in the taste buds and convey information about the five main tastes: sour, sweet, salty, bitter, and umami. The signal for each taste is triggered differently and these signals are conveyed to the brain via two different nerves—the glossopharyngeal nerve and the facial nerve—depending on what region of the tongue the receptor is coming from. Tastes help individuals determine what is and is not suitable to eat. For example, bitterness indicates highly alkaline food, which often can be harmful or poisonous to the consumer. Additionally, sweet is an indicator of a high carbohydrate content, which is a very useful source of energy for most individuals.

Olfaction

The olfactory system is responsible for a sense of smell. Signals are conveyed by free nerve endings (cilia) within the nostril that convert chemical odorants into electrical signals that can be transduced to the brain. The trigeminal nerve conveys the information back to the olfactory bulb where the signal then proceeds to the olfactory cortex via the olfactory tract. Errors in the olfactory system can result in partial or complete loss of smell (anosmia), distorted smell (dysosmia), and phantom smells (phantosmia).

Somatosensation

Touch is relayed through the somatosensory system. There are four main types of sensory receptors for touch: Meissner's corpuscles (respond to moderate vibration and light touch), Pacinian corpuscles (respond to high vibrations and gross touch), Merkel nerve endings (respond to low vibrations and sustained touch), and Ruffini corpuscles (respond to sustained skin stretch—which helps maintain the pressure needed to hold objects). Information from these receptors is conveyed to the brain and mapped to the cortex based on the region it comes from. This mapping is called a homunculus. The somatosensory system also conveys information about temperature, pain, and contact with chemicals.

Nociception

Nociception is the sensory system responsible for pain. "Free" nerve endings respond to noxious stimuli such as excessive heat, excessive cold, and some chemicals. The signals produced by these stimuli are conveyed down the spinothalamic pathway and the trigeminal pathway to the brain depending on the location of the stimuli. Both pathways have synapses at many levels along the spinal cord, brainstem, and cerebral cortex, allowing for both a fast and slow response to the stimulus. The synapses within the spinal cord and brainstem are why you pull your hand away from a hot stove before your brain realizes it was hot.

Thermoception

Thermoception is achieved by thermoreceptors that are nonspecific and react to relative changes. In humans there are two main types of thermoreceptors: those that respond to decreases in temperature (cold receptors) and those that respond to increases in temperature (heat receptors). The information picked up by these receptors is sent to the thalamus. Receptors for temperature are located in the skin, cornea, and urinary bladder.

Equilibrioception

Balance is conveyed by equilibrioception and is a complex integration of information from three other sensory systems: visual, proprioceptive, and vestibular. The vestibular system consists of specialized organs within the inner ear: the utricle, the saccule, and three semicircular canals. These organs provide information about vertical position (which way is down), linear movement, and rotational movement. Each of the organs is filled with fluid and it is the motion of the fluid that provides information. Information from the vestibular system is conveyed via the vestibulocochlear nerve to the brain.

Riannon C. Atwater

See also: Auditory System; Balance; Interoception; Nociception; Olfactory System; Proprioception; Somatosensory System; Taste System; Thermoreceptors; Visual System

Further Reading

Purves, Dale, George J. Augustine, David Fitzpatrick, William C. Hall, Anthony-Samuel LaMantia, James O. McNamara, & Leonard E. White. (2008). *Neuroscience* (4th ed.). Sunderland, MA: Sinauer Associates.

EYE PROTECTION

Protecting the eyes is essential to maintaining a healthy visual system. The eyes are the receptive organs for sight, and damage to them can cause severe vision loss and/ or permanent blindness. Several daily activities both in work environments and in leisure events can increase the risk of eye injuries. Threats that may cause eye injuries include but are not limited to (1) particles (e.g., dust or insects) in the air or water, (2) light from the sun or lasers, (3) explosive chemical reactions, (4) working at a construction site, (5) sports equipment (e.g., ball, Frisbee, etc.), and (6) pellets/ bullets shot from a firearm (CO_2 gun, paintball gun, or a regular handgun). Wearing adequate eye protection devices can prevent most eye injuries. Today, there are many different types of eye protection that have different attributes in order to provide maximum protection depending on the activity. For best results, consult the regulations of the industry you are working in to help you determine the correct eye protective gear to wear.

Types of Eye Protection

There are three main groups of eye protection: (1) glasses—such as safety glasses, sunglasses, welding glasses, and solar eclipse glasses; (2) goggles—such as general safety goggles, swim goggles, and lab goggles; and (3) shields—mainly face shields including the gold-impregnated face shield of a spacesuit, blood-splatter face shields for use in the medical and dental fields, and facemasks on a football, hockey, or baseball helmet.

Glasses are devices that have plastic lenses (not glass) that cover the front of the eyes. The lenses are held in place by a frame that wraps around the ears. Glasses are best worn if the threat to the eye comes only from the front, as the lenses do not wrap around to the peripheral vision. If the lenses are tinted or darkened, they are used to protect the eyes from sunlight. However, most safety glasses have a clear lens so that visual acuity is not affected. When determining the best type of safety glasses, the strength and the heat protection of the lenses should be noted, particularly if you will be working with explosive devices that can produce heat and/or shrapnel. Studies have shown that attractively designed safety glasses are more likely to be worn than if they are not considered attractive. As the goal is to wear the safety glasses, purchase glasses that you like so that you will wear them (Eppig et al., 2014).

Goggles are similar to glasses, but the main differences are that (1) the lenses will also cover the peripheral portions of the face, and (2) the frame is held onto the head by an elastic band. Thus, the lens wraps around toward the temples and the frame makes a seal with the face. Swim goggles are intended to have strong suction so that the seal around the eyes is tight and resistant to water leakage. In science laboratories, particularly chemistry labs, goggles are necessary as chemical explosions may occur. These goggles may or may not have small holes surrounding the lenses to allow the goggles to "breathe" and not fog up.

Face shields are a type of eye protection that also protects the nasal and oral openings. This provides more complete coverage when hazardous activities are being performed, protecting against potential blood splatter from medical emergencies, severe chemical reactions from welding, or contact with the face from the ball or puck when playing sports. Face shields used in the medical field are made of plastic that wraps around the entire face and may be flipped up and down, like a visor. The bottom of the visor is open to the air so that the face shield does not fog up. Face shields used for welding must be heat resistant and provide protection from the bright light. Finally, in sports, face shields are designed to also protect the bones of the face.

Jennifer L. Hellier

See also: Blindness; Retina; Visual Fields; Visual System

Further Reading

Eppig, T., A. Speck, B. Zelzer, & A. Langenbucher. (2014). [Protective glasses. Personal eye protection for professional use]. [Article in German]. *Der Ophthalmologe: Zeitschrift der Deutschen Ophthalmologischen Gesellschaft, 111*(7), 681–690. http://dx.doi.org/10.1007/s00347-014-3094-0

Lee, Rachel, & Douglas Fredrick. (2015). Pediatric eye injuries due to nonpowder guns in the United States, 2002–2012. *Journal of AAPOS: American Association for Pediatric Ophthalmology and Strabismus, 19*(2), 163–168.e1. http://dx.doi.org/10.1016/j.jaapos.2015.01.010

Rosen, Edward. (1956). The invention of eyeglasses. *Journal of the History of Medicine and Allied Sciences, 11,* 13–46 (part 1), 183–218 (part 2).

EYE-HAND COORDINATION: *See* Visual Motor System

EYESIGHT: *See* Visual System

F

FACIAL NERVE

The facial nerve is the seventh of 12 paired cranial nerves. Thus it is also called cranial nerve VII. The facial nerves are mixed nerves, meaning they carry both motor and sensory information to the head and face. Thus, cranial nerve VII is involved with a variety of different functions in the head and face including facial movement and expression, transmission of taste sensation from the tongue, and some parasympathetic innervation to the head—which involves the autonomic nervous system. Specifically, the parasympathetic nerves stimulate the salivary (producing saliva) and lacrimal (producing tears) glands as well as the nasal mucosa. The nerve emerges from the brainstem at the junction of the pons and medulla oblongata. From its points of origin in nuclei in the pons, cranial nerve VII splits into two divisions: the motor root and the intermediate nerve. The larger motor root innervates many of the muscles in the face, and the smaller intermediate nerve carries taste, somatic sensory fibers, and parasympathetic fibers.

General Functional Components

The facial nerve has four components: branchial motor, visceral motor, general sensory, and special sensory. This entry will focus on the sensory portions of the nerve. The general sensory component brings information to the brain about the ear—particularly the skin near the ear, the wall of the acoustic meatus, and the external tympanic membrane. The special sensory portion brings sensory information to the brain regarding taste from the anterior two-thirds of the tongue as well as from the hard and soft palates of the mouth.

Anatomy and Physiology

Within the skull and inferior to the external ear, the facial nerve passes through an opening in the petrous portion of the temporal bone called the internal acoustic meatus. It travels a short distance, then turns sharply and runs along the wall of the tympanic cavity, where the bones of the middle ear are located. At the point where the nerve turns is the sensory ganglion of the facial nerve called the geniculate ganglion. The term *genu* is a Latin word for "knee" or "bend," thus the geniculate ganglion is L-shaped and houses the neurons involved with motor, sensory, and parasympathetic activities.

The lingual nerve is part of the trigeminal nerve that sends sensory information of the tongue to the central nervous system. It also carries fibers from the facial nerve. Thus, the chorda tympani piggybacks with the lingual nerve on its way to the tongue and conveys taste sensation from the anterior two-thirds of the tongue and soft palate. Finally, parasympathetic innervation of the facial nerve also drops off branches to the sinuses and nasal cavity. A few motor fibers from the facial nerve innervate a small muscle, the stapedius, which stabilizes the stapes (one of the bones used for hearing) in the middle ear.

Clinical Symptoms, Diseases, and Treatments

The facial nerve is one of the most frequently damaged of the cranial nerves, especially during its passage through the temporal bone. Viral infections can cause inflammation and even swelling of the nerve. This may lead to paralysis of several muscles, but in most cases the paralysis disappears after the infection resolves.

Certain infections have been identified as causing acute swelling (inflammation) of the facial nerve such as the varicella-zoster and Epstein-Barr herpes viruses as well as Lyme disease. Reactivation of the latent (dormant) viruses can cause Bell's palsy, particularly during cold weather, emotional stress, or trauma to the face. Bell's palsy has a rapid onset: a person may go to bed without symptoms and wake with partial or complete paralysis. To reduce inflammation, corticosteroids have shown to be effective if provided near the onset of the palsy. Most acute cases of Bell's palsy will recover completely after a month or so, but during the condition patients must protect the affected eye from drying out, as the eyelid will not be able to close.

Jennifer L. Hellier and Robin Michaels

See also: Bell's Palsy; Cranial Nerves; Nerves; Trigeminal Nerve

Further Reading

Liang, Barbara. (2012). *The 12 cranial nerves.* Retrieved from http://www.wisc-online.com/objects/ViewObject.aspx?ID=AP11504

Moore, Keith L., Anne M. R. Agur, & Arthur F. Dalley (Eds.). (2010). *Essential clinical anatomy* (4th ed.). Baltimore, MD: Williams and Wilkins.

Yale University School of Medicine. (1998). *Cranial nerves.* Retrieved from http://www.yale.edu/cnerves/

FAINTING

Fainting (medically known as syncope) is a short loss of consciousness with spontaneous recovery, typically due to inadequate delivery of oxygen or blood to the brain. The collection of symptoms that occurs at the onset of fainting is referred to as "presyncope" and includes lightheadedness, fatigue, muscle weakness, and blurred vision. There are three major classes of syncope: neurally mediated (reflex) syncope, cardiac syncope, and syncope due to orthostatic hypotension (European Society of Cardiology, 2009).

Reflex Syncope

Neurally mediated syncope is fainting as a response to a neural stimulus. Extreme emotion such as stress or fear may cause an individual to faint, as well as exercise, hyperventilation (fast breathing), low blood sugar, and even coughing or sneezing. Reflex syncope takes place when the nervous system cannot initiate an appropriate response to a stimulus and causes a change in heart rate or blood pressure. An individual is in danger of fainting if blood pressure or heart rate is too low to meet the oxygen demands of the brain. An example of this is hyperventilation. When an individual breathes too quickly, there is a dramatic tightening of blood vessels resulting in constricted flow to the brain and fainting occurs. Reflex syncope is the most common form of fainting and may affect healthy individuals. Neurally mediated fainting may happen a single time or be reoccurring.

Cardiac Syncope

Cardiac syncope can result from problems arising in the function or structure of the heart, blood vessels, or lungs. Arrhythmia (irregular heartbeat) is the most common cause of cardiac-related fainting. Certain conditions or medications can cause the heart to beat too quickly (tachycardia), too slowly (bradycardia), or too irregularly to meet the needs of the brain. Cardiac syncope can also be the result of structural defects in the cardiac system, though it is a much rarer cause of fainting.

Syncope Due to Orthostatic Hypotension

Orthostatic hypotension syncope, or postural hypotension, is a condition resulting from a sudden change in posture. When an individual stands up quickly, blood pooling in the lower body (due to gravity) must be pumped to the brain to maintain consciousness. If vessels fail to move blood from the body to the brain fast enough, blood pressure in the brain drops and the individual may faint. Orthostatic hypotension commonly occurs in individuals with low blood pressure and the elderly, but it has been known to occur in individuals with diabetes or as a side effect of certain pharmaceuticals. The onset of fainting may be slower in some individuals, and presyncope symptoms may allow the individual to intervene before fainting occurs.

Diagnosis

Lack of consciousness is always a cause for concern and, while fainting itself is not particularly dangerous, it may be a symptom of a more serious underlying condition. A doctor will consider a patient's medical history as well as perform a medical examination in order to properly diagnose the cause of fainting. Individuals who faint frequently may experience a reduction in mobility and self-care and an increase in depression and pain (due to injuries). Fainting is particularly hazardous for elderly individuals, as falls are the fifth leading cause of death for older adults (Rubenstein & Josephson, 2002).

Preventive measures for fainting will vary between individuals, but there are a few tactics that health professionals agree on: first, dehydration makes one more liable to faint, so proper hydration is vital. Second, eating regular meals will prevent fainting caused by low blood sugar. Third and most importantly, syncope sufferers need to recognize their own warning signs, as different individuals will experience unique presyncope symptoms (Syncope Trust and Reflex Anoxic Seizures, 2009). This self-awareness can provide an individual with enough warning to prevent an episode or seek help before losing consciousness.

Kendra DeHay

See also: Aura; Baroreceptors; Diplopia; Dizziness; Reflex; Seizures

Further Reading

European Society of Cardiology. (2009). Guidelines for the diagnosis and management of syncope. *European Heart Journal, 30*, 2631–2671. http://dx.doi.org/10.1093/eurheartj/ehp298

Rubenstein, Laurence Z., & Karen R. Josephson. (2002). The epidemiology of falls and syncope. *Clinics in Geriatric Medicine, 18*, 141–158. http://dx.doi.org/10.1016/S0749-0690(02)00002-2

Soteraides, Elpidoforos S., Jane C. Evans, Martin G. Larson, Ming Hui Chen, Leway Chen, Emelia J. Benjamin, & Daniel Levy. (2002). Incidence and prognosis of syncope. *New England Journal of Medicine, 347*(12), 878–885.

Syncope Trust and Reflex Anoxic Seizures (STARS). (2009). Reflex syncope (Vasovagal syncope). Retrieved from http://www.nhs.uk/ipgmedia/national/syncope%20trust%20and%20reflex%20anoxic%20seizures/assets/reflexsyncope(vasovagalsyncope).pdf

FAMILIAL DYSAUTONOMIA

Familial dysautonomia, also called hereditary sensory and autonomic neuropathy, type III and also known as Riley Day syndrome, is a genetic disorder that affects the development and survival of certain nerve cells. It disturbs cells in the autonomic nervous system, which is responsible for things including but not limited to digestion, breathing, tear production, and the regulation of blood pressure and body temperature. Familial dysautonomia also affects the sensory nervous system, particularly those responsible for the sense of taste, the perception of pain, and the perceptions of heat and cold. Thus, persons with familial dysautonomia often have a form of congenital insensitivity to pain. Familial dysautonomia affects about 1 in every 3,700 individuals and is primarily found in central or eastern European Jewish populations. It is extremely rare in the general population.

Familial dysautonomia is an autonomic recessive disease, meaning both copies of the gene in each cell must have the mutation. Parents are called "carriers" for the disorder, as the mother and father carry one copy of the affected gene. Carriers typically do not have any of the signs of the disease. As of now, the average life expectancy for an individual with familial dysautonomia is age 20, with about 60 percent of the population with the disorder surviving to that age.

Signs and Symptoms

The first signs and symptoms of familial dysautonomia are most often seen within the first few months of birth. Early signs and symptoms include but are not limited to feeding difficulties, poor growth, lack of tear production, and difficulty maintaining body temperature. Older infants are likely to hold their breath for prolonged periods of time, causing a bluish appearance of the skin (cyanosis) or fainting. This behavior will typically stop by the age of six years old. Normal developmental milestones are usually delayed; however, some children with familial dysautonomia may develop on time and not show any signs of delay.

In school-aged children, symptoms may include bed-wetting, poor balance, and poor bone quality. Additionally these children may have kidney and heart problems. They could experience orthostatic hypotension—which is a drop in blood pressure upon standing—and could have episodes of high blood pressure when they get nervous or excited. About 33 percent of children with familial dysautonomia experience learning disabilities, such as having a short attention span.

By adulthood, most symptoms of familiar dysautonomia have been overcome except for balance and walking difficulties. Thus, adults may need assistance for balance and/or walking. As a person with familiar dyautonomia ages, he or she may experience frequent lung infections and worsening of vision because the optic nerves shrink.

Treatment and Management

As of today, there is no cure for familial dysautonomia. The only treatment is supportive and preventive care. These treatments include but are not limited to medications to maintain the cardiovascular, respiratory, and digestive functions, and surgical interventions such as (1) placing a gastrostomy feeding tube into the stomach to reduce aspiration of food, which can cause lung infections; (2) fusing spinal vertebrae together to provide more stability for the person when walking; and (3) cauterizing the tear ducts so that the tears produced by the eye stay on the eye longer and do not drain away. Finally, persons with familial dyautonomia may have therapy to help with speech development.

Research

At the Dysautonomia Center at the New York University School of Medicine, there is a state of the art clinical research lab that is fully equipped to perform neurophysiological tests of sensory and autonomic nerve functions. The Dysautonomia Foundation funds this center as it is the only treatment and clinical research center in the world. Past clinical research has led to the development of new treatments, which have altered the prognosis of the disease as well as enhanced the quality of life for individuals with the disease. Started in 1990, genetic research focused on identifying the familial dysautonomia gene with a goal of developing a treatment and cure. Trials using kinetin are currently under way at the Dysautonomia Center in patients with familial dysautonomia thanks to the research of Drs. James Gusella and Susan Slaugenhaupt when they identified the gene with the mutation in 2001.

Renee Johnson

See also: Autonomic Nervous System; Congenital Insensitivity to Pain; Somatosensory System

Further Reading

Dysautonomia Foundation. (n.d.). Dysautonomia Foundation Research. Retrieved from http://www.familialdysautonomia.org/facts.htm
Dysautonomia Foundation. (n.d.). FD Fact Sheet. Retrieved from http://www.familialdysautonomia.org/facts.htm
Palma, Jose-Alberto, Lucy Norcliffe-Kaufmann, Cristina Fuente-Mora, Leila Percival, Carlos Mendoza-Santiesteban, & Horacio Kaufmann. (2014). Current treatments in familial dysautonomia. *Expert Opinion on Pharmacotherapy, 15*(18), 2653–2671. http://dx.doi.org/10.1517/14656566.2014.970530.

FARSIGHTEDNESS: *See* Hyperopia

FOVEA CENTRALIS

The fovea centralis is a very specialized section of the retina, which is the photosensitive lining of the eye. Based on its name, it is located in the center of the retina and has a pit shape. It is an avascular region of the retina and is responsible for the central vision of each eye. Lastly, the fovea centralis contains the highest number of cones—light-sensitive receptors that are responsible for the ability to see colors—within its region compared to the rest of the retina.

Anatomy and Physiology

The visual system's external organ is the eye, and light entering the eye begins the process of sight. The eye is a complex organ that acts like a camera as it uses the laws of optics, which are based in physics. The eye uses light from an external object to focus an image onto its photoreceptors—rod and cone cells. These photoreceptors are found at the posterior portion of the eye in the retina. To help focus the light and project the image, the eye will refract the incoming light first through the cornea. The light then passes through the pupil and is refracted again via the lens. Together, the cornea and the lens act like a compound lens to project the image upside down onto the retina.

The definition of central vision or the central visual field is the central 10 degrees of a visual angle. Basically, it is the visual field that is seen when a person is looking straight ahead and does not move the eyes. For mapping images to the retina, scientists have measured that 1 degree of a visual angle maps to about 0.3 millimeter (mm) of the retina. Thus, 10 degrees would map to about 3 mm of the central retina or the area within a 1.5 mm radius from the exact center—0 degree eccentricity. This 3 mm region contains the macula, which looks yellow in color under an ophthalmoscope. Within the middle of the macula is where the fovea centralis is located. It is about 1 mm in diameter and forms a depression or pit within the macula. This depression occurs because there are no blood vessels in the fovea centralis. Instead it is densely packed with cone cells and contains the majority of cone cells within the entire retina. The number of cones drastically decreases in number as you move away from the fovea centralis and toward the periphery of the retina.

Macular Degeneration

Cone cells have a faster response time to light stimuli compared to rod cells, thus allowing details of objects to be viewed and/or perceived. Because activation of cone cells is used to identify details of an object, they need plenty of light to be stimulated. In rare cases, cones can be damaged, resulting in a type of cone dystrophy, which is a general term to describe rare disorders that affect cone cells.

Today, macular degeneration is the leading cause of central vision loss and blindness among Americans who are age 65 and older. Symptoms start with center vision becoming blurred and colors may become muted in this region. Over time, gray spots may appear in the central vision.

Jennifer L. Hellier

See also: Blind Spot; Color Blindness; Cones; Hubel, David H.; Retina; Rods; Sensory Receptors; Visual Fields; Visual Perception; Wiesel, Torsten N.

Further Reading

Bear, Mark F., Barry W. Connors, & Michael A. Paradiso. (2007). *Neuroscience exploring the brain* (3rd ed.). Baltimore, MD: Lippincott Williams & Wilkins.

Provis, Jan M., Adam M. Dubis, Ted Maddess, & Joseph Carroll. (2013). Adaptation of the central retina for high acuity vision: Cones, the fovea and the avascular zone. *Progress in Retinal and Eye Research, 35*, 63–81.

FREE NERVE ENDINGS

A sensory receptor is the first component of a sensory system, which is activated by a specific stimulus from the internal or external environment or an organism. Well-known and well-studied sensory receptors include those that detect pressure (mechanoreceptors in the skin), light (photosensitive receptors in the retina), chemicals (chemoreceptors in the nose and tongue), and temperature (thermoreceptors in the skin). Once the receptor is activated it begins sensory transduction, which is a conversion of a sensory stimulus from one form (e.g., chemical) to another (e.g., electrical). Activated sensory receptors create action potentials or graded potentials in the same neuron or in an adjacent cell. Receptors involved in taste and smell have specific receptor molecules that respond and bind to different chemicals. For example, in the olfactory system, odor receptors found in the olfactory sensory neurons are activated by the interaction of molecular structures on the odor molecule. Free nerve endings, however, are commonly used to detect pain and temperature. This is because these sensations need to be sent to the brain quickly so that a reaction can be processed.

Anatomy and Physiology

A free nerve ending is an unspecialized afferent neuron and is used by vertebrates to detect pain or temperatures of the external and internal environments. They have no complex sensory structures and are the most common type of nerve ending found mostly in the skin. Free nerve endings resemble the small roots of plants. They go through the epidermis and end in the stratum granulosum, which is a thin layer of cells in the epidermis. Free nerve endings are classified based on their rate of adaptation, stimulus modalities, and their fiber types.

In the sensation of taste, free nerve endings are used to sense the temperature of the tongue and the food placed in the mouth. These free nerve endings also sense pain that is caused by spicy foods, particularly capsaicin. Capsaicin comes from plants and vegetables that are in the genus *Capsicum*. These plants contain molecules that are collectively called capsaicinoids, which are the molecules responsible for hot (not temperature) and spicy flavors. The only plant in the *Capsicum* genus that does not contain capsaicinoids is *Capsicum annum*, which is also known as the bell pepper. Scientists have been researching capsaicin activation in taste receptors and discovered the transient receptor potential (TRP) vanilloid subfamily member

Spearmint Experiment

Foods and beverages provide calories and nutrients that are essential for humans to survive. There are five basic tastes—bitter, salty, sour, sweet, and umami—that help humans find the foods that their bodies need, particularly those required for nutrition. In general, the bitter sensation detects possibly poisonous foods. Most people will spit out bitter foods, which is a survival mechanism. Salty sensation is important to control salt (NaCl or KCl) balance within the body. Sodium (Na^+), potassium (K^+), and chloride (Cl^-) are necessary chemicals for most cellular functions, such as propagating action potentials in neurons. Similar to salty sensation, sour detection helps maintain acid balance of the body. The sweet sensation helps a person find calorie-rich foods. These are needed when energy is depleted and needs to be replenished quickly. Finally, umami—which is a Japanese word for "savory"—detects protein-rich foods. These are needed to keep muscle health as well as the desire to eat essential amino acids that the human body cannot make.

Spicy and minty foods are often mistaken for additional taste sensations. These, however, are sensations that stimulate pain or temperature receptors on free nerve endings within the mouth. For pain sensations, these nerve endings are stimulated by capsaicin found in spicy food, while menthol—found in mint oils—activates the transient receptor potential cation channel subfamily M member 8 (TRPM8) for temperature sensation.

Materials:

1–2 mint candies (like Tic-Tac®, Lifesavers®, or Altoids®)
1 small paper cup
2 to 4 tablespoons of soda (such as a cola type)

Directions:

Pour the soda into the paper cup. As a control for this experiment, take a sip of the soda to determine its temperature. Next, for about 1 to 2 minutes, chew/dissolve, swish, and coat your mouth with the mint. You want to ensure that the spearmint oils are bound to your free nerve endings, which are located on the tongue, cheeks, and the roof of the mouth. For best results, ensure you take your time with this step. Swallow the chewed candy with your saliva.

Next, purse your lips and suck in. Your mouth should instantly feel very cool or cold. This is because the spearmint oils are stimulating the free nerve endings even though the temperature in your mouth did not significantly drop. Next, drink some of the soda. The spearmint should make the soda feel much colder than it did during the control taste.

Jennifer L. Hellier

1 (TRPV1). It is this receptor that is activated by capsaicin and is part of the super-family of TRP receptors, which sense stimuli from external events.

The Scoville scale measures the "heat" of capsaicin, which has a range of 0 (bell peppers) to 15 million Scoville units (pure capsaicin). In the United States, pepper sprays have a range of 2 to 5.5 million Scoville units. Capsaicin is not water soluble, thus drinking water after eating a hot pepper will not alleviate the pain. Capsaicin is lipid soluble and can be unbound from the TRPV1 receptor by dairy-based products like milk, sour cream, yogurt, or ice cream. This is why many Mexican foods are served with sour cream.

Types of Free Nerve Endings

Free nerve endings can be rapidly adapting, intermediately adapting, or slowly adapting. Rapidly adapting nerve endings react and adapt quickly to a stimulus. This means after a relatively short amount of time, a person will no longer feel the stimulus. These are generally called Meissner's corpuscles. There is no response to continued pressure, unless there is a change in pressure. Conversely, slowly adapting nerve endings react and adapt slowly to a stimulus. Thus, it will take longer for the feeling to go away. These receptor types are also called Ruffini corpuscles. There will continue to be a response to pressure for as long as it is sustained. Intermediate adapting free nerve endings fall somewhere in between.

Free nerve endings are also classified based on the type of modality they can detect. Types of modalities include but are not limited to temperature (thermoreceptors), mechanical stimuli (mechanoreceptors), and pain (nociceptors). Because of this, free nerve endings have polymodality, meaning they can respond to different types of stimuli.

The final classification of free nerve endings is based on their fiber types. The majority of free nerve endings contain (1) A delta fibers, also known as group III fibers, and (2) C-fibers, also known as group IV fibers. A delta fibers are sensory nerve fibers that carry cold, pressure, and some pain signals. They are myelinated and therefore carry signals much faster than C-fibers. C-fibers are unmyelinated with a small diameter and slow conduction velocity. These fibers include but are not limited to postganglionic fibers in the autonomic nervous system and nerve roots in the dorsal root ganglia. They are also sensory nerve fibers that respond mostly to pain.

Renee Johnson

See also: Taste System; Thermoreceptors

Further Reading

O'Neill, Jessica, Christina Brock, Anne Estrup Olesen, Trine Andresen, Matias Nilsson, & Anthony H. Dickenson. (2012). Unravelling the mystery of capsaicin: A tool to understand and treat pain. *Pharmacological Reviews, 64*(4), 939–971.

Schepers, Raf J., & Matthias Ringkamp. (2010). Thermoreceptors and thermosensitive afferents. *Neuroscience and Biobehavioral Reviews, 34,* 177–184.

FUNGIFORM PAPILLAE

Fungiform papillae are structures found on the tongue that play an important role in gustation or taste. Fungiform papillae get their name because they are shaped very much like mushrooms. They are found primarily on the tip of the tongue and run down the lateral aspect of the tongue. Taste buds, which are important in distinguishing between various tastes of food and liquids, are found within fungiform papillae, which then transmit information about taste to the brain via cranial nerve VII, also called the facial nerve.

Papillae Anatomy

There are four major types of papillae found on the human tongue. There is some disagreement among scientists as to whether all four types of papillae have taste buds associated with them. There is general agreement that fungiform papillae do have taste buds capable of sensing the five major tastes (sweet, sour, salty, bitter, and umami) to varying degrees.

The four major papillae found on the tongue include (1) filiform papillae, which are found in highest density on the anterior two-thirds of the tongue. There is general agreement that these papillae most likely do not have taste buds associated with them. (2) Fungiform papillae are found in highest density on the tip of the tongue and along the lateral aspects or sides of the tongue. These papillae tend to have a high concentration of taste buds associated with them. (3) Foliate papillae are found in highest density along the posterior lateral aspect of the tongue and in the back of the tongue. (4) Circumvallate papillae (or vallate) are found in highest density in the back of the tongue and down the middle or medial aspects of the tongue.

Anatomy and Innervation of Fungiform Papillae

Fungiform papillae are found on the tip of the tongue and along the lateral aspects of the tongue. It is estimated that the average human tongue has approximately 200 papillae in total. The papillae located at the tip of the tongue tend to have a greater number of taste buds associated with them (range of 1–18), while the fungiform papillae along the sides of the tongue generally have 1–9 taste buds associated with them. These papillae often appear as raised red spots on the tongue. It is possible for a person to determine the number of fungiform papillae on the tongue by using various dyes such as food coloring. A person who has a high density of these papillae on the tongue is considered to be a "supertaster."

Taste receptors of the tongue follow a complex pathway to the brain for integration within the central nervous system. In summary, when taste buds within the fungiform papillae are stimulated, that information is then sent by the gustatory axons associated with the taste buds through cranial nerve VII to a specialized region in the brainstem called the gustatory nucleus. The gustatory nucleus is actually part of a larger structure known as the solitary nucleus. From this nucleus, information is carried to the primary sensory integration center of the brain, the thalamus, and then on to the primary sensory cortex within the cerebral hemispheres. This information is then acted upon and an appropriate response, if any is needed, is generated by the primary motor cortex.

Pathology of the Papillae

There are a number of common pathologies of the papillae of the tongue including transient lingual papillitis, which often affects the fungiform papillae. In this condition, the papillae are abnormally enlarged and individuals affected by this, depending on the density of the papillae on their tongue, may experience a burning or tingling sensation. Benign enlargement of the papillae is often caused by excessive smoking, canker sores, acid reflux (GERD), or irritation caused by excessively spicy or hot foods. In some rare cases, exposure to environmental toxicants such as insecticides or excessive alcohol can also cause enlarged papillae. Some vitamin B deficiencies can cause enlarged papillae in some individuals. A relatively rare condition known as depapillation can affect some individuals. In this case, the papillae of the tongue are damaged or lost, creating a condition that is also known as "bald tongue." Bald tongue is often the result of nutritional deficiencies. Treatment for these conditions often consists of treating the underlying cause of the inflammation or loss of papillae.

Charles A. Ferguson

See also: Circumvallate Papillae; Facial Nerve; Taste System

Further Reading

Mistretta, Charlotte M., & Hong-Xiang Lieu. (2006). Development of fungiform papillae: Patterned lingual gustatory organs. *Archives of Histology and Cytology, 69*(4), 199–208.

Sollars, Suzanne I., Peter C. Smith, & David L. Hill. (2002). Time course of morphological alterations of fungiform papillae and taste buds following chorda tympani transection in neonatal rats. *Journal of Neurobiology, 51*, 223–236. http://dx.doi.org/10.1002/neu.10055

Srur, Ehab, Oliver Stachs, Rudolf Guthoff, Martin Witt, Hans Wilhelm Pau, & Tino Just. (2010). Change in the human taste bud volume over time. *Auris Nasus Larynx, 37*, 449–455.

G

GANGLIA

Within the central nervous system and the peripheral nervous system, there are regions where cell bodies or somas of neurons and their vast dendritic arbors group together. These can make very distinct "bumps" within the nervous systems. In the central nervous system, collections of somas and dendrites are called nuclei (plural; nucleus, singular form). In the peripheral nervous system, these collections are called ganglia (plural; ganglion, singular form). This distinction is used to help scientists and anatomists identify the location of the cells.

The term *ganglion* is derived from Greek meaning a "cyst-like tumor." In the nervous system, ganglia may interconnect with other ganglia forming a complex structure called a plexus. The inputs and outputs of a ganglion can form a nerve, a collection of fibers and/or axons that travel relatively together. In general, a ganglion will be the interconnection between the peripheral and central nervous systems. For example, the cranial nerves that supply motor and sensory function to the head, neck, and face are part of the peripheral nervous system. Their sensory ganglia are located within the brainstem, which is part of the central nervous system.

Anatomy and Physiology

In the mammalian nervous system, there are two main types of ganglia: the dorsal root ganglia and the autonomic ganglia. The dorsal root ganglia are located just outside of the spinal cord. They are the collection of cell bodies for the sensory nerves (afferent nerves) and lack any motor neurons. The dorsal root ganglia are sometimes called the spinal ganglia and are located in the intervertebral foramina (openings between two spinal vertebrae). They attach to the spinal cord by the posterior (or dorsal) roots. Along the length of the spinal cord, there are 31 bilaterally symmetrical pairs of spinal nerves with each having two divisions. The dorsal division carries sensory information from the skin, muscles, and visceral organs, while the ventral portion transmits motor information. At each level of the spinal cord—cervical, thoracic, lumbar, and sacral—the dorsal root ganglia contain the cell bodies of the neurons that serve that region of the body.

The axons of the dorsal root ganglia neurons are called afferent nerves or just afferents. This is because they transmit information to the central nervous system. Sensory neurons within the dorsal root ganglia are classified as pseudo-unipolar, where the axon has two branches that act as a single axon. These distinct axon branches are named based on their location: distal process and proximal process.

These dorsal root ganglia pseudo-unipolar neurons are unique as they can initiate an action potential in the distal process. These action potentials will then bypass the soma and continue to transmit to the proximal process, where they will enter and synapse in the spinal cord's dorsal horn.

The autonomic ganglia are part of the autonomic nervous system and are located between the spinal cord and the target organ. The autonomic nervous system has two divisions and hence there are two types of ganglia: the sympathetic ganglia and the parasympathetic ganglia. The sympathetic ganglia house about 20,000 to 30,000 neurons that signal distress or possible danger for the person, providing the "fight-or-flight" response. These ganglia are found next to and on both sides of the spinal cord, forming bilaterally symmetric long chains from the upper neck to the coccyx. However, the coccygeal ganglion is unpaired. The parasympathetic ganglia are small compared to the sympathetic ganglia and are located close to the organs or effectors that they innervate. The four paired parasympathetic ganglia that supply the head and neck (the ciliary, pterygopalatine, submandibular, and otic ganglia), however, do not follow this rule.

Of important note, the basal ganglia are part of the central nervous system and are a collection of deep neurons within the cerebrum that are associated with movement. These nuclei were misnamed when anatomy was beginning to develop as a science. Today, anatomists are using the term *basal nuclei* more often than the previous name, basal ganglia.

Jennifer L. Hellier

See also: Autonomic Nervous System; Central Nervous System; Peripheral Nervous System

Further Reading

Kandel, Eric R., James H. Schwartz, Thomas M. Jessell, Steven A. Siegelbaum, & A. J. Hudspeth (Eds.). (2012). *Principles of neural science* (5th ed.). New York, NY: McGraw-Hill.

Purves, Dale, George J. Augustine, David Fitzpatrick, William C. Hall, Anthony-Samuel LaMantia, James O. McNamara, & Leonard E. White. (2008). *Neuroscience* (4th ed.). Sunderland, MA: Sinauer Associates.

Yasuchika Aoki, Yuzuru Takahashi, Seiji Ohtori, Hideshige Moriya, & Kazuhisa Takahashi. (2004). Distribution and immunocytochemical characterization of dorsal root ganglion neurons innervating the lumbar intervertebral disc in rats: A review. *Life Science,* 74(21), 2627–2642.

GLOSSOPHARYNGEAL NERVE

The glossopharyngeal nerve is a pair of cranial nerves that contain both motor and sensory fibers. It is the ninth of the 12 paired cranial nerves and therefore is also known as cranial nerve IX. As its name implies, it serves both the tongue and the pharynx (throat). The sensory fibers originate at many different sites including the pharynx, middle and outer ear, internal carotid artery, and the posterior one-third of the tongue, which contains taste buds. These nerve fibers terminate in the brainstem, specifically at the medulla oblongata (generally called the medulla). The motor fibers originate at the medulla and end at the parotid salivary gland in the cheek just in front of the ear, posterior tongue glands, and the stylopharyngeal muscle, which moves the pharynx up and down.

Anatomy

The glossopharyngeal nerve has six distinct branches: tympanic, stylopharyngeal, tonsillar, carotid sinus nerve, lingual branches, and branch to the vagus tympanic. The tympanic nerve or nerve of Jacobson is found near the ear. The stylopharyngeal branch goes to the stylopharyngeus muscle. The tonsillar branches supply the palatine tonsils. The branch to the carotid sinus runs down to the internal carotid artery. The lingual branches have two nerves: one supplies the base of the tongue and the other supplies part of the tongue, which also meets with the lingual nerve. And finally, the pharyngeal branches have three or four filaments that meet with the pharyngeal branches of the vagus nerve.

The glossopharyngeal nerve consists of five components: branchial motor, visceral motor, visceral sensory, general sensory, and special sensory. This entry will focus on the sensory portions of the nerve.

The visceral sensory component of the glossopharyngeal nerve originates in the carotid sinus where the common carotid artery splits into two. It travels up in the sinus nerve and joins the other components of the glossopharyngeal nerve at the inferior hypoglossal ganglion. From here they enter the skull via the jugular foramen, which is an opening through which multiple arteries and veins travel. The visceral sensory fibers enter the brainstem at the level of the medulla between distinct bumps called the olives and the inferior cerebellar peduncles. The fibers then travel downward within the tractus solitarius to communicate with neurons located in the nucleus solitarius. From here, the fibers continue and synapse in the reticular formation of the brainstem and hypothalamus.

The general sensory component of the glossopharyngeal nerve originates in several different places. General sensory fibers from the skin of the external ear and middle ear, as well as general sensory fibers from the upper pharynx and posterior one-third of the tongue meet at the superior or inferior glossopharyngeal ganglion. Next, the fibers of the general sensory neurons need to pass through the skull via the jugular foramen. Just like the visceral sensory fibers, the general sensory fibers enter the medulla and then connect to neurons in the caudal spinal nucleus of the trigeminal.

The special sensory component of the glossopharyngeal nerve originates from the back one-third of the tongue and travels through the pharyngeal branches of the glossopharyngeal nerve to the inferior glossopharyngeal ganglion. Again these fibers enter the brainstem at the level of the medulla but on the rostral end and follow the tractus solitarius to synapse in the caudal portion of the nucleus solitarius. In addition, taste fibers from cranial nerves VII and X (facial and vagus nerves, respectively) synapse here. From the nucleus solitarius, the nerves travel bilaterally to the ventral posteromedial nuclei of the thalamus. Finally, they reach the lower one-third of the primary sensory cortex, which is the gustatory cortex of the parietal lobe and where the sense of taste is processed in the brain.

Physiology

The visceral sensory component of the glossopharyngeal nerve receives important information about blood pressure from the carotid sinus and helps the autonomic nervous system during a "fight-or-flight" response. Specifically, the visceral sensory component detects the amount of stretch within the blood vessel walls (determines blood pressure) and sends the signal to the hypothalamus in response to the stretch. This nerve also transmits information from the carotid body about oxygen and carbon dioxide levels in the blood.

The general sensory component of the glossopharyngeal nerve carries general sensory information from the skin of the external ear, the internal surface of the tympanic membrane, the walls of the upper pharynx, and the posterior one-third of the tongue to the medulla. This information includes pain, temperature, and touch signals.

The special sensory component of the glossopharyngeal nerve provides taste and touch signals from the posterior one-third of the tongue to the taste centers of the brain.

Diseases

The glossopharyngeal nerve, if damaged, can have several effects on the human body. Because this nerve is involved in the functions of tasting, swallowing, and maintenance of blood pressure, any damage or injury affects these functions. These effects include loss of bitter and sour taste as well as impaired swallowing. In one-sided damage to the sensory component of the glossopharyngeal nerve, there is no gag response when touching the back wall of the mouth on the same side of the damaged nerve. Other signs include speech impediments and loss of taste on the posterior one-third of the tongue.

The most common disorder of this cranial nerve is glossopharyngeal neuralgia. Glossopharyngeal neuralgia is a condition in which there is severe pain in the tongue, throat, ears, and tonsils. This pain can last from a few seconds to a few minutes. These pain symptoms can be triggered by swallowing, drinking cold liquids, sneezing, coughing, talking, clearing the throat, or even touching the gums or inside of the mouth. It is considered to be a rare disorder and usually begins after the age of 40, occurring more often in men. There are several causes of glossopharyngeal neuralgia, but generally it is caused by compression of the glossopharyngeal nerve from a blood vessel or tumor. Glossopharyngeal neuralgia may also be associated with multiple sclerosis.

Mario J. Perez

See also: Cranial Nerves; Taste System

Further Reading

Liang, Barbara. (2012). *The 12 cranial nerves.* Retrieved from https://www.wisc-online.com
/learn/general-education/anatomy-and-physiology1/ap11504/the-12-cranial-nerves
Yale University School of Medicine. (1998). *Cranial nerves.* Retrieved from http://www.yale
.edu/cnerves/

GOLGI TENDON ORGANS

The human skeletal muscle system is critical for movement and locomotion. In order for this system to function properly, the relationship between various muscles at all the joints of the body must be maintained so that one muscle group does not overpower others or prevent other muscle groups needed for movement from functioning. This interplay is accomplished by the Golgi tendon organs found throughout the skeletal system in humans. This structure is important in preventing hyperextension or hypercontraction of muscles and allows for the movement associated with joint motions.

Anatomy

The anatomy of the Golgi tendon organ (GTO) is complex and multifaceted. It requires a very integrated interplay between the muscles and tendons of a joint as well as the nervous system via the spinal cord. In summary, the role of the GTO is to signal the nervous system how strong a muscle is in contracting and then to let the nervous system send a signal back to the muscle to regulate its continued contraction and relaxation as well as to regulate the muscles that are antagonistic or agonistic to the contracting muscle. For example, in order to flex the arm, the bicep muscle must contract, while at the same time, the tricep muscle on the back of the arm must relax and stretch. The GTO is integral in this coordinated movement.

Physiology

A more detailed look at the physiology of the GTO reveals this interplay. The body of the GTO is composed of collagen (a protein) and is embedded within the tendon connecting the muscle to the bone associated with a specific muscle and joint. By being embedded in the tendon, the GTO is able to sense the strength of a muscle contraction as the muscle is stimulated to shorten. What is unique is that the GTO is able to respond in a graded way depending on the speed of muscle contraction as well as the strength of the contraction. The more rapidly a muscle contracts and the harder it contracts, the tighter the tendon becomes and the more simulated the GTO becomes. This results in action potentials being sent to the spinal cord (the intensity of the action potentials is directly proportional to the speed and strength of the muscle contraction), which then determines how to further regulate muscle contraction. Should the speed or intensity of the muscle contraction be too great, the GTO signals the spinal cord to send action potentials to the primary muscle as well as the surrounding agonistic and antagonistic muscle to relax or lengthen and protect the joint (https://www.youtube.com/watch?v=7T4NI_2qDEM).

The Tendon Reflex

The tendon reflex, one that many people are familiar with (knee reflex), is a way to test and determine how well the nervous system is working, and how well the reflex arc is functioning. The tendon reflex is very different from what is called the stretch reflex, which regulates muscle contraction. The tendon reflex is a feedback mechanism that causes muscle relaxation before damage is done to overcontracted or stretched muscles. This reflex arc has a very specific pathway. Once tension is applied to the tendon, the GTO is stimulated and sends signals to the spinal cord. Through a series of neurotransmitters including glutamate and glycine, action potentials are sent back to the tendon/muscle, causing relaxation.

Pathology

While there are not a significant number of diseases that affect the GTO, the obvious, most significant issue involving the GTO is muscle damage as a result of the GTO failing to prevent hyperextension or overcontraction of the muscle. As stated earlier, the role of the GTO is to inhibit further tension if a muscle becomes overstimulated. Failure of the GTO to prevent this overstimulation could result in tearing of the muscle fibers.

A second disease that has been shown to affect the GTO function of some individuals is Parkinson's disease. In this disease the effectiveness of the GTO in preventing overcontraction or overstimulation is decreased and could be a contributing component to the tremor and rigidity often seen in this disease process.

Charles A. Ferguson

See also: Meissner's Corpuscles; Pacinian Corpuscles; Reflex

Further Reading

Moore, J. C. (1984). The Golgi tendon organ: A review and update. *American Journal of Occupational Therapy, 38*(4), 227–236.

Prochazka, A., D. Gillard, & D. J. Bennett. (1997). Positive force feedback control of muscles. *Journal of Neurophysiology*, 77(6), 3226–3236.

G PROTEINS

A neurotransmitter is a chemical that is released into the synaptic cleft, the space between a presynaptic neuron and its target cell or organ, and that binds to specialized proteins called receptors on the postsynaptic target. Some of these specialized receptors are G proteins, also known as guanosine nucleotide-binding proteins. G proteins are a group or family of proteins or GTPases (enzymes that hydrolyze guanosine triphosphate, GTP) that sense chemical stimuli outside of its cell. Once this external stimulus occurs, it results in the G protein changing its shape and activating molecular pathways or second-messenger cascades within the cell. This means a G protein can be thought of as a molecular switch.

History

In the 1960s through the early 1970s, American biochemists Alfred Goodman Gilman (1941–) and Martin Rodbell (1925–1998) were studying the process of how adrenaline stimulated cells. During their research, they discovered that G proteins were the target receptor for adrenaline. Specifically, with the binding of adrenaline to a G protein, the G protein would undergo a conformational change and stimulate another protein or enzyme (such as adenylate cyclase that makes the second messenger cyclic adenosine monophosphate or cAMP) located within the cell. This would start a cascade of other molecular signaling inside the cell, thus changing its activity. For this contribution to science, Gilman and Rodbell won the 1994 Nobel Prize in Physiology or Medicine.

Anatomy and Function

G proteins are named because of their ability to bind GTP and break apart (hydrolyze) GTP to guanosine diphosphate (GDP), which releases some energy within the cell. A G protein is considered active when GTP is bound to the complex and is inactive when GDP is bound. G proteins are divided into two classes based on their function: monomeric small GTPases and heterotrimeric G protein complexes. The latter class consists of several different subunits including alpha (α), beta (β), and gamma (γ). G proteins are generally located just beneath the cell membrane within the cytoplasm and are coupled with a receptor that spans the membrane. This makes up a G protein-coupled receptor (GPCR) that can be found in many cell types. Within the central nervous system, these GPCRs are usually associated with sensory systems like olfaction and gustation or with producing longer lasting or modulated responses in neurons. For instance, the G protein G_{olf} is necessary for odorant signal transduction and is found in olfactory neuroepithelium

(Jones & Reed, 1989) while other G proteins (TAS1Rs) are necessary for taste transduction of sweet, bitter, and umami in taste cells (Sanemastu et al., 2014). Lastly, G proteins and GPCRs are known to regulate many cell activities such as cell contractility and motility, controlling transcription, and secretion, which can lead to regulating larger functions like embryonic development, learning and memory, and homeostasis, to name just a few.

Jennifer L. Hellier

See also: Bitter Sensation; Olfactory Sensory Neurons; Olfactory System; Sensory Receptors; Sweet Sensation; Taste System; Type I Taste Cells; Type II Taste Cells; Type III Taste Cells; Umami

Further Reading

Jones, D. T., & R. R. Reed. (1989). Golf: An olfactory neuron specific-G protein involved in odorant signal transduction. *Science, 244*(4906), 790–795.

Lans, Hannes, & Gert Jansen. (2006). Multiple sensory G proteins in the olfactory, gustatory and nociceptive neurons modulate longevity in *Caenorhabditis elegans. Developmental Biology, 303*(2), 474–482.

Sanematsu, Keisuke, Ryusuke Yoshida, Noriatsu Shigemura, & Yuzo Ninomiya. (2014). Structure, function, and signaling of taste G-protein coupled receptors. *Current Pharmaceutical Biotechnology, 15*(1), 1–11. http://dx.doi.org/10.2174/1389201015666140922105911

GRAPHEME-COLOR SYNESTHESIA

Synesthesia, or "joined perception," is a condition in which sensations from one sense are simultaneously perceived by one or more additional senses. Those who have this condition, called synesthetes, can hear, smell, or taste in colors or shapes. Synesthesia is estimated to occur in anywhere from 1 in 20,000 people to 1 in 200. One of the most common forms of synesthesia involves seeing letters, digits, and words in unique colors. This is grapheme-color synesthesia. The word "grapheme" means a unit (as a letter or digraph—a single sound) of a writing system.

Characteristics

Synesthetes with this condition almost always see a certain color in response to a specific letter, digit, or word. For example, these synesthetes could see the word "library" as brown, the number "2" as orange, or the letter "f" as bright green. These perceptions are specific to each individual, and different synesthetes experience the same number in completely different colors—one person may see the digit "8" as green while others may see it as yellow or blue. Grapheme-color synesthesia, however, does not translate across meaning. The written word "five" is blue but the actual number "5" may be olive green, and "3" may be red but "three" is bright yellow. Plus synesthetes report seeing both the synesthetic color and the color it is printed in ("five" is both blue, the printed color, and bright red, the synesthetic color).

Since digits, letters, and words take on unique colors, synesthetes report having an unusually good memory for passwords, phone numbers, and addresses. However, sometimes they run into issues if colors clash (for example, within a name) or are the same. Colors seem to be stronger when there is a high contrast in printed letters against the background. Color distribution shows some regularities: shorter figures seem to be lighter, in general, than taller ones; the numbers zero and one are often black or white; and the letter "A" is seen as red by 43 percent of synesthetes. A grapheme can also have a gender or character: "L" is an intelligent blue woman and "4" is an ornery chartreuse little boy. When deciding if a name is male or female, synesthetes will answer more slowly if they feel the name is composed of male-like letters.

Anatomical Markers

Functional brain imaging studies show that synesthetic color activates the central visual areas of the brain thought to be involved in color perception. It has been proven that grapheme-color synesthetes seem to have thicker areas of gray matter in certain areas of the brain as well. Additionally, people with synesthesia require only one-third the stimulation of their visual cortex to experience transient flashes of light compared to subjects without synesthesia. It is also known that synesthetes lose their synesthetic perceptions if they experience brain damage. The exact neural mechanism by which colors are automatically linked to alphanumeric characters is still not known. One theory is that synesthesia might result from some kind of cross-wiring between digit and letter processing areas and neighboring color processing areas.

Research

This type of synesthesia is the most widely studied form and research has documented its reality. Synesthetes are not people with overactive imaginations who take metaphorical speech too literally. Two groups of synesthetes with grapheme-color synesthesia have been identified: "projector" synesthetes and "association" synesthetes. "Projector" synesthetes see synesthetic color appearing directly in front of their eyes as if on a projection screen. "Association" synesthetes see the colors in their "mind's eye" and not outside their bodies.

Synesthetic colors are perceived in the same way that real colors are perceived by those people who do not experience synesthesia. A variety of traditional visual perception tasks show this:

1. When given the task of saying the color of ink a word is printed in as quickly as possible, responses are fast if the synesthetic color matches the ink color and slow if there is a mismatch. This seems to indicate that the synesthete needs to resolve a conflict over which color name to use and demonstrates that synesthesia is automatic.
2. Searching for a "2" among "5"s is difficult due to the visual similarity until color is used. A synesthete has less difficulty because he or she already differentiates using color, so the digits stand out.
3. Arrays of equally spaced letters and digits organize themselves into distinct rows or columns for synesthetes depending on whether they are the same synesthetic color. This is similar to the perceptual grouping nonsynesthetes experience with real colors.

Carolyn Johnson Atwater

See also: Auditory-Tactile Synesthesia; Color Perception; Lexical-Gustatory Synesthesia; Mirror-Touch Synesthesia; Synesthesia; Visual System

Further Reading

Chudler, Eric H. (2016). Synesthesia. Retrieved from https://faculty.washington.edu/chudler/syne.html

Palmeri, Thomas J., Randolph B. Blake, & Ren Marois. (2006). What is synesthesia? *Scientific American*. Retrieved from http://www.scientificamerican.com/article/what-is-synesthesia/

Than, Ker. (2005). Rare but real: People who feel, taste and hear color. *Livescience.com*. Retrieved from http://www.livescience.com/169-rare-real-people-feel-taste-hear-color.html

GUSTATORY SENSE: *See* Taste System

H

HEARING: *See* Auditory System

HEIGHTENED SENSES

It has been well documented that some people's senses are heightened, meaning that they see many more hues of a color compared to others, while another person may have significantly increased hearing acuity. Heightened senses are commonly found in individuals with a sense that is lost or not developed in the brain, such as in blindness or deafness. It has been hypothesized that the brain region that normally is used for perception and integration of a specific sense, like the occipital lobe for vision, will be developed to increase another sense such as hearing. Finally, senses can be heightened for short periods of time under the influence of the autonomic nervous system, such as during the fight-or-flight response.

Highly Sensitive People

Having heightened senses does not equate to being highly sensitive, meaning that a subtle stimulus can be amplified by a person's sensory system(s), making the stimulus almost unbearable. It is estimated that about 20 percent of the population is highly sensitive, with men and women having this sensitivity equally, and that it is innate and not learned. Persons who are highly sensitive may have emotional experiences or responses that are significantly intensified, which may affect their social life, job performance, and intimate relationships. In fact, a single negative comment or the clicking of a pen can be internalized so much that the person may become confrontational or withdrawn.

Highly sensitive individuals may have a heightened sense of smell or touch, where the smell of hand lotion on another person can be extremely irritating just as much as an itchy fabric on their skin. These people tend to have zero tolerance for such stimuli.

Synesthesia as a Type of Heightened Senses

Synesthesia, or "joined perception," is a condition in which sensations from one sense are simultaneously perceived by one or more additional senses. The two main categories used to classify synesthesia are (1) perceptual—triggered by sensory stimuli such as sights and sounds, and (2) conceptual—involving abstract concepts such as time and calendars. Those who have this condition are called synesthetes and their experiences are involuntary, with the associations being unique to the individual. For instance, synesthetes can hear, smell, or taste in colors or shapes. Synesthesia is estimated to occur in anywhere from 1 in 20,000 people to 1 in 200. One of the most common forms of synesthesia involves seeing letters, digits, and words in unique colors and is called grapheme-color synesthesia, while one of the more rare forms of synesthesia involves words being experienced as strong tastes, a type called lexical-gustatory synesthesia.

Loss of One Sense Resulting in Another Heightened Sense

In 2004, Gougoux and colleagues studied whether people who were born blind or lost their eyesight had a better sense of hearing. They found that blind people develop superior abilities in auditory perception and are significantly better at orienting themselves toward sound than persons who are sighted. In fact, many blind persons are better at identifying voices and pitch change between sounds compared to controls (persons with vision). However, this depended on the age at which the person became blind. Gougoux et al. found that the younger the onset of blindness (that is, from birth to two years of age), the better the person's hearing sense was developed. They hypothesized that this increase was due to the plasticity of the brain at early ages. Additionally, people who lost their eyesight at an early age might not have increased nonspatial hearing compared to persons born with blindness.

Jennifer L. Hellier

See also: Auditory-Tactile Synesthesia; Blindness; Grapheme-Color Synesthesia; Lexical-Gustatory Synesthesia; Mirror-Touch Synesthesia; Spatial Sequence Synesthesia; Supertaster; Synesthesia

Further Reading

Bartz, Andrea. (2011). Sense and sensibility. *Psychology Today*. Retrieved from https://www.psychologytoday.com/articles/201107/sense-and-sensitivity
Gougoux, Frédéric, Franco Lepore, Maryse Lassonde, Patrice Voss, Robert J. Zatorre, & Pascal Belin. (2004). Pitch discrimination in the early blind. *Nature, 430,* 309.
Sole-Smith, Virginia. (2015). This is what it's like to have extraordinarily heightened senses. *Prevention*. Retrieved from http://www.prevention.com/health/heightened-senses

HOLMES-ADIE SYNDROME

Holmes-Adie syndrome is a condition that affects the eye, more specifically the pupillary parasympathetic innervation that is responsible for constriction and dilation of the pupils, as well as the dorsal root ganglion involved in the reflexes of the autonomic nervous system. In an individual with Holmes-Adie syndrome, the pupil of the affected eye (or eyes) is larger than normal at all times and very rarely, if ever, constricts in response to increased exposure to light.

Causes

The exact cause of Holmes-Adie syndrome is unknown; however, it is widely believed that it is typically caused by a viral infection, which leads to subsequent damage to the ciliary ganglion. The ciliary ganglia are in direct control of pupil constriction and dilation in response to changing exposure to light. This etiology is also present in the form of peripheral neuropathy of the dorsal root ganglion of the spinal cord, which is responsible for responses in the autonomic nervous system. This damage to the dorsal root ganglion and subsequent impairment of the autonomic nervous system is responsible for the associated areflexia, or absence of deep tendon reflexes. Another hypothesis for the cause of this condition is through the inheritance of an autosomal dominant trait. The largest demographic for the onset of the condition is women between the ages of 25 and 45.

Diagnostic Characteristics

Holmes-Adie syndrome is easily characterized by a symptom known as "Adie pupil," which describes a dilated pupil in one or both eyes that does not constrict quickly in response to light. This inability to constrict the pupil can be problematic and may lead to damage of the retinal cells in the afflicted eye(s). Another common characteristic that is used in identifying Holmes-Adie syndrome is known as anisocoria, which is the process in which the pupil of one eye is larger than normal and constricts very slowly when exposed to bright light. This diagnostic anisocoria can be seen in the onset of Holmes-Adie syndrome, in which the symptoms begin in one eye, or in the reflexes on one side of the body, before gradually spreading to the other side to take effect on the body bilaterally. Visual and reflexive symptoms may develop at different times. Case study–based research has also identified a chronic dry cough associated with the disease, which is believed to be caused by a number of stimuli including neoplasms, inflammatory lung disease, respiratory tract infections, asthma, or even gastroesophageal reflux disease, although the exact onset of the chronic cough is still unknown.

Associated Symptoms

Holmes-Adie syndrome can also be characterized through a number of associated symptoms such as orthostatic hypotension, segmental and generalized anhidrosis (inability to sweat, also known as Ross's syndrome), carotid gustatory syndrome, impaired cardiovascular reflexes, and chronic diarrhea. Although Holmes-Adie syndrome is known to be a benign diagnosis, failure to treat it can lead to other troublesome symptoms as a result of the autonomic dysfunction, including hyperhidrosis (compensatory mechanism that causes excessive sweating), the inability to tolerate heat normally, and syncope (the loss of consciousness). Studies on patients afflicted with Holmes-Adie syndrome revealed that the patients' chronic cough was exacerbated upon taking deep breaths or through hyperventilation, which is indicative of increased cough reflex sensitivity.

Treatment and Prevention

Because of the largely unknown etiology of this condition, there are no known preventive measures to protect from its onset. However, there are numerous treatment options for those who are diagnosed, including the use of reading glasses and pilocarpine drops to be applied three times per day in order to help constrict the overly dilated pupil. Unfortunately, the loss of deep tendon reflexes is permanent, so there is no treatment for this symptom of the ailment. Holmes-Adie syndrome is not life-threatening and does not cause any notable severe disability.

Gage Williamson

See also: Autonomic Nervous System; Blindness; Consensual Pupillary Light Reflex; Reflex; Visual System

Further Reading

Kimber, J., D. Mitchell, & C. Mathias. (1998). Chronic cough in the Holmes-Adie syndrome: Association in five cases with autonomic dysfunction. *Journal of Neurology, Neurosurgery, and Psychiatry*, 65(4), 583–586.

Millichap, J. Gordon. (2013). Holmes-Adie syndrome. In *Neurological syndromes: A clinical guide to symptoms and diagnosis* (p. 96). New York, NY: Springer.

National Institute of Neurological Disorders and Stroke (NINDS). (2011). NINDS Holmes-Adie syndrome information page. Retrieved from http://www.ninds.nih.gov/disorders/holmes_adie/holmes_adie.htm

Siddiqui, Aazim A., Jonathan C. Clarke, & Andrzej Grzybowski. (2014). William John Adie: The man behind the syndrome. *Clinical Experiment Ophthalmology*, 42(8), 778–784.

HOMUNCULUS

In mammals, and particularly in humans, the cerebral cortex receives sensory information from and sends out motor information to the head and body. These processes are performed by the primary sensory and motor cortices of the brain. The primary somatosensory cortex is the region of the brain directly responsible for the exchange of sensory information of the body, while the primary motor cortex is responsible for voluntary movement. To be able to determine the location of the sensory or motor signals, the brain has a pictorial map of the head and body "on" these cortices. It is a map in the sense that certain parts of the body's sensory or motor information are connected to certain neuron groups located in a specific region of the corresponding cortex. This anatomical map is called a cortical homunculus, or homunculus, which is Latin meaning "little man." *Somatotopy* is another term that is used to describe the point-for-point connection of a body region to a specific part of the cerebral cortex.

History

In the late 1940s to the early 1950s, Canadian neurosurgeon Wilder Graves Penfield (1891–1976) was a leader in his field as he was performing brain surgery on humans with epilepsy to destroy the neurons that were primarily involved in generating seizures. To ensure that he did not damage important sensory or motor functions for the patient, Penfield stimulated the motor and sensory cortices while the person was under local anesthesia but awake to answer questions about what was felt during the stimulation. From this information, Penfield was able to map out regions of the sensory and motor cortices that were connected to the different parts of the limbs and organs of the body. Penfield, along with Canadian psychologist and neurologist Herbert Henri Jasper (1906–1999), published these cortical homunculi in 1951 and again in 1954 (second edition) in their book titled *Epilepsy and the Functional Anatomy of the Human Brain*. These maps are still used today without much change from the originals.

Location and Orientation of the Homunculi

There are two types of homunculi: sensory and motor. Each type has a homunculus on the left and the right cerebral hemispheres; thus, there are four total homunculi—two sensory and two motor. The primary somatosensory cortex is the postcentral gyrus (the ridges of the cerebral cortex), and the primary motor cortex is the precentral gyrus. The maps wrap along these gyri from the medial (toward the midline) to the lateral (toward the side) surfaces. It is important to note that because the afferent and efferent pathways cross over (decussate) either in the spinal cord or brainstem, the right postcentral and precentral gyri contain information for the left side of the body and vice versa.

For the sensory homunculus, the most medial and deep portion of the postcentral gyrus maps to the genitals. Just superior to that are the toes and foot. At the gyrus's bend, the leg is represented. From the medial superior surface moving laterally the following are mapped: hip, trunk, neck, head, shoulder, arm, elbow, forearm, and wrist. The hand and fingers come next, but these are connected to a much larger area of the sensory cortex than any other previously described body part. This is because humans have significantly large numbers of sensory receptors in their hands and fingers, which helps produce discriminative touch. The specific mapping continues: hand, little finger, ring finger, middle finger, index finger, and thumb. Now on the lateral surface superior to the temporal lobe, the next body regions are recorded: eye, nose, and face. As with the hands and fingers having a largely mapped region of the sensory cortex, so do the lips. This is because humans have many sensory receptors around the mouth that are mainly used for sensing taste, temperature, and proprioception (position in space). Thus, the following are represented: upper lip, lips, and lower lips. Nearing the final downward mapping are the teeth, gums, tongue, and pharynx. The very last body region that is demarcated, where the postcentral gyrus meets the temporal lobe, is the intraabdominal. It is important to note that the viscera are not mapped to the postcentral gyrus.

The motor homunculus is mapped relatively similar to the sensory homunculus, but the proportions are slightly different based on the amount of controlled movements a body regions has. For instance, the hand and fingers are mapped to almost twice the region that they were in the sensory cortex. This is because humans have significantly large numbers of motor fibers in their hands and fingers, which give them finely controlled movements that are needed to play a piano, knit, write, or throw a ball.

Jennifer L. Hellier

See also: Discriminative Touch; Phantom Pain; Somatosensory Cortex; Somatosensory System

Further Reading

Kell, Christian A., Katharina von Kriegstein, Alexander Rösler, Andreas Kleinschmidt, & Helmut Laufs. (2005). The sensory cortical representation of the human penis: Revisiting somatotopy in the male homunculus. *Journal of Neuroscience, 25*(25), 5984–5987.

Saladin, Kenneth S. (2012). *Anatomy and physiology.* New York, NY: McGraw-Hill.

HORNER SYNDROME

Horner syndrome is a relatively rare syndrome that affects the eye, eyelid, pupil, and face of those with this syndrome. It is characterized by three major symptoms including abnormal constriction of the pupil (miosis), a weak droopy eyelid (ptosis), and a decrease or lack of sweating on the surface of the skin of the face on the side affected. These symptoms arise when the sympathetic nerve supply to the eye is decreased or interrupted. The causes of Horner's syndrome are extensive and can include other medical disease processes, trauma/surgical procedures, and a very long list of medications. Treatment is directed to the initial cause of the interruption of the sympathetic nerve supply, and success will depend on the primary or initial cause of symptoms.

Symptoms

Patients with Horner's syndrome can present with varying symptoms and a varying severity of symptoms. The most common symptoms include (1) a constricted pupil (miosis) on one side of the face, (2) delayed opening of the pupil affected, (3) drooping of the upper eyelid on the side of the face affected (ptosis), (4) a mild elevation of the lower eyelid on the side of the face affected (reverse ptosis), and (5) a decrease in sweating on the side of the face affected (anhidrosis).

Other clinical symptoms an individual with Horner's syndrome may experience include (1) impaired vision, particularly difficulty focusing or maintaining depth perception because of the unequal pupil size, (2) dizziness, (3) perceived muscle weakness in the face, particularly on the side of the face affected, and (4) significant headaches or neck pain.

Anatomy

Horner's syndrome is a result of decreased nerve impulses coming into the face through the sympathetic pathway of the head and neck. The nerves of this system are part of a larger system known as the autonomic nervous system. The specific nerves involved in this syndrome come off the spinal cord at the level of the shoulder and chest and then continue upward to supply the neck, head, and face with sympathetic innervation. This pathway is composed of three distinct parts called the first-order neurons, second-order neurons, and third-order neurons, and depending on which aspect of this pathway is affected, the condition could create varying symptoms in a patient.

The first-order neurons connect the hypothalamus of the brain with the cervical region of the spinal cord. Secondary pathologies such as multiple sclerosis, brain tumors, or encephalitis could affect this neuron pathway, creating the symptoms seen in Horner's syndrome. The second-order neurons connect the spinal cord with the muscles and other anatomy of the neck. They pass across the chest to get to the neck. Secondary pathologies such as thyroid cancers, tumors of the top or apex of the lung (Pancoast tumor—see https://www.youtube.com/watch?v=c7LD9 bdw9ag), trauma to the chest, or a thoracic aortic aneurysm could affect this neuron pathway. The third-order neurons pass from the neck into the face including the skin, muscles, and vessels that supply the face with blood in innervation. Secondary pathologies such as middle ear infections, carotid artery aneurysms or clots, or cluster headaches (Horton's headaches) can cause the symptoms of Horner's syndrome.

Treatment

Treatment for Horner's syndrome depends on determining which neuron in the pathway may be affected, and then treating the underlying pathology. There are three primary tests used to help determine which neurons in this pathway may be affected. In the cocaine drop test, cocaine drops are placed in the eye. Under normal conditions, this would cause a dilation of the pupil. In Horner's syndrome this will have no effect on the pupil. The Paredrine test is similar to the cocaine drop test and helps determine if the cause of the pupil constriction is damage to the third-order neurons. The third test is the dilation lag test. When a slit lamp is turned off or removed from the eyes, the affected pupil will dilate at a slower rate or lag compared to the unaffected eye. These tests help to narrow down where the problem may be within the sympathetic pathway. However, treatment still depends on what other pathology may be causing a decrease in nervous system function in this system.

Charles A. Ferguson

See also: Autonomic Nervous System; Dizziness; Ptosis

Further Reading

Bardorf, Christopher M., Enrique Garcia-Valenzuela, & Gregory Van Stavern. (2015). Horner syndrome: Overview, anatomy, pathophysiology. Retrieved from http://emedicine.medscape.com/article/1220091-overview

Ropper, Allan H., & Robert H. Brown. (2005). Disorders of ocular movement and pupillary function. In A. H. Ropper & R. H. Brown, *Adams and Victor's principles of neurology* (8th ed., pp. 222–245). New York: McGraw-Hill Professional.

HUBEL, DAVID H.

In 1981, Canadian neuroscientist David Hunter Hubel became a Nobel laureate and earned this award for his pioneering work in the visual system with Dr. Torsten N. Wiesel (1924–). Together, Drs. Hubel and Wiesel are considered the fathers of the visual system. They investigated how visual information is transmitted to and processed in the visual system as well as the structure and function of the visual cortex. In their most famous experiment, performed in 1959, Hubel and Wiesel placed electrodes in the primary visual cortex to record the brain activity of an anesthetized cat. They found that certain neurons were activated when specific patterns of light or light intensities were presented in front of the cat's visual field. In addition, other sets of neurons would be activated when the edge of the light or moving light occurred in the visual field. From their experiments, Hubel and Wiesel were able to classify the different cell types as simple or complex cells as well as identify ocular columns in the visual cortex. Their results showed that simple stimuli (light, intensity, and movement) are processed in the visual cortex as a complex system used by all mammals. Hubel and Wiesel continued to work together for more than 20 years. Their research has improved our knowledge of how the senses, specifically sight, are processed in the brain. In fact, their partnership is discussed in their book titled *Brain and Visual Perception: The Story of a 25-Year Collaboration* (2005).

Hubel was born in Windsor, Ontario, Canada, in 1926. He became interested in science at a young age and was influenced by his father's profession—electrical engineering. As a child, Hubel performed many chemical and engineering experiments, which eventually led him to study mathematics and physics at McGill University in Montreal, Quebec. In 1954, Hubel graduated from McGill University School of Medicine and became a resident in neurology at Johns Hopkins University School of Medicine in Baltimore, Maryland. A few years later, Hubel was drafted into the army and served his term at Walter Reed Hospital, where he performed his first experiments in the visual cortices of cats. Then in 1958, he returned to Johns Hopkins and met Wiesel. This is when they began their collaboration. In Hubel and Wiesel's next set of famous experiments, they blocked a kitten's vision in one eye to learn how the developing brain processes vision. They found that the visual cortices of these cats had adapted so that the unaffected eye developed ocular columns in regions that would normally be developed by the blocked eye. In addition, they were able to better understand the irreversible critical period required for the development of binocular vision and ocular dominance in the primary visual cortex. This led to developing treatments for babies born with cataracts and strabismus (crossed eyes).

In 1959, Hubel joined the faculty at Harvard University. He was the John Franklin Enders University Professor of Neurobiology at Harvard Medical School for most of his career. Hubel died in Lincoln, Massachusetts, on September 22, 2013.

Jennifer L. Hellier

See also: Visual System; Wiesel, Torsten N.

Further Reading

Hubel, David H., & Torsten N. Wiesel. (2005). *Brain and visual perception: The story of a 25-year collaboration*. New York, NY: Oxford University Press.

HUNGER

Hunger is the physical sensation and processes that signal our bodies and brains to eat. It can be perceived by low energy levels, rumblings in the stomach, and cravings for food. The cycle of hunger begins with the hormone ghrelin, which communicates with the hypothalamus in the brain, responsible for governing metabolism and regulating the basic body functions such as thirst, sleep, and sex drive. Receiving the message from ghrelin, the hypothalamus triggers the release of neuropeptide Y, which then stimulates appetite. When the brain perceives ghrelin it also signals the hindbrain, which controls the body's automatic, unconscious process, and the mesolimbic reward center in the midbrain, where feelings of pleasure and satisfaction are processed. In contrast, satiety is the absence of hunger; it is the sensation of feeling full, while appetite is the desire to eat food.

The Biology of Hunger

The hunger cycle is experienced throughout the body. The center of the brain, known as the mesolimbic region, is the area that processes pleasure. The vagus nerve is responsible for signaling the stomach, which secretes digestive acids. The pancreas produces insulin and the liver works to process the sugar and fat and starch coming in. This complex process involves taste, smell, sight, texture, brain chemistry, gut chemistry, metabolism, and psychology.

The change in the levels of the hormone leptin results in the motivation to consume food. Upon eating, adipocytes trigger the release of leptin into the body. Increasing levels of leptin result in a reduction of motivation to eat. After hours of nonconsumption, leptin levels drop significantly, beginning the cycle once again.

Introception and Hunger

Though the body is designed to operate regularly and efficiently, circumstances such as genetic and psychological disorders, over- and underabundance of food, and cultural norms affect how individuals interface with hunger. Most of us learn along the way that even after we have had enough to eat, it can take a while for the brain to get the message. For some, the message of satiety, or fullness, is not received loud and clear. These individuals may have issues with interoception.

Interoception is the perception of the internal state of the body so that an individual recognizes sensations of being full or hungry, hot or cold, itchy or in pain. People who have problems processing sensory information, a condition called sensory processing disorder (SPD), may have impaired interoception and not recognize feelings of hunger or fullness. As a result, they overeat. Further, impaired interoception leads to emotional eating as being aware of the body's internal state underlies self-awareness and emotional experience.

The peptide cholecystokinin (CCK) increases the feeling of heavy satisfaction, signaling fullness. Glucagon-like peptide-1 (GLP-1) and pancreatic polypeptide (PYY), which are produced in the lower gut, tell the brain the body has had enough and also tell the stomach to stop what it is doing and not move anything further along into the intestines. GLP-1 adjusts blood chemistry, stimulating the pancreas to release more insulin, which soaks up sugars released into the blood by the inrushing food and stores them in the body's fat deposits.

Mistaken Hunger

Thirst occurs when the body needs water. When it does not drink enough water, the body receives mixed signals on hunger. Dehydration causes the brain to believe it needs to eat when the body really needs liquid intake. Hunger is the result because the body incorrectly thinks it needs food for energy. As people get older, they lose their thirst sensation and tend to confuse thirst with hunger. People often mistake hunger for thirst because the adult thirst mechanism is weak. Misdiagnosing the sensation of thirst can easily mislead the body into thinking it needs food when what it is really asking for is water.

Candida overgrowth in the intestines can make the body feel tired and irritable and cause a foggy head and poor concentration. It can also cause intense carbohydrate cravings. *Candida* is a type of yeast that is naturally present in everyone's digestive tract; however, if the immune system is weak and digestion is poor, *Candida* levels can get out of control. Because it is a type of yeast, it needs sugar in order to grow. The overabundance of *Candida* in the system wants to be fed and its preferred food is sugar. This often results in an individual mistaking such sensations for true hunger.

Lin Browning

See also: Brain Anatomy; Interoception; Thirst

Further Reading

Heller, Sharon. (2014). Flunked intuitive eating? You may not know when you are hungry or full. *Natural News.* Retrieved from http://www.naturalnews.com/043766_interoception _fullness_hunger_signals.html#ixzz3wmeCfGzy

How Stuff Works Science. (n.d.). Stomach hunger—How food cravings work. Retrieved from http://science.howstuffworks.com/innovation/edible-innovations/food-craving1 .htm

Kluger, Jeffrey. (2007). The science of appetite. *Time.* Retrieved from http://content.time .com/time/specials/2007/article/0,28804,1626795_1627112_1626670,00.html

HYPERGEUSIA

Hypergeusia, also known as gustatory hyperesthesia, is a disorder of the taste receptors in which the sense of taste is abnormally heightened. Often, hypergeusia is associated with a lesion in the posterior fossa of the skull, or with Addison's disease. Addison's disease is a rare disorder that may develop when a person's adrenal glands do not produce enough steroid hormones. Thus, those experiencing hypergeusia in correlation with Addison's disease will experience a great craving for salty flavors in order to accommodate the abnormally high amount of ions lost in their urine.

Hypergeusia may present itself in a generalized manner, in which the sense of all tastes is heightened, or it may be limited to specific tastants, which are chemicals or substances that stimulate the sense of taste, such as salt or sugar. This disorder does not affect a person's ability to detect certain tastes; rather it makes each taste drastically magnified far beyond what the normal response or taste should be.

Causes

Although the exact mechanism of contracting hypergeusia is unknown, the most commonly associated causes of the ailment are lesions to the posterior fossa of the skull, and often Addison's disease. Additionally, people suffering from multiple sclerosis and diabetes mellitus have also commonly reported a new onset of hypergeusia with disease progression.

Lesions or tumors to the posterior fossa of the skull often will damage local structures such as cranial nerves that are associated with the sense of taste. For example, hypergeusia was associated with a posterior fossa lesion as noted in a case study of a 73-year-old male patient. The man reported that his wife's cooking seemed about two to three times sweeter than normal, while his wife had not made any alterations to her recipes to add more sugar. Although many hypotheses were made in the case, the only ailment that could account for his newfound heightened sense of taste was a mass lesion present in his posterior fossa (Noda et al., 1989).

Due to the etiology of Addison's disease, patients suffering from the disease suffer a large loss of ions in their urine, and therefore crave salty tastes to replace the lost ions. These patients often report a heightened sense of taste when it comes to salty items, leading to the belief that hypergeusia is often associated with Addison's disease.

In other diseases like multiple sclerosis, hypergeusia can present unilaterally if the progression of the disease is only affecting cranial nerves on one side (Rollin, 1976).

Treatments

Because of the unknown etiology of the onset of hypergeusia, there are no currently known treatments. Researchers continue to work to find an underlying cause so they can develop treatments and prevention measures, but until that has been accomplished, there are no current treatments for hypergeusia.

Gage Williamson

See also: Ageusia; Dysgeusia; Hypogeusia; Taste System

Further Reading

Noda, S., K. Hiromatsu, H. Umezaki, & S. Yoneda. (1989). Hypergeusia as the presenting symptom of a posterior fossa lesion. *Journal of Neurology, Neurosurgery & Psychiatry, 52*(6), 804–805. Retrieved from http://www.ncbi.nlm.nih.gov/pmc/articles/PMC1032046/?page=1

Rollin, H. (1976). [Gustatory disturbances in multiple sclerosis]. [Article in German]. *Laryngologie, Rhinologie, Otologie (Stuttgart), 55*(8), 678–681.

Virtual Worldlets Network. (2007). Sensory malfunction: Taste. Retrieved from http://www.virtualworldlets.net/Resources/Hosted/Resource.php?Name=SensoryMalfunctionTaste

HYPEROPIA

Hyperopia or farsightedness affects 5–25 percent of the population. People with hyperopia see objects in the distance clearly but have difficulty seeing up close. If not corrected, hyperopia can cause amblyopia (lazy eye) or strabismus (crossed eye). Treatment for hyperopia includes eyeglasses, contacts, or surgery.

History

Hyperopia has a genetic component, can be passed down in families, and exists in all races. Evidence of hyperopia can be found as early as the 1200s in Italy where early eyeglasses were created. These early glasses had lenses that were convex-shaped disks, which would be appropriate for correcting hyperopia.

A convex lens corrects hyperopia by compensating for the eye structures that are not focusing images correctly. Light rays must be focused by the structures of the eye in order to project a clear image on the retina. The cornea and lens of the eye focus light as it travels to the retina. A hyperopic eye is too short to allow the light rays to bend enough to arrive focused at the retina. Alternatively, a hyperopic eye may have a flatter cornea or insufficient lens power. If corrective lenses are not used to focus the image, the image would be in focus behind the retina.

Advances in the past two centuries have improved the early convex lenses to allow precise calibration. The amount of correction needed is measured in diopters. A person who is farsighted needs a convex lens denoted by a plus sign preceding the diopter strength. Digital aspheric lenses minimize distortion and make eyeglasses lighter.

Types and Symptoms

The AOA (American Optometric Association) divides hyperopia into three clinical categories: simple hyperopia, pathological hyperopia, and functional hyperopia (Moore et al., 2008). Simple hyperopia results from an eye that is too short, a flattened cornea, or an abnormal lens. Pathological hyperopia results from changes in eye anatomy caused by developmental problems, eye diseases, or eye injury. Functional hyperopia results when muscles in the eye become paralyzed.

Additionally, hyperopia can be categorized by severity: low hyperopia, moderate hyperopia, and high hyperopia. Low hyperopia can be corrected with lenses of 2 diopters or less. Patients with low hyperopia may be able to accommodate on their own without correction. Moderate hyperopia requires +2.25 to +5 diopters of correction. While patients with moderate hyperopia may be able to function with uncorrected vision, they may have difficulty with close work and experience eye fatigue and headaches. High hyperopia requires greater than 5 diopters of correction and working at near distances without correction becomes difficult for these patients.

Symptoms of hyperopia include difficulty seeing clearly up close, eyestrain, eye fatigue, headaches, and squinting. Young children may have asymptomatic hyperopia, called developmental or age-appropriate hyperopia. Most children have some degree of farsightedness, which often self-corrects as the eyes grow.

Treatment

Glasses or contact lenses are common treatment options for hyperopia. Digital aspheric lenses have been developed that provide less distortion and thinner lenses. Contact lenses can be placed directly on the cornea to bend light rays and help the image focus on the retina.

More recently, surgical techniques have been developed to correct hyperopia. During LASIK (laser-assisted in situ keratomileusis) surgery a flap of corneal tissue is removed, the cornea is reshaped, and the flap is replaced. PRK (photorefractive keratectomy) surgery also uses a laser to reshape the cornea, but the laser is applied directly to the cornea without creating a flap. Phakic intraocular lens surgery places a new lens in front of the existing lens, whereas refractive lens exchange surgery replaces the patient's lens entirely.

Outcomes

Hyperopia treatment with glasses, contacts, or surgery leads to positive outcomes as measured by restored vision in most cases. Surgical outcomes for hyperopia vary depending on the severity, cause, and techniques used.

In contrast to patients with successfully treated hyperopia, children with untreated hyperopia are at risk for amblyopia (lazy eye) and strabismus (crossed eye), two conditions that can lead to permanent vision loss. Patients with hyperopia also have an increased risk for acute angle-closure glaucoma, which can cause optic nerve damage and blindness.

Future

Research is ongoing to discover additional therapies and interventions for patients with hyperopia. Just as digital aspheric lenses have created thinner, lighter eyeglasses with less distortion, additional advances may provide better lenses. Contacts also continue to improve with extended-wear and disposable lenses now available. Surgical outcomes may be developed for farsighted patients. Additional screening methods may be developed to identify children with significant hyperopia so that fewer children develop complications that compromise vision.

Lisa A. Rabe

See also: Accommodation; Amblyopia; Blindness; Strabismus

Further Reading

Moore, Bruce D., et al. (2008). Care of the patient with hyperopia. *American Optometric Association*. Retrieved from http://www.aoa.org/documents/optometrists/CPG-16.pdf

HYPOGEUSIA

Individuals with hypogeusia have a reduced ability to taste bitter, salty, sour, sweet, and umami. Hypogeusia is a type of dysgeusia, which means a distorted sense of taste. A person who has no sense of taste has a disorder called ageusia.

Signs, Symptoms, and Causes

The main symptom of hypogeusia is complaining that food and beverages are not as flavorful, meaning candy may not taste as sweet or popcorn not as salty. It is common for a person with hypogeusia to oversalt or oversweeten food and beverages to intensify the flavor of meals and drinks. Usually, a change in taste perception is a side effect of an underlying disease or cause. Since the sense of taste is interrelated with the sense of smell, a person with allergies, a cold, or flu may suffer from hypogeusia. This is because the nasal passage is congested, resulting in decreased ability to sense smells through retronasal olfaction. This cause of hypogeusia is short term and lasts for the duration of the condition. Other acute conditions that may cause hypogeusia are gum disease, dental plaque, and some medications.

Common treatments for cancers, chemotherapy, and radiation (particularly to the head and neck region), can often cause hypogeusia. Chemotherapy and radiation can affect the normal mucosal layer of the mouth, resulting in sores and decreased saliva production, and thus resulting in hypogeusia. Saliva is important for the gustatory system as it brings the tastants to the taste cells—within taste buds—for binding. Reduced saliva decreases the ability of tastants to bind to taste cells.

Treatment

In most acute cases of hypogeusia, the symptoms will improve as the underlying cause heals. However, if the cause is from a prescribed medication that reduced saliva production, then patients can increase their saliva by sucking on hard candies, lozenges, or breath mints. Chewing gum—particularly sugarless gum—can also increase saliva production. If these over-the-counter treatments are not successful, a health care provider can prescribe artificial saliva or other drugs that can increase saliva production, such as pilocarpine. In some cases of drug-induced hypogeusia, decreasing the medication's dose or substituting for another drug is an alternative treatment.

Jennifer L. Hellier

See also: Ageusia; Bitter Sensation; Dysgeusia; Salty Sensation; Sour Sensation; Sweet Sensation; Taste Aversion; Taste System; Umami

Further Reading

Cowart, Beverly J. (2011). Taste dysfunction: A practical guide for oral medicine. *Oral Diseases, 17,* 2–6.

Halyard, Michele Y. (2009). Taste and smell alterations in cancer patients—Real problems with few solutions. *Journal of Supportive Oncology, 7*(2), 68–69.

Malaty, John, & Irene A. C. Malaty. (2013). Smell and taste disorders in primary care. *American Family Physician, 88*(12), 852–859.

INFERIOR COLLICULUS

The inferior colliculus, Latin for "little hills," is a midbrain nucleus or a complex cluster of neurons consisting of two small rounded elevations situated on the back aspect of the midbrain, just below the superior colliculus. The inferior colliculi are relay centers for auditory (sense of hearing) fibers and serve as a principal auditory center for the body as well as for both auditory and visual reflexes.

Anatomy

There are four physical bumps located on the posterior surface of the midbrain. The upper two bumps are the superior colliculi, which are involved in visual processing and the control of eye movements. The lower two bumps are the inferior colliculi. Together, the two superior and two inferior colliculi form the corpora quadrigemina or quadruplet bodies. The inferior colliculus is organized into three distinct parts: the central nucleus, the external nucleus, and the dorsal cortex.

The incoming auditory data to the inferior colliculus involve links to many brainstem nuclei. All the connections between the central nucleus of the inferior colliculus and the brainstem nuclei have connections on both sides of the brain, with the exception of one. It is the nucleus of the lateral lemniscus, a tract of axons that carry sound information. In addition, the inferior colliculus receives input from three sources: the auditory cortex, the medial division of the medial geniculate body, and deep layers of the superior colliculus.

The inferior colliculus consists of a compact cluster of gray matter nerve cells. These clusters are made up of large and small multipolar nerve cells. They are almost completely surrounded by nerve fibers from the lateral lemniscus. Most of these fibers end in the gray nucleus of the same side, but some cross over the middle line and end in the opposite side. From the gray nucleus cells, fibers stretch through the brachium of the inferior colliculi into the midbrain tectum. From here, they are carried to the thalamus and then to the cortex of the temporal lobe. Other fibers cross the middle line and end in the opposite inferior colliculus.

Physiology

The inferior colliculus is a part of the midbrain that serves as a principal auditory center for the body; each inferior colliculus receives auditory signals from both ears. Most signals sent by the right ear cross over to the left inferior colliculus of the human brain, and vice versa for the left ear. Like a radar system, one colliculus compares a given signal with its counterpart on the opposite side. The colliculi then determine if there are differences in the signal such as time lag and find the source of the sound within three-dimensional space.

The inferior colliculus receives input from somatosensory nuclei (neurons that contain sensory information of the body), which are involved in auditory-somatosensory interaction. This multisensory interaction leads to the ability to ignore "self-induced" sounds that are caused by vocalization, chewing, or breathing. Furthermore, the function of the inferior colliculus can be compared to a computer, acting to unify all the data about sound location. It is also responsible for pitch discrimination, ramping frequency recognition, and the startle reflex. Because of its complex functions in both vision and hearing, this part of the brain shows a higher rate of metabolic activity than other areas of the brainstem.

Diseases

Since the main function of the inferior colliculus is to process sound information, one of the main effects of damage to this structure is hearing loss. Hearing loss can be categorized by what part of the auditory system is damaged. There are three basic types of hearing loss: sensorineural (problems with the vestibulocochlear nerve, the inner ear, or central processing centers of the brain), conductive (problems with sound getting into the ear), and mixed (both sensorineural and conductive) hearing loss. There is also a fourth, less common type referred to as a central hearing loss, which involves damage to the inferior colliculus.

In central hearing loss, the ears work just fine but some function in the central nervous system (mainly the brainstem, including the inferior colliculus) is lost so that the person cannot mentally understand what is being heard. There are four subtypes of central hearing disorders or central deafness: central auditory processing disorder, auditory agnosia, pure word deafness, and cortical deafness. In central auditory processing disorder, the person finds it hard to understand or interpret what is being said, making communication very difficult. Because this condition involves a mental aspect, people tend to be diagnosed as having a learning disorder. They are thought to have trouble understanding people, ideas, and concepts, but actually they have central auditory processing disorder. Learning disorder is an incorrect diagnosis because the person's hearing works just fine; he or she just cannot make any sense of what is being heard because of some loss of function in the auditory cortex.

Mario J. Perez

See also: Auditory System; Cochlea; Deafness; Vestibulocochlear Nerve

Further Reading

MedlinePlus. (2012). *Hearing disorders and deafness.* Retrieved from http://www.nlm.nih
.gov/medlineplus/hearingdisordersanddeafness.html

INFERIOR SALIVATORY NUCLEUS

The inferior salivatory nucleus is a structure associated with cranial nerve IX or the
glossopharyngeal nerve that innervates the parotid salivary gland and is important
in the secretion of saliva for digestion. It works together with the superior salivatory nucleus to allow for full function of the parotid gland.

Anatomy

The major salivary glands in humans are responsible for the synthesis and secretion of saliva, a product that helps with the initial steps of digestion of food. There
are three major paired salivary glands that make up this system. The sublingual
glands are the smallest of the major salivary glands and are located under the
tongue. They secrete saliva into the floor of the mouth through the duct of Rivinus.
The submandibular glands are somewhat larger than the sublingual glands and are
located under the mandible (or jaw bone) and also secrete saliva into the floor of
the mouth. The parotid glands are the largest of the salivary glands and are located
just below and behind the ear. The parotid glands are the glands that become inflamed when a person has the mumps. Saliva is secreted into the mouth from the
parotid gland through the Stensen duct (or parotid duct). The parotid gland is
regulated by sensory and autonomic nerves including cranial nerve IX which is
composed in part by the inferior and superior salivatory nuclei.

Autonomic Innervation of the Parotid Gland

The peripheral nervous system in humans is composed of the somatic nervous
system, which sends nerves to many of our muscles that we control voluntarily and
exits the central nervous system from the spinal cord, and the autonomic nervous
system, which regulates the organs and structures of our body that we do not voluntarily control. In the autonomic nervous system there are two neurons that are
important to the function of this system. The preganglionic neuron passes from the
spinal cord or brain to a peripheral autonomic "ganglion," where a synapse is
formed with the second neuron, known as the postganglionic neuron, which
passes from the autonomic ganglion after forming a synapse with the preganglionic
neuron to the organ or other structure innervated by the nerve.

Cranial nerve IX is responsible for the innervation of the parotid gland. It is
composed of two neurons, both a preganglionic and a postganglionic neuron. The
first neuron, or the preganglionic neuron, originates in the region of the brain

known as the medulla oblongata from a collection of neurons called the inferior salivatory nucleus. This nerve passes through the base of the skull through the jugular foramen and forms a synapse with the postganglionic nerve in the otic ganglion. The postganglionic nerve then goes on to innervate the secretory cells of the parotid gland, forming saliva and secreting it when stimulated to do so by the process of early digestion in the mouth.

Pathology

There are a number of medical conditions that can affect the parotid gland and indirectly affect the ability of the inferior salivatory nucleus to perform properly. One of the more common conditions is parotitis, or an inflammation of the parotid gland. This is more commonly known as the mumps. Today it is possible to receive a vaccination to prevent this inflammation/infection. In severe cases, the swelling associated with this inflammation can block the salivary ducts, and when these ducts are stimulated to contract by the inferior salivatory nucleus, they most likely contribute to the pain many patients feel with this disease. It is also possible to form stones within the ducts of the parotid gland, which again can cause significant pain and discomfort when the ducts are stimulated to contract. In both of these instances, clinical treatment is available that in most cases resolves the issues being experienced by the patient.

Charles A. Ferguson

See also: Autonomic Nervous System; Glossopharyngeal Nerve; Superior Salivatory Nucleus; Taste Bud; Taste System

Further Reading

Holsinger, F. Christopher, & Dana T. Bui. (2007). Anatomy, function, and evaluation of the salivary glands. In *Salivary gland disorders*, Eugene N. Myers & Robert L. Ferris (Eds.) (pp. 1–16). Berlin and Heidelberg: Springer-Verlag.

Kiernan, John A. (2005). *Barr's the human nervous system: An anatomical viewpoint*, p. 150. Baltimore, MD: Lippincott Williams & Wilkins.

INHIBITION

The main function of the central nervous system (CNS) is to receive sensory signals and send out the appropriate motor responses. This integration is mainly done by interneurons. The CNS receives thousands of inputs every minute. Interneurons decide which signals are important and propagates them, and which signals are not important to respond to. These signals are inhibited, meaning that the signal does not continue on to generate a response to the stimulus. Inhibition can occur by two major mechanisms: lateral inhibition—where excited neurons can inhibit their neighbors to prevent cross-activation, and inhibitory postsynaptic potentials

(IPSPs)—where the postsynaptic neuron (second neuron) is inhibited by the release of certain neurotransmitters that prevents the signal from continuing onward. It is important to note that most neurons are responding to an intricate balance of excitatory and inhibitory signals to respond in the proper way that allows individuals to function at "normal." If not enough signals are inhibited, it can result in neurologic disease. Similarly, patients are adversely affected if too many signals are inhibited (possibly an individual would not be able to feel pain in certain body parts).

Lateral Inhibition

Lateral inhibition is the ability of an electrically excited neuron to inhibit the neurons around it. This is important because if lateral inhibition were not in place, it is possible that cross-excitation would occur. Cross-excitation is the excitation of neighboring neurons by the transduction of an action potential down one neuron. Lateral inhibition also is incredibly important in sensory perception such as touch, sound, and sight. This is because it allows a contrast to be made between strong, light, and nonexistent senses. The retina is a major region where lateral inhibition is used. This mechanism increases sharpness and contrast of images captured by the retina. This is because rods that pick up light dampen the rods surrounding them, causing their signal to indicate darkness. There is also some evidence of a link between color perception and lateral inhibition. For the most part, the cells that utilize lateral inhibition are located in the cerebral cortex and the thalamus.

Inhibitory Postsynaptic Potential

IPSPs are utilized to inhibit the propagation of neural signals by most neurons. IPSPs can happen at any synapse that utilizes neurotransmitters to pass the electrical signal to the next neuron. This is a type of synaptic potential, which makes it less likely that the postsynaptic neuron will be able to generate an action potential. The neurons that use IPSPs inhibit the postsynaptic neuron by releasing neurotransmitters that bind to postsynaptic receptors and change the electrical current that the postsynaptic cell experiences. The binding of these neurotransmitters to the postsynaptic receptor increases the negative postsynaptic potential of the second neuron. This means that when the generation of an action potential in the postsynaptic neuron occurs, it must depolarize more than it would normally do to overcome the inhibitory response. Depolarization from the resting threshold has to go further to get to the action potential threshold—the electrical potential has to become more positive than normal. This type of inhibition is very similar to what occurs in a hyperpolarization event after the generation of the action potential. Each postsynaptic neuron receives signals via neurotransmitters from both ISPSs and ESPSs. It is the intricate balance between the two signals that allows the nervous system to function as well as it does.

There are two main type of inhibitory receptors used in ISPSs: ionotropic receptors and metabotropic receptors. The two receptors are classified by the way that they function after binding of the neurotransmitter to the receptor. Ionotropic receptors take advantage of ion channels nearby in the membrane. When a neurotransmitter binds to an ionotropic receptor, it signals the nearby ion channels to open, allowing ions to flow into the postsynaptic neuron's intracellular compartment. The influx of ions polarizes the cell's potential, making it take longer for an action potential to be generated. This type of receptor is important in modulating the speed and size of action potentials generated in the postsynaptic neuron. Ionotropic receptors can act fairly quickly since they are in more direct contact with the ion channels.

Metabotropic receptors have two major regions or domains—the extracellular domain and the intracellular domain. Neurotransmitters bind to the extracellular domain of the metabotropic receptor. The intracellular domain is coupled to a G protein. When the neurotransmitter binds to the extracellular domain, it sends a signal down the receptor to activate the G protein within the cell. This activates a pathway within the cell that interacts with ion channels to close them. By closing ion channels, the cell prevents a depolarization event and thus an action potential event from occurring. Metabotropic receptors generate a long response because of the time it takes for the G protein pathway to be complete before any interactions with ion channels can occur.

Riannon C. Atwater

See also: Action Potential; Excitation; Membrane Potential: Depolarization and Hyperpolarization; Retina

Further Reading

Bear, Mark F., Barry W. Connors, & Michael A. Paradiso. (2007). *Neuroscience exploring the brain* (3rd ed.). Baltimore, MD: Lippincott Williams & Wilkins.
Grobstein, Paul. (2003). *Tricks of the eye, wisdom of the brain.* Retrieved from http://serendip.brynmawr.edu/bb/latinhib.html

INTEROCEPTION

Interoception is the perception of sensation originating from within the body, especially the visceral organs. Together with exteroception, it comprises the senses of the body for animals and humans. Most of interoception comes from sensory receptors within visceral organs. However, there are a large number of receptors that reside in the blood vessels called baroreceptors. These baroreceptors help with monitoring levels of chemicals, oxygen, carbon dioxide, and noxious stimuli within the body. These signals are then translated into an appropriate response to help maintain homeostasis (a constant internal state at which the organism functions the most efficiently) within the body.

Stretch Receptors

Stretch receptors are one of the largest types of receptors that originate from visceral organs. When these stretch receptors are activated, the receptors will send signals to the brain for an action to take place. For instance, stretch receptors help play a role in the sensations of hunger and the need for defecation and diuresis. When these receptors are stretched tightly in the urinary bladder, the brain interprets the signal as needing to relieve the pressure and as such you urinate. Similarly in the rectum and anus, when stretch receptors are under high stretch, they indicate that the bowels need to be voided. However, in the stomach, low stretch in these receptors plays a role in letting the brain know that the body needs to eat more food. Hunger is one of the biggest sensations that arises from the visceral organs, but it is also strongly affected by some of the external senses such as sight, smell, and taste.

Other examples of stretch receptors are those that exist in the lungs, esophagus, and pharynx. Stretch receptors in the lungs help to control and regulate breathing rates. The level of stretch, either high or low, indicates how full of air the lungs are and if a deep breath is required. These receptors work with baroreceptors (a type of chemoreceptor) to help keep the oxygen (O_2) to carbon dioxide (CO_2) ratio stable. The esophagus and pharynx both contain stretch receptors that send signals to the brain that there are objects within the space. Within the esophagus, the receptors play a role in the sensation of swallowing and vomiting. The stretch receptors within the pharynx alert the brain that there is a foreign object within the pharynx. This creates the response of gagging to clear the foreign object from the pharynx.

Chemoreceptors

Chemoreceptors are another type of interoceptor and are found in many of the visceral organs to help maintain proper function. Chemoreceptors within the small intestine help the body determine how much pancreatic amylase (a key digestive enzyme) needs to be released to create the correct pH within the small intestine for proper absorption of nutrients. Additionally, chemoreceptors within the brain determine if noxious chemicals have breached the blood-brain barrier and will tell the body to vomit to remove them from itself. These receptors reside in the chemoreceptor trigger zone in the medulla. Other chemoreceptors reside within the brain and play a key role in determining carbon dioxide levels in the blood. When carbon dioxide levels reach a high concentration, the brain feels starvation of oxygen and tells the lungs to breathe more to increase the amount of oxygen within the blood.

Chemoreceptors also exist within blood vessels and measure levels of sugars and salts. If the level of sugar or salt is too low, the response to these receptors is often a craving for the foods that will provide more of the sugar or salt. High concentrations of salts in the bloodstream prompt thirst in the individual to help reduce the concentration to an acceptable level. Receptors in the esophagus and pharynx respond to noxious chemicals and produce a vomiting response to help rid the body of the harmful chemical.

Riannon C. Atwater

See also: Autonomic Nervous System; Baroreceptors; Exteroception; Sensory Receptors

Further Reading

Craig, A. D. (2002). How do you feel? Interoception: The sense of the physiological condition of the body. *Nature Reviews: Neuroscience, 3*(8), 655–666.

Craig, A. D. (2013). Cooling, pain, and other feelings from the body in relation to the autonomic nervous system. *Handbook of Clinical Neurology, 117,* 103–109.

D'Alessandro, Giandomenico, Francesco Cerritelli, & Pietro Cortelli. (2016). Sensitization and interoception as key neurological concepts in osteopathy and other manual medicines. *Frontiers in Neuroscience, 10,* 100. Retrieved from http://www.ncbi.nlm.nih.gov/pmc/articles/PMC4785148/

INTERRELATEDNESS OF TASTE AND SMELL

The nervous system helps an organism understand the environment around it and helps the organism respond and interact within its world. The most fundamental portion of the nervous system is its sensory system. This system consists of the five main senses—audition (hearing), gustation (taste), olfaction (smell), touch, and vision (sight). However, since foods and beverages provide calories and nutrients that are essential for survival, the senses of smell and taste are highly interrelated. In fact, this is how flavor is identified or perceived. For example, a person can determine if a strawberry is ripe by using only one sense: vision or touch. When you look at a strawberry, you can tell by its color if it is ripe—red in color—or not—green in color. Additionally, using only the sense of touch, if a strawberry is tender or gives when handled, it is another sign that the strawberry is ripe. However, we do not know what the strawberry's flavor is or perceive its flavor without using both the sense of taste and the sense of smell.

Only using the sense of taste, the ripe strawberry will be sweet, but if it is unripe there is no taste. Only using the sense of smell, the ripe strawberry will smell sweet, but we cannot tell what its chemical signature truly is that makes "strawberry." This is because a person who sniffs is using orthonasal olfaction. However, an individual who is eating and chewing is using retronasal olfaction where odors trapped in the food enter the nose via the pharynx. This is why food does not taste as flavorful when a person has a stuffy or runny nose from a head cold, flu, or sinusitis. Now, when you bite into the strawberry (with a clean nose), the flavor of strawberry is more complex; it is not just sweet. The strawberry's tastants along with its odorants work together so that our brain perceives the uniqueness that makes a strawberry—which is different from a raspberry, blueberry, or cherry.

Jennifer L. Hellier

See also: Ageusia; Anosmia; Odor Intensity Scale; Odor Threshold; Olfactory System; Supertaster; Taste Aversion; Taste System

Further Reading

Finger, Thomas E., & Sue C. Kinnamon. (2011). Taste isn't just for taste buds anymore. F1000 Biology Reports. Retrieved from http://www.ncbi.nlm.nih.gov/pmc/articles/PMC3169900/

Gire, David H., Diego Restrepo, Terrence J. Sejnowski, Charles Greer, Juan A. De Carlos, & Laura Lopez-Mascaraque. (2013). Temporal processing in the olfactory system: Can we see a smell? *Neuron, 78*(3), 416–432.

Society for Neuroscience. (2012). Senses and perception: Taste and smell. BrainFacts.org. Retrieved from http://www.brainfacts.org/sensing-thinking-behaving/senses-and-perception/articles/2012/taste-and-smell/

JOINT POSITION SENSE: *See* Proprioception

K

KELLER, HELEN

Helen Keller was a famous blind and deaf author, speaker, and activist known worldwide. She dedicated her life to help improve the lives of others, especially those like herself. Helen Adams Keller was born completely healthy on June 27, 1880, in Tuscumbia, Alabama. At 19 months old, Helen contracted an unknown illness that left her blind and deaf. Experts today think the illness might have been meningitis or scarlet fever. When Helen was six, her parents brought her to see Alexander Graham Bell, who at the time had been working with the deaf. Per his advice, they contacted the Perkins Institute for the Blind in Boston, Massachusetts. Through the Perkins Institute the Keller family met Anne Mansfield Sullivan, who became Helen's teacher. Sullivan, a 21-year-old graduate from the Perkins Institute for the Blind, was also visually impaired. She began teaching and communicating with Keller by physically spelling words in her hands. Helen was a quick learner and was able to master the manual alphabet and braille.

In 1890, Sullivan took Keller to Sarah Fuller at the Horace Mann School for the Deaf where she learned to speak, after Helen expressed the desire. Keller continued her education at many different institutes. She attended the Perkins School for the Blind, the Wright-Humason School for the Deaf, and the Cambridge School of Young Ladies in order to prepare for college. Helen then went on to attend Radcliffe College and graduated cum laude in 1904 with a bachelor of arts degree. She became the first deaf-blind person to do so. Sullivan accompanied Keller to all of her classes throughout the years, interpreting for her. She remained with Helen until she died on October 20, 1963.

Throughout her life, Keller had many achievements. In 1903, at the age of 22, she published her autobiography, *The Story of My Life*. The book is still in print today and has been translated into numerous languages. She went on to publish 13 more books as well as many articles. Some of her other published works include "Optimism," *The World I Live In*, *My Religion*, *Let Us Have Faith*, *Teacher, Anne Sullivan Macy*, and *The Open Door*. Helen also wrote many essays and speeches on topics such as preventing blindness, birth control, and faith, which can be found in the Helen Keller Archives. Keller's greatest passion was helping others like herself. In 1921 she joined the American Foundation for the Blind (AFB) where she worked for more than 40 years. Keller worked to improve the treatment and quality of life of the blind and deaf, both in the United States and other countries. She was able to empathize with so many people and brought inspiration to many. She visited military hospitals and helped provide hope to the injured soldiers. In 1915 she founded Helen Keller International. Not only was Helen involved in helping others with disabilities, she was also a Socialist and advocated for many causes such as civil rights and women's suffrage. She was also a member of the American Civil Liberties Union. Helen Keller received many awards throughout her life. She was awarded the Presidential Medal of Freedom, several honorary doctoral degrees, the Lions Humanitarian Award, and received many other awards for her accomplishments. Helen Keller died on June 1, 1968, in her sleep at 87 years old.

Shannen McNamara

See also: Blindness; Deafness; Sullivan, Anne

Further Reading

American Foundation for the Blind (AFB). (2015). Helen Keller biography and chronology. Retrieved from http://www.afb.org/info/about-us/helen-keller/biography-and-chronology /123

Helen Keller Foundation. (n.d.). Helen Keller. Retrieved from http://www.helenkellerfoun dation.org/helen-keller/

Perkins School for the Blind. (n.d.). Helen Keller. Retrieved from http://www.perkins.org /history/people/helen-keller

KINESTHESIA: *See* Proprioception

KLÜVER-BUCY SYNDROME

Klüver-Bucy syndrome is a very rare disease of the brain in which there is damage bilaterally to the temporal lobes of the cerebral cortex. Individuals with this syndrome often experience a number of different symptoms including issues with short-term memory, significant issues with appropriate social and sexual function, and myriad other idiosyncratic behaviors. At this time, there is no treatment available to stop or reverse the symptoms of this syndrome. Treatment is based on treating the ameliorating symptoms.

History

This syndrome was first described in 1937 by Heinrich Klüver (1897–1979) and Paul Bucy (1904–1992) after they performed temporal lobectomies on rhesus monkeys and looked at the postsurgical effects. Symptoms exhibited by the monkeys very closely resemble those seen in humans today including (1) docility, (2) hyperorality (the tendency to put things in the mouth to identify them), (3) visual agnosia (lack of the ability to recognize the names or functions of familiar objects), (4) disconnection of the visual system from the limbic system, and (5) hypersexuality demonstrated through an increased sex drive and inappropriate sexual behavior toward others.

The first case in humans was reported in 1975 in a 22-year-old male who had been diagnosed with bilateral temporal lobe damage after contracting herpes simplex meningoencephalitis. Other human cases have been reported in patients diagnosed with Todd's palsy (neurocysticercosis), neurotuberculosis, temporal atrophy, cerebral atrophy, or hydrocephalus. While there is no known treatment at this time, and this disease appears to be irreversible, managing symptoms, particularly those that are behavioral in nature, appears to have some positive effects for patients.

Pathology

Very little is known about the pathophysiology of this disease. Some studies reported by Jha and Patel (2004) suggest that lesions of Ammon's horns, parts of the hippocampi, as well as the medial lobes of the temporal lobe may be contributing to the symptoms seen in this syndrome. In addition, some evidence exists that compression of the hippocampi bilaterally may play a role. But it is important to stress that at this time, there is not a clear understanding of the relationship between injury/damage to the temporal lobes and the symptoms observed with this syndrome.

Related Disorders

There are a number of disorders that are very similar to Klüver-Bucy syndrome and are easily confused with this disease. They include Pick disease (frontotemporal dementia), which is another very rare progressive nervous system disease that affects primarily the frontal and temporal lobes. While early symptoms of this disease do not mimic Klüver-Bucy syndrome well, as the disease progresses, its symptoms more closely resemble Klüver-Bucy syndrome. Korsakoff's syndrome is the result of a deficiency in vitamin B_1. This leads to cardiovascular issues as well as problems with both the peripheral and central nervous systems. Again, the early symptoms of this disease including fatigue, irritation, memory loss, and poor appetite do not necessarily closely resemble those of Klüver-Bucy syndrome, but as the disease progresses, symptoms more readily mimic Klüver-Bucy syndrome. There are a number of other diseases that also share similarities with Klüver-Bucy syndrome including Alzheimer's disease, Huntington's disease, tuberculosis, meningitis, shigellosis, and acute intermittent porphyria. Care must be taken to accurately make this diagnosis.

Charles A. Ferguson

See also: Agnosia; Brain Anatomy; Limbic System; National Organization for Rare Disorders; Proprioception Deficit Disorders; Sacks, Oliver Wolf; Visual System

Further Reading

Deginal, Amaresh, & Siddling Changty. (2011). Post traumatic Kluver-Bucy syndrome: A case report. *Indian Journal of Neurotrauma, 8*(1), 41–42.

Jha, Sanjeev, & R. Patel. (2004). Klüver-Bucy syndrome—an experience with six cases. *Neurology of India, 52*(3), 369–371.

National Organization for Rare Disorders (NORD). (2015). Klüver-Bucy syndrome. Retrieved from http://rarediseases.org/rare-diseases/kluver-bucy-syndrome/

Weisberg, Leon A. (2002). Kluver-Bucy syndrome after minor brain injury. *Southern Medical Journal, 95*(8), editorial.

LAZY EYE: *See* Amblyopia

LEXICAL-GUSTATORY SYNESTHESIA

There are more than 60 known types of synesthesia, a condition in which two or more of the senses are joined and result in mixed sensations. Synesthetes' experiences are involuntary and the associations are unique to the individual. One of the rarer forms of synesthesia involves words being experienced as strong tastes. This type is called lexical-gustatory synesthesia. People with lexical-gustatory synesthesia can taste a word even before they speak it or write it, and it seems to be the word's meaning that triggers the taste sensation. For example, the word "bed" could trigger the taste of apples, and the name "Jim" could result in the taste of ice cream. There is even a female synesthete who chose her husband because she loved the taste of his name. Of course, often food names taste like the food named: "garlic" tastes like garlic, "banana" tastes like a banana. However, many other words also have distinct tastes, and synesthetes with lexical-gustatory synesthesia taste many types of words.

Synesthetic Experience

Another type of lexical-gustatory synesthesia, occurring rarely, happens when the synesthete not only experiences a strong taste but experiences a sense of touch because of the taste. For example, a strong, spicy flavor of jalapeno causes a rush of warmth down the leg. This indicates that a third sensory cortex has been crossed, the parietal lobe area of the brain that deals with touch. Some synesthetes even taste and see colors when they have an orgasm. Some have lists of words with terrible taste associations that they cannot handle hearing, writing, or reading.

Research on lexical-gustatory synesthetes has yielded some interesting information about the condition. Many of these synesthetes associate similar tastes for the same words—evidence that seems to indicate that it is not the whole word but certain sounds within words that are related to tastes. For example, many of the lexical-gustatory synesthetes find that words with the sounds "mmm" or "eh" taste of mint, the sound "aye" tastes like bacon, words with "x" sounds taste like eggs, and the sound "tony" tastes like macaroni. Plus most of these synesthetes are influenced, to some extent, by the language they speak—which means that the word associations are different in a different language. This suggests that the experience of the condition might change depending on the language in which an individual is conversing.

Lexical-Gustatory Synesthesia Research

Recent studies have shown that lexical-gustatory synesthesia might go even deeper than words. In an experiment, synesthetes with this type of synesthesia were shown images of objects that were familiar but not regularly encountered—a sextant, a gazebo, an artichoke, a platypus, and a phonograph. They were asked if they knew the word or any part of it for the object and what it tasted like. Even when they could not identify the object, they still sometimes experienced taste sensations, and these word-taste combinations persisted even years later.

Researchers theorize that word-taste associations are developed at a young age. These associations in nonsynesthetes stop being experienced perceptually as the individual grows. Nonsynesthetes make the same types of word and taste associations if they are required to make a judgment. For example, the word "onion" is linked to the taste of onion in those who have eaten onions and know what they are. One hypothesis suggests that all humans begin life as synesthetes and the connections between different sensory areas become blocked or pruned as a person matures. This is a part of the process called synaptic pruning that plays a role in neuroplasticity. For synesthetes, it is proposed that the process of pruning does not occur completely and some of these connections are left intact and active, causing the experiences that synesthetes have. This might explain lexical-gustatory synesthesia where the region just behind the temporal lobe in the forebrain and the area of the brain that controls auditory and specifically lexical cognition are crossed.

Carolyn Johnson Atwater

See also: Auditory-Tactile Synesthesia; Grapheme-Color Synesthesia; Mirror-Touch Synesthesia; Proprioception; Synesthesia; Taste Aversion; Taste System

Further Reading

Colizoli, Olympia, Jaap M. Murre, & Romke Rouw. (2013). A taste for words and sounds: A case of lexical-gustatory and sound-gustatory synesthesia. *Frontiers in Psychology, 4,* 775. http://dx.doi.org/10.3389/fpsyg.2013.00775

Inglis-Arkell, Esther. (2011). Lexical-gustatory synesthesia: When people taste words. *Gizmodo.* Retrieved from http://io9.gizmodo.com/5847521/lexical-gustatory-synesthesia-when-people-taste-words

Than, Ker. (2006). New insight into people who taste words. *Live Science.* Retrieved from http://www.livescience.com/1141-insight-people-taste-words.html

LIMBIC SYSTEM

The limbic system is not just one part of the brain but is a group of several brain regions with similar functions. Playing a critical role in emotions and long-term memory, the limbic system is referred to as the "old brain" because it evolved in mammals prior to the neocortex. This evolutionary progression affects the way that the brain responds to threatening stimuli and is responsible for managing the fight-or-flight response. The limbic system also serves as the emotional core of the human brain. Emotions in this context are best described as "a group of inter-related superior cerebral functions, resulting from states of reward and punishment" (Roxo et al., 2011). Mechanisms of motivation, learned behavior, and classical conditioning are all rooted in this part of the brain. However, there is some debate as to which particular structures are included in the limbic system.

Generally, parts of the diencephalon, the cerebral cortex, and the rhinencephalon (the part of the brain used for smell) are commonly included in the limbic system. Connecting these structures is a fiber tract called the fornix. The diencephalon comprises the thalamus, the epithalamus, and the hypothalamus. Though not directly involved in emotional processes, the thalamus is the relay station for information while the epithalamus functions to regulate sleep. Fear, anger, and pleasure are all processed by basal nuclei in the hypothalamus. Connecting the hypothalamus to the pituitary gland is the infundibulum. The cingulate gyrus and the parahippocampal gyri are part of the cerebral cortex, and the closely associated hippocampus indexes information for future retrieval. The rhinencephalon's original purpose was olfactory sensation and processing; however, in humans, only the olfactory bulbs and tracts are still used for this purpose. The remaining structures factor into the emotion and memory functioning of the limbic system. The strong link between olfaction and memories is due to this evolutionary pathway. In conjunction with the olfactory bulbs and tracts, the fornix and uncus make up the rhinencephalon. Though anatomically separate, the orbitofrontal cortex is also considered a part of the system.

History

The first true pioneer of the limbic system was Paul Pierre Broca, a renowned anatomist who identified the area of speech known as Broca's area. Although he did not determine the function of the limbic system, he laid its foundation. The discovery of Broca's area in 1861 was an important event in the history of neuroscience because it was the first time that a specific area of the brain was proven to have a specific function. Broca's second major contribution was in 1878 when he described the cortical aspect of the limbic system based on its morphological features. Broca's limbic lobe comprised the parahippocampal and cingulate gyri encircling the corpus callosum. The parahippocampal gyrus surrounds the hippocampus and has a role in memory, specifically in scene recognition and understanding social cues. Both of these structures make up the limbic association area of the cortex and enable the emotional influence of decision making.

Almost a century later, in 1952, John D. MacLean coined the modern term "the limbic system" and included Broca's limbic lobe and its associated subcortical nuclei in his definition. MacLean is also credited with the triune brain hypothesis, which divides the brain into three phylogenetic metastructures; the most primitive is the reptilian complex, followed by the limbic system, and finally the neocortex. It is important to note that the term "neocortex" is not interchangeable with "cerebral cortex," as the former specifically refers to this triune concept. The anatomy of the triune layers is consistent with the evolutionary trend of cephalization in which the neurons of the central nervous system gradually develop toward the rostral end of the organism. The reptilian complex is responsible for the most basic survival instincts, notably the fight-or-flight response; and the neocortex processes the more advanced, logical, and conscious thoughts. MacLean proposed that the limbic system initially evolved in mammals to manage the fight-or-flight response by learning how to react to environmental stimuli. Emotional memories are created from truly threatening stimuli, and when the stimuli are encountered again, the fight-or-flight response from the reptilian complex is activated. This mechanism allows humans to better learn and adapt to their environments by quickly responding to threats and not wasting metabolic resources on stimuli that are startling but harmless.

Current Standing

Under nonstressful conditions the limbic system is moderated by the neocortex. However, distress causing the fight-or-flight response bypasses the neocortex and decisions are made by the limbic system. According to John Bowlby's theory of attachment, infants who fail to develop secure attachments to their primary caregivers do not learn how to process social situations in healthy ways. Children's styles of attachment develop internal working models that create frameworks through which they view the world. Children who have developed an attachment disorder either learn to distrust other people completely, or simply do not learn how to deal with the fear and anxiety of interacting with strangers. They often find social situations to be unnecessarily stressful, triggering a fight-or-flight response. This accounts for the impulsive and aggressive behaviors and poor social skills endemic to the insecurely attached. These symptoms are readily identifiable as the product of the limbic system.

Even when not embroiled in the fight-or-flight response, the limbic system plays an important role in decision making. It is intimately connected to the neocortex via the cingulated gyrus. Thus, many psychologists argue that to bring about fundamental change in a person's beliefs or behavior, such as eating habits, the limbic system must be involved. This means that to influence behavior, one must make an emotional appeal because the logic being processed by the neocortex is insufficient to permanently influence decision making. This is evident in the emotional appeals made in advertisements and political campaigns. Logical factual data do matter, but emotions have the potential for more impact.

Erin Slocum

See also: Autonomic Nervous System; Brain Anatomy; Central Nervous System; Olfactory System; Thalamus

Further Reading

Chudler, Eric H. (2015). *Milestones in neuroscience research.* Retrieved from http://faculty
.washington.edu/chudler/hist.html

Dubuc, Bruno. (2002). *The brain from top to bottom.* Retrieved from http://thebrain.mcgill
.ca

Roxo, M., et al. (2011). The limbic system conception and its historical evolution. *Scientific
World Journal, 11,* 2428–2441.

M

MECHANORECEPTORS

Mechanoreceptors are sensory neurons that are active in response to mechanical stimuli. Outside forces cause a temporary physical deformity in the mechanoreceptor, which in turn initiates a nerve impulse in response to the stimulatory input. These outside forces generating stimulation include, but are not limited to touch, pressure, stretching, vibration, sound waves, and motion. There are four main types of mechanoreceptors, each responding to different types of mechanical stimuli: Pacinian corpuscles, Meissner's corpuscles, Merkel cells, and Ruffini corpuscles. Other less specific forms of mechanoreceptors include muscle spindles and their function in the stretch-reflex arc, and various free nerve endings in the form of cutaneous receptors. Mechanoreceptors are known as low-threshold receptors due to their very high sensitivity, allowing even very weak mechanical stimulation of the skin to induce the generation of an action potential.

Pacinian Corpuscles

Pacinian corpuscles are deep touch and vibration receptors found primarily in the skin. They are relatively large in size, leading to the ability of scientists to isolate a single Pacinian corpuscle and study its properties and mechanism of sensory reception. The corpuscle reacts to physical deformity through creating a generator potential in the sensory neuron within the corpuscle, and the response of the generator potential is proportional to the degree of deformity; the greater the deformity, the greater the generator potential. If the generator potential reaches a certain threshold, it creates action potentials at the node of Ranvier of the sensory neuron, and thereby releases its action potential down the length of the axon, leading to a sensation of pressure being felt. With continuous pressure, the frequency of action potentials decreases and comes to a halt; this response is known as adaptation. Pacinian corpuscles are located in the subcutaneous tissue and in the deep layers of the interosseous membranes and mesenteries of the gastrointestinal tract.

Meissner's Corpuscles

Meissner's corpuscles are often called "tactile corpuscles" due to the fact that they receive tactile information from stimuli. Meissner's corpuscles are more sensitive to movement across the skin than Pacinian corpuscles. This is because after

Receptor-Building with Clay

Receptors, also called channels, are specialized proteins embedded within membranes of cells, particularly neurons. They act as gates through the membrane that selectively allow only certain molecules to travel through. The protein's conformation (shape) exists in the closed state for the majority of the time. When a neurotransmitter or other chemical binds to the receptors located on the channels, the protein's conformation changes to open, allowing molecules to pass through. This binding is crucial to ensuring the changes in membrane voltage so that neurons are able to transmit neural impulses. Without proper levels of neurotransmitters, neurons do not function properly. There are many different types of receptors for sensory function, including but not limited to mechanoreceptors (that activate when it is physically moved), olfactory sensory receptors (that activate when a volatile odorant binds to the receptor), and thermoreceptors (that activate when heat is applied). For this sidebar, the receptor being made is the most common type that is associated with an ion channel.

Materials:

Three colors of clay (brown, yellow, red), waxed paper, tabletop, and paper towels

Directions:

Take a walnut-sized piece of yellow clay and roll it on the waxed paper to protect the tabletop. Form the clay into a worm, approximately one-fourth of an inch in diameter. Cut this worm into three pieces, each an inch-and-a-quarter long. These pieces will represent one subunit of the channel. Clean your hands with the paper towels between each color of clay.

Repeat this process with brown clay, only cutting two pieces of clay. These pieces will represent the other subunit of the channel. Lay the subunits next to each other lengthwise, alternating colors. Gently push the pieces together so they will stick but not mix. Wrap the pieces into a hollow tube. This represents the channel.

Finally, take two pea-sized pieces of the red clay and roll them into balls. These pieces will represent neurotransmitters that act as an agonist for the channel. Stick the pieces of red clay on to the channel gently. This is a receptor-bound channel that is open, allowing molecules to pass through the channel to the other side of the cell membrane. Remove the red clay from the receptor and gently twist the channel so that it is closed. When the channel is not bound by a neurotransmitter, molecules cannot pass through.

Riannon C. Atwater

adaptation to a sustained stimulus, they are also activated when the stimulus is removed. Meissner's corpuscles lie between the dermal papillae just beneath the epidermis in regions such as the palms, fingers, and soles of the feet.

Merkel Cells

Merkel cells are transducers of pressure and are activated in response not only to the mechanical stimulus, but also to the edges, textures, and shapes of the objects that come in contact with the skin. Merkel cells are also specialized in their ability to differentiate in point localization and to discriminate between the applied pressures at two distinct points. Merkel cells do not undergo rapid adaptation to stimuli as Pacinian and Meissner's corpuscles do; instead they will continue to generate the nerve impulse in the form of action potentials for as long as the stimulus remains in contact with the skin. Often, Merkel cells are found in the skin close to hairs. Merkel cells are located in the epidermis, primarily in the fingertips, lips, and external genitalia.

Ruffini Corpuscles

Ruffini corpuscles are responsible for the sense of deep pressure and the stretching of the skin. Like Merkel cells, Ruffini corpuscles are slow-adapting, spindle-shaped cells located deep in the skin, in tendons, and in ligaments. The functions of Ruffini corpuscles are much less well understood than those of the other mechanoreceptors, but it is believed that they respond to stretching, particularly through digit or limb movement.

Muscle Spindles

Muscle spindles are responsible for reflexes in a mechanism known as proprioception, or the sense of relative position of body parts, and are activated in response to stretching; this is known as the stretch-reflex arc. The mechanism of nerve impulse generation is seen when the tendon of a muscle undergoes deformity, leading to the stretching of the muscle to which it is attached. This stretching of the muscle leads to the subsequent stretching of muscle spindles, which are made up of sensory nerve endings that are wrapped around spindle fibers. Stretching the spindle fibers sends a nerve impulse through the sensory neurons all the way up to the spinal cord, which then returns the stimulus through motor neurons to cause the contraction of the muscle, thus completing the stretch reflex.

Gage Williamson

See also: Meissner's Corpuscles; Pacinian Corpuscles; Reflex; Sensory Receptors; Touch

Further Reading

Johnson, Kenneth O. (2001). The roles and functions of cutaneous mechanoreceptors. *Current Opinion in Neurobiology, 11,* 455–461. Retrieved from http://www.cns.nyu.edu/~david/courses/sm12/Readings/Johnson%20Curr%20Biol%202001.pdf

Purves, Dale, et al. (Eds.). (2001). Mechanoreceptors specialized to receive tactile information. *Neuroscience* (2nd ed.). Sunderland, MA: Sinauer Associates. Retrieved from http://www.ncbi.nlm.nih.gov/books/NBK10895/

Wayne State University Department of Health Care Sciences. (n.d.). Receptor types and function. *Somatosensory examination and evaluation study guide introduction.* Retrieved from http://healthcaresciencesocw.wayne.edu/sensory/1_5.htm

MEISSNER'S CORPUSCLES

Also known as tactile corpuscles, Meissner's corpuscles are a type of mechanoreceptor and a type of nerve ending responsible for the sensitivity of light touch. Meissner's corpuscles are found in hairless skin (glabrous skin) and within the dermal papillae. Meissner's corpuscles are the most common type of mechanoreceptor in the hand, providing about 40 percent of sensory information. They are rapidly adaptive receptors, meaning the cells respond maximally but briefly to a stimulus and then if the stimulus is maintained, the response will decrease. Meissner's corpuscles are most commonly found in thick, hairless skin, predominantly on the finger pads and the lips. The number of corpuscles on the fingertips, however, drops during aging. Studies have found that by the age of 50 years old the number of Meissner's corpuscles are generally four times lower than the number observed at the age of 12 years old.

Meissner's corpuscles are enclosed unmyelinated nerve endings consisting of flat (laminar), supportive cells in a horizontal arrangement and surrounded by a connective tissue capsule. The Meissner's corpuscles contain primary afferent terminal fibers that are situated between the flattened cells.

Function

Meissner's corpuscles are very sensitive to shape and textural changes in touch. They help provide the neural basis for reading braille by the blind. Particularly sensitive to touch and vibrations at low frequencies (30–50 hertz), they are still limited in their detection as they can only sense that something is touching the skin. When pressure is applied to the skin, the laminar cells slide past one another and distort the membranes of the axon terminals in the cells. A deformation in the corpuscle will cause an action potential (firing of a neuron), causing you to sense the change but to rapidly adapt and stop feeling things like the clothes you are wearing. Due to the discharge of a low-frequency vibration, the primary afferent neuron can detect and signal very small movements across the skin.

Renee Johnson

See also: Braille; Chemoreception; Discriminative Touch; Mechanoreceptors; Merkel Cell; Pacinian Corpuscles; Somatosensory System

Further Reading

Dougherty, Patrick, & Chieyeko Tsuchitani. (2015). Somatosensory systems. In *Neuroscience online* (Chap. 2). John H. Byrne (Ed.). Retrieved from http://neuroscience.uth.tmc.edu/s2/chapter02.html

Purves, Dale, et al. (2008). *Neuroscience* (4th ed.). Sunderland, MA: Sinauer Associates.

MELKERSSON-ROSENTHAL SYNDROME

Melkersson-Rosenthal syndrome (MRS) is a neurological disorder and is quite rare. The disorder was first referred to as Melkersson-Rosenthal syndrome in 1949. Ernst Melkersson first described the link between facial swelling and paralysis of the face in 1928. Curt Rosenthal then acknowledged that the symptoms could be correlated with a fissured tongue. MRS is characterized by three main features that are often recurring: (1) swelling of the face and/or lips, which is also known as cheilitis granulomatosa, (2) facial paralysis or weakness, and (3) folds or creases in the tongue. Individuals can be affected with all three characteristic features at the same time, or can only have one or two of them at a time. Often, all three of the characteristic features are not seen together or at the same time. All three features are found in approximately 25 percent of the cases of MRS, while in 42 percent of cases, swelling of the face is the presenting feature and main finding. Facial paralysis or weakness is found in approximately 30 percent of individuals (Kang & Gaillard, n.d.). In 40 percent of cases, folds or creases in the tongue are seen (Scully, 2015). Facial paralysis or weakness can be on one or both sides of the face and may be permanent or temporary. MRS is a recurrent disease, and attacks can last from days to several years. MRS typically starts in childhood or early adulthood. Females are slightly more prone to being affected than males.

Causes

The exact cause of MRS is unknown; however, genetics, infectious agents, environmental factors such as allergies, and autoimmune diseases may play a role in the cause of MRS. In some cases, MRS is thought to be genetic, as the characteristic folded tongue has been described as a characteristic of these families. However, no specific gene has been recognized as causing MRS.

Signs and Symptoms

The signs and symptoms of MRS include the characteristic features previously described: facial swelling, facial paralysis or weakness, and folds or creases in the tongue. Typically, swelling is the first symptom that occurs and most often affects the upper lip. It is also usually the most prevailing sign. Other symptoms may include a reduced sense of taste and diminished secretion from the salivary glands. The lips also may become cracked and painful and might become discolored. Other symptoms including headaches, fever, and vision troubles are sometimes associated with MRS.

Diagnosis

Diagnosing MRS can be difficult, as the signs and symptoms may not always point toward MRS, and the characteristic findings do not always occur together. MRS can also emulate other diseases and conditions. A variety of tests are used to help diagnose MRS. These tests include the physical exam, history, laboratory tests, patch tests, imaging studies, histological studies, and biopsy. Many of these tests are performed to help rule out other diseases and conditions. Disorders related to MRS include Crohn's disease, sarcoidosis, orofacial granulomatosis, and Bell's palsy. History and physical examination can help to rule out other causes, as can many of the other tests. Imaging tests include radiographs, endoscopy, and positron emission tomography (PET) scans. Patch tests are used to rule out reactions to various substances such as metals and other antigens. Probably one of the most important tests to help exclude other causes and to conclusively diagnose MRS is a biopsy.

Treatment

Treatment for MRS is based mostly on symptoms. It can be hard to treat MRS, as no specific cause has been identified. The most common form of treatment is medication. Medications include nonsteroidal anti-inflammatory drugs (NSAIDS), corticosteroids, antibiotics, and immunosuppressants. The NSAIDS and corticosteroids are used to help reduce swelling. One study reported success in treatment by using intralesional triamcinolone (Rachisan et al., 2012). Surgery and radiation may also be necessary and recommended for treatment. These treatments are aimed toward swelling reduction. Surgery can be used to help facial paralysis or weakness by surgically decompressing the nerves. The efficacy of surgery and radiation has yet to be recognized. If MRS is left untreated, the attacks may start to last longer and occur more often. More research is needed to determine the best course of treatment for MRS. Research currently focuses on increasing awareness and knowledge of MRS. It also focuses on treatment and prevention of the disease as well as trying to find a cure.

Shannen McNamara

See also: Bell's Palsy; Facial Nerve; National Organization for Rare Disorders; Taste System

Further Reading

Kang, Owen, & Frank Gaillard. (n.d.). Melkersson-Rosenthal syndrome. *Radiopaedia Online*. Retrieved from http://radiopaedia.org/articles/melkersson-rosenthal-syndrome

National Institute of Neurological Disorders and Stroke. (2011). *NINDS Melkersson-Rosenthal syndrome information page*. Retrieved from http://www.ninds.nih.gov/disorders/melkersson/melkersson.htm

National Organization for Rare Disorders (NORD). (2015). *Melkersson-Rosenthal syndrome*. Retrieved from http://rarediseases.org/rare-diseases/melkersson-rosenthal-syndrome/

Rachisan, Andreea L., et al. (2012). Granulomatous cheilitis of Miescher: The diagnostic proof for a Melkersson-Rosenthal syndrome. *Romanian Journal of Morphology and Embryology, 53*(3), 851–853. Retrieved from http://www.rjme.ro/RJME/resources/files/531312851853.pdf

Scully, Crispian. (2015). *Cheilitis granulomatosa*. Retrieved from http://emedicine.medscape.com/article/1075333-overview

MEMBRANE POTENTIAL: DEPOLARIZATION AND HYPERPOLARIZATION

In an animal's nervous system, brain cells called neurons are unique in the fact that they transmit electrical signals or action potential down their axons. It is this action potential that brings the sensory information from the body to the brain. The word *depolarization* means in physiological terms any reduction in the voltage difference across the cell membrane, which can mean a graded potential as well as an action potential. Hyperpolarization or repolarization is the opposite of depolarization, meaning the increase in the voltage difference across the cell membrane, which results in "preventing" depolarization. In relation to an action potential, depolarization is the first phase, or rising phase, of an action potential, while hyperpolarization is the last phase, or falling phase, of an action potential. In general, depolarization and action potentials occur in unidirectional motor neurons, meaning that the action potential travels away from the neuron's cell body and down its axon. An action potential is a short-lasting electrical impulse on the plasma membrane of cells.

Resting Membrane Potential

A neuron has fingerlike projections surrounding the soma known as dendrites as well as a single axon. The dendrites capture the electrical or chemical signals being sent from other neurons. If the signal is large enough, the dendrite will conduct the impulse to other parts of the cell. More specifically, the signal is transferred from the dendrites to the soma. Once it reaches the soma, the signal continues to an area known as the axon hillock. If the signal is large enough to elicit an action potential, it will conduct this electrical potential down the axon and finally to the axon's terminal branches.

When neurons are at rest they present an uneven distribution of ions across the plasma membrane. This means that the inside of a neuron is more negatively charged than the outside of a neuron. This phenomenon is known as resting membrane potential, which is essentially the voltage difference between the inside and outside of a cell. The main ions that create this uneven distribution of charges across the plasma membrane are sodium (Na^+), which has a significantly higher concentration (both chemically and electrically) outside the cell, and potassium (K^+), which is significantly more abundant inside the cell. Even though both of these are cations, the degree of positivity is greater outside the cell compared to the inside, with the inside of the cell having a net charge that is negative. Thus, a charge difference or electric gradient is created across the cell's plasma membrane. It is important to note that the majority of a neuron's cytoplasm and the extracellular fluid that surrounds the outside of the neuron are electrically neutral. The charge difference only occurs across the cell membrane where the cations line the plasma membrane on both sides.

Membrane Potential

One way of modifying the distribution of ionic charges is through facilitated diffusion. Facilitated diffusion is the process of allowing the ions to flow from areas of high concentration gradients to areas of low concentration gradients. There are specific channels or pumps that allow this to occur. Many different types of channels exist that allow this exchange to happen, but most are Na^+, K^+, and/or chloride (Cl^-) channels. The channels are made of specific proteins that are bound to the plasma membrane. The first type of ion channel is known as a leakage channel. These channels are always open, allowing ions to freely flow into and out of the neuron; however, they do conduct the flow of ions in one direction if a certain voltage difference is reached across the membrane.

A second type of ion channel, which is not always open, is known as a gated channel. A ligand-gated channel is a type of channel that opens upon chemical stimulation. These channels bind to specific types of neurotransmitters (natural and/or manmade chemicals) in order for them to open. Once they open, because there is a greater distribution of Na^+ outside the cell, diffusion will occur down the electrochemical gradient, creating an inflow of Na^+ inside the cell. While this is happening, there is also an outflow of K^+ outside the cell. The result of this chemical transfer causes a local depolarization of the plasma membrane, known as a graded potential.

Depolarization

Depolarization occurs when there is more positive charge inside the cell than outside. The greater the stimulus, specifically what is received at the dendrites, the greater the depolarization will spread throughout a given neuron. Therefore the more neurotransmitter that is dumped onto the ligand-gated channels, the more channels will open. In turn, increased amounts of Na^+ will flow into the cell, resulting in a greater depolarization. The depolarization of a cell membrane decays with distance from the stimulus. This means that the depolarization will be much greater around the dendrites and the soma of a neuron versus the axon terminal branches.

If a stimulus is strong enough, it will depolarize a neuron all the way to the axon hillock. The majority of neurons at rest usually have a voltage of –70 mV. They depolarize when Na^+ flows inward and changes the voltage inside the cell to be more positive. When a neuron's membrane potential is depolarized by a 15 mV threshold, which is –55 mV for a resting membrane potential of –70 mV, the production of an action potential will occur. This is because action potentials follow the "all-or-none" law, which is defined by a neuron responding to a stimulus completely or not at all. For most neurons, the membrane potential must reach a threshold between –60 mV and –45 mV to overcome this all-or-none phenomenon.

Once the local current reaches the axon hillock and the membrane potential is at or above the threshold, voltage-gated channels along the axon open. These channels will allow more Na^+ to enter the cell's axon at their location, which allows the action potential to be elicited and conducted. These specialized proteins are called voltage-gated channels because the –55 mV threshold generates enough voltage to open the channels.

There are two main types of voltage-gated channels: fast-opening Na^+ channels and slow-opening K^+ channels. The first ones to open are the Na^+ voltage-gated channels, allowing all the Na^+ present on the outside of the cell to flow into the axon through normal diffusion. This causes the neuron to be depolarized at the axon level. The more Na^+ that enters the axon hillock, the more adjacent Na^+ voltage-gated channels open up, creating a positive feedback loop. This phenomenon progresses throughout the entire length of the axon, causing the inside of the cell to change from –55 mV to +30 mV almost instantaneously. This radical shift of opening Na^+ channels shows how the neuron's membrane changes its permeability so that Na^+ can rush down its electrochemical gradient and quickly depolarize a cell.

Hyperpolarization

Once the voltage reaches between +30 mV and +50 mV, the depolarization phase of an action potential hits its peak. Immediately, the voltage-gated Na^+ channels close and the voltage-gated K^+ channels open. This is the beginning of the hyperpolarization phase or the falling phase of an action potential, which brings the membrane potential back toward the cell's resting membrane potential. Repolarization occurs when the voltage-gated K^+ channels open, causing K^+ to flow down its electrochemical gradient and exit the cell. Again, this radical shift of closing Na+ channels and opening K^+ channels shows how the neuron's membrane changes its permeability quickly so that K^+ ions can rush out of the cell.

During the falling phase, Cl^- channels also open and allow these anions to enter the cell. This makes the membrane potential to become even more negative. Since the K^+ channels are slow at opening and closing, the membrane potential will go past (or undershoot) the resting potential. This makes the neuron hyperpolarized as well as making it more difficult for another action potential to occur. This more negative membrane potential is called the refractory period, which makes the neuron physiologically unable to generate another action potential until this period is over. Eventually, through the leakage channels and pumps, the neuron's membrane voltage returns to its resting membrane potential of –70 mV. This process occurs over and over again and is the primary way neurons and their target cells communication with each other.

Michael Romani and Jennifer L. Hellier

See also: Action Potential; Axon; Sensory Receptors

Further Reading

Hall, John E., & Arthur C. Guyton. (2011). *Guyton and Hall textbook of medical physiology.* Philadelphia, PA: Saunders/Elsevier.

Kandel, Eric R., James H. Schwartz, Thomas M. Jessell, Steven A. Siegelbaum, & A. J. Hudspeth (Eds.). (2012). *Principles of neural science* (5th ed.). New York, NY: McGraw-Hill.

Marieb, Elaine N., Patricia B. Wilhelm, & Jon B. Mallatt. (2011). *Human anatomy* (6th ed.). San Francisco, CA: Pearson Education.

Thibodeau, G. A., C. P. Anthony, & K.T. Patton. (2007). *Anthony's textbook of anatomy & physiology.* St. Louis, MO: Mosby.

MENIERE'S DISEASE

Meniere's disease is a disease of the inner ear named after the French physician Prosper Meniere (1799–1862), who first described this disease in 1861. Symptoms often include (1) loss of hearing, particularly in the lower-frequency bands, (2) tinnitus or ringing in the ears, and (3) vertigo, which is described as a "whirling" or spinning movement where patients feel as if they are moving when in fact they are not. It is often accompanied by nausea and/or vomiting as well as problems with balance and equilibrium. This is often the most severe presenting symptom of this disease.

At this time, there is no known definitive cause of Meniere's disease. There is evidence it may be related to a buildup of excess fluid in the inner ear, and further studies are being done to determine other causes, if any. Diagnosis is often established through a review of patient symptoms. There are currently no reliable objective diagnostic tools available to determine if a patient has this disease. Treatment is aimed at decreasing the prevailing symptoms a patient might have.

Pathology

Meniere's disease is thought to be linked to changes in quantity and pressure of the fluids found within the inner ear. Current data suggest that individuals with Meniere's disease have an excess of fluid in the inner ear and that this fluid "escapes" the inner ear proper and enters other areas of the cochlea. This condition is called hydrops of the inner ear. Under normal conditions, this fluid is constantly being produced and recycled. With hydrops, this fluid is unable to recycle, resulting in a pressure buildup within the cochlea, which is thought to cause swelling of the tissues of the vestibular and auditory systems of the ear. This pressure buildup is then thought to interfere with the normal function of the semicircular canals, which results in the nausea and vertigo that many patients exhibit.

Diagnosis

Diagnosis of Meniere's disease is difficult at best. It is considered an idiopathic disease, meaning there is at this time no known cause for the disease. There are currently no reliable diagnostic tests or imaging studies that can be done to definitively diagnose this disease. Physicians often make this diagnosis after ruling out other diseases such as bacterial/viral inner-ear infections, or nervous system tumors such as a vestibular schwannoma. This means that the diagnosis of Meniere's disease is often a diagnosis of exclusion. It is diagnosed when as many other diseases/pathologies as possible are ruled out.

The American Academy of Otolaryngology has made an attempt to establish some minimal criteria that may help with the diagnosis of Meniere's disease. These criteria were first introduced in 1972 and amended in 1985. They include (1) a fluctuating, progressive loss of hearing over an unspecified period of time, (2) incidents of vertigo lasting 20 minutes to 24 hours with no loss of consciousness and the presence of vestibular nystagmus, and (3) the onset of tinnitus or a ringing in the ears.

Management

While there are currently no recognized medical treatments for Meniere's disease, research has found some dietary and pharmacologic treatments that seem to help some patients to varying degrees. A growing body of evidence suggests that diets high in salt could be an exacerbating factor in the onset of Meniere's disease as high salt concentrations in the body fluid tend to cause retention of fluid. Patients are often advised to maintain a low-sodium diet in an attempt to prevent fluid buildup within the inner ear. In addition to a low-salt diet, some patients have been prescribed medications called diuretics, which are designed to increase the frequency of urination and keep the buildup of body fluids to a minimum.

Individuals affected by this disease are also advised to avoid consuming significant quantities of alcohol or caffeine, and to avoid tobacco products, all of which have been shown to increase the severity of the symptoms of Meniere's disease.

Prognosis

Currently, the prognosis for the successful treatment and elimination of the symptoms of Meniere's disease is not very positive. While this disease often starts out only affecting one ear, most patients eventually develop symptoms in both ears. Many patients will eventually become disabled to the point of being unable to function normally in society. It is important to remember that the severity of symptoms is quite variable and that the differences between individuals as to the extent of disability are quite extreme.

Charles A. Ferguson

See also: Auditory System; Cochlea; Dizziness; Vestibular System

Further Reading

Bear, Mark F., Barry W. Connors, & Michael A. Paradiso. (2001). *Neuroscience: Exploring the brain*. Philadelphia, PA: Lippincott Williams and Wilkins.

Greenberg, Simon L., & Julian M. Nedzelski. (2010). Medical and noninvasive therapy for Meniere's disease. *The Otolaryngologic Clinics of North America, 43*(5), 1081–1090.

Horner, K. C. (1991). Old theme and new reflections: Hearing impairment associated with endolymphatic hydrops. *Hearing Research, 52*, 147–156.

MERKEL CELL

The human sense of touch is complex and relies on several types of cells in the skin to detect different types of stimuli. Touch receptors can be divided into two categories: mechanoreceptors, which detect pressure or movement, and thermoreceptors, which detect changes in temperature. Most touch receptors are specialized nerve cells. The cells responsible for the sensation of light touch or pressure are known as Merkel cells, named after the German anatomist Friedrich Sigmund Merkel (1845–1919) who discovered them in the late 19th century. Friedrich Merkel originally named them "tastzellen" or "touch cells" before other types of touch receptors had been discovered. It has been more than 100 years since their discovery and the origin and role of Merkel cells are not yet fully understood; in fact, it was only recently that scientists discovered that Merkel cells are highly specialized epithelial (skin) cells rather than neural receptor cells. It is also thought that Merkel cells can detect texture and shape of stimuli in addition to faint touch sensations, although there is ongoing research to confirm these functions.

Location

Skin is a complex organ made of three distinct tissue layers. The outermost layer (the one we are able to see and feel) is called the epidermis; the middle and thickest layer is called the dermis; and at the bottom is a layer of fat known as the subcutaneous tissue. The epidermis contains five of its own distinct layers, and Merkel cells are located near the bottom of the epidermis in the stratum basale (basal layer). Interestingly, this is the same layer where melanocytes, or skin pigment cells, are located. This location is vital to the functional success of Merkel cells; the stratum basale is deep enough to provide adequate protection of sensory cells but close enough to the surface that light touch can be detected. Other types of touch receptor cells are located deeper in the skin and are responsible for sensation of stronger stimuli, such as pain and temperature. Merkel cells have been found to cluster around sweat glands and hair follicles and are present in certain mucosal tissues.

Pathology

The most common disease that affects Merkel cells is Merkel cell carcinoma, an aggressive but rare skin cancer. The first signs are small, painless, firm nodules in the skin that grow rapidly after detection. Merkel cell carcinoma usually appears on areas of the skin that face the most sun exposure, such as the head, face, and neck, and can spread aggressively to many other tissues and organs. It most commonly affects adult Caucasian males and individuals with weakened immune systems. It is often confused with other carcinomas and may be misdiagnosed, but the treatment procedure for Merkel cell carcinoma is similar to that for other skin cancers. Once diagnosed, it is crucial to receive treatment as soon as possible.

Up to 80 percent of Merkel cell carcinomas are caused by Merkel cell polyomavirus (MCV), which is one of the few known human oncoviruses (cancer-causing viruses). The mode of transmission of MCV is unknown; fortunately, a person infected with MCV is not contagious and will not transmit the virus further. The remaining 20 percent of Merkel cell carcinomas have unknown origins. Health care providers suggest that Merkel cell carcinoma may be avoided by taking the same precautions one would take for other skin cancers: limit sun exposure and use sunscreen if exposure cannot be avoided.

Kendra DeHay

See also: Discriminative Touch; Meissner's Corpuscles; Mirror-Touch Synesthesia; Pacinian Corpuscles; Touch

Further Reading

Lumpkin, Ellen A., Kara L. Marshall, & Aislyn M. Nelson. (2010). The cell biology of touch. *Journal of Cell Biology*, 191(2), 237–248. Retrieved from http://jcb.rupress.org/content/191/2/237.full

Moll, Ingrid, Marion Roessler, Johanna M. Brandner, Ann-Christin Eispert, Pia Houdek, & Roland Moll. (2005). Human Merkel cells—aspects of cell biology, distribution and functions. *European Journal of Cell Biology*, 84(2–3), 259–271.

National Cancer Institute. (2015). Merkel cell carcinoma treatment. Retrieved from http://www.cancer.gov/types/skin/patient/merkel-cell-treatment-pdq

MICROPHTHALMIA

Microphthalmia, also known as microphthalmos, is an eye abnormality that arises before birth. This condition can affect one or both eyeballs, causing them to be abnormally small. The eyeball could appear to be completely missing, but eye tissue is still present. This condition is often confused with anophthalmia, in which no eyeball forms at all before birth. Microphthalmia may or may not result in significant vision loss. A condition called coloboma often accompanies microphthalmia. Colobomas are missing pieces of the tissue structures from the eye. There could be an appearance of notches or gaps in the iris (the colored part of the eye), the retina, the choroid (blood vessel under the retina), or the optic nerve. They could be present in one or both eyes and could affect a person's vision.

Many other eye abnormalities may accompany microphthalmia. These abnormalities include but are not limited to clouding of the lens (cataract), narrowing of the eye opening (narrowed palpebral fissure), and microcornea.

Causes

Microphthalmia occurs in approximately 1 in every 10,000 individuals. It may be caused by changes or mutations in genes involved in early development of the eye. Many of these gene mutations have not yet been identified. It could also result from a chromosomal abnormality (Trisomy 13) that affects one or more genes. Most genetic changes related to microphthalmia have only been identified in a small number of affected individuals. Environmental factors may also cause microphthalmia. Factors affecting the early development of the eye include but are not limited to vitamin deficiency, radiation, infections (rubella, herpes, or cytomegalovirus), or exposure to substances (alcohol or drugs) that cause birth defects (teratogens). Microphthalmia has an autosomal recessive pattern of inheritance. This means that both copies of the mutated gene in each cell must be present, meaning both parents carry one copy of the mutated gene. Parents typically do not show signs or symptoms of the condition. Microphthalmia is often not inherited and only affects one individual in a family.

Fetal Alcohol Syndrome

Microphthalmia is sometimes associated with fetal alcohol syndrome. It is important to understand that there is no safe amount of alcohol to use during pregnancy and as a result, there is a wide range of effects such as microphthalmia based on the dose and timing of the alcohol exposure. The timing of the alcohol exposure will determine the variations of the anatomical effects in the developing fetus. Because the fetal development occurs over the course of several months, critical structures may be affected at various periods. In addition, the dose or amount of alcohol consumed also plays a critical role in the damage that can occur. If you have a critical period of development, timing, and a dose high enough to cause damage, the fetus will be impacted by the prenatal alcohol exposure. One example of this is the facial development of the fetus. This occurs during the embryonic period of gestation or around the third and fourth weeks after conception. Drinking alcohol during this time may result in damage to the face, causing the dysmorphic facial features including short palpebral fissures (small eye opening), microphthalmia, smooth philtrum (area under the nose that typically has a ridge is now smoothed and flattened), and thin upper lip. An individual who has the dysmorphic face will also have some degree of brain injury due to the prenatal alcohol exposure.

Treatment

Treatments of microphthalmia are very limited. Most of the treatments just involve support. A doctor may patch the better eye to encourage the poorer eye to develop better vision. If other issues like glaucoma or cataracts arise, treatment could include using drops or performing operations. Family members and friends can support the affected individual in wearing glasses or contact lenses. The corrective lenses ensure that the vision regions of the brain will grow and develop correctly. Prescription eye drops should also be used regularly.

Renee Johnson

See also: Amblyopia; Anophthalmia; Visual Fields; Visual System

Further Reading

Blaikie, Andrew. (n.d.). *Medical information on microphthalmia*. Scottish Sensory Centre. Retrieved from http://www.ssc.education.ed.ac.uk/resources/vi&multi/eyeconds/Micro.html

Genetics Home Reference. (2011). Microphthalmia. Retrieved from https://ghr.nlm.nih.gov/condition/microphthalmia

Minnesota Department of Health. (n.d.). Anophthalmia and microphthalmia. Retrieved from http://www.health.state.mn.us/divs/cfh/topic/diseasesconds/anophthalmia.cfm

MIRROR-TOUCH SYNESTHESIA

Individuals with mirror-touch synesthesia (also known as vision-touch synesthesia) experience the sensations that they observe in others. For instance, if a mirror-touch synesthete saw an individual slap their knee, they would feel the sensation as if they had hit their own knee.

History and Indicators

Synesthesia has been known to exist for the past 300 years and was thought to be quite rare, mainly because people with the condition maintained silence about their experiences when they realized theirs were not typical. However, Blakemore and colleagues recorded the first official report of a single case of mirror-touch synesthesia in 2005. Vision-touch synesthesia is very unique as it is the tactile sensation or feeling that the synesthete is being touched when he or she sees another person being touched in the same manner. There are two variants of vision-touch synesthesia: body-centered reference frame and viewer-centered reference frame. In body-centered reference frame, the sensation of touch may be mirrored by the synesthete. For instance, if the synesthete saw a person being touched on the left side of her face, the synesthete would experience a tactile sensation on the right side of his or her face, hence the name mirror-touch synesthesia. Other synesthetes will feel the touch sensation on the same side of the face as the actual person being touched (using the same example, both will feel the touch on the left side of the face). This type of vision-touch synesthesia is called viewer-centered reference frame.

Prevalence of Vision-Touch Synesthesia

It is estimated that 1.6 percent of people have some sort of vision-touch synesthesia, with the body-centered reference frame (or mirror-touch) being more common. There are a few vision-touch synesthetes who also have the ability to feel touch on their body or hands when they see an object being touched. Testing vision-touch synesthesia for those who have sensations when objects were touched, researchers touched a mannequin or dummy to see if this would induce a response. For some of these synesthetes, seeing a human-related object (like the head or foot) being touched induced fewer or less intense viewer-centered or body-centered reference frame responses. However, in a very few vision-touch synesthetes, seeing a rubber hand being touched had a greater response; in fact these synesthetes actually felt as if their own hand had been replaced by the rubber hand. This is called rubber hand illusion, which can occur even when another person is not touching the rubber/mannequin's hand. No other body part elicits the same type of illusion. To date, research has observed that only an object that has the form of a human hand is associated with rubber hand illusion.

Theories of Vision-Touch Synesthesia

Currently there are two theories of mirror-touch synesthesia: threshold theory and self-other theory. Threshold theory states that this type of synesthesia is the extreme end-point of normal brain mechanisms, meaning that the somatosensory system has crossed a threshold of awareness of others being touched that the majority of people's somatosensory systems have not crossed. Self-other theory states that the synesthetes are not able to distinguish self from others, meaning that this atypical self-other representation in the brain is amplified when seeing another person being touched.

Jennifer L. Hellier

See also: Auditory-Tactile Synesthesia; Grapheme-Color Synesthesia; Lexical-Gustatory Synesthesia; Synesthesia

Further Reading

Bolognini, Nadia. (2015). Causal mechanisms of mirror-touch synesthesia: Clues from neuropsychology. *Cognitive Neuroscience, 6*(2–3), 137–139.

Heyes, Cecilia, & Caroline Catmur. (2015). A task control theory of mirror-touch synesthesia. *Cognitive Neuroscience, 6*(2–3), 141–142.

Meier, Beat, Katrin Lunke, & Nicolas Rothen. (2015). How mirror-touch informs theories of synesthesia. *Cognitive Neuroscience, 6*(2–3), 142–144.

Ward, Jamie, & Michael J. Banissy. (2015). Explaining mirror-touch synesthesia. *Cognitive Neuroscience, 6*(2–3), 118–133.

MISOPHONIA

One of the least beneficial forms of synesthesia is misophonia or the "hatred of sound." This condition is extremely rare and results in strong, specific, negative adverse emotions in response to the specific sounds of other people breathing and eating. Repetitive sounds typically produced by other people like chewing, pen clicking, or tapping trigger misophonia. During a trigger event, the person may become defensive or offensive, agitated, and possibly act out and express anger or rage at the offending sound's source in an actual fight-or-flight reflex. The reaction to these sounds makes the misophone (person with misophonia) avoid situations where these sounds may be produced and limits the misophone's ability to interact professionally and socially.

Causes and Symptoms

Misophonia, also referred to as selective sound sensitivity syndrome, may be caused by faulty or hyperconnectivity between the limbic system and the auditory cortex. This condition may be hereditary with at least one family relative suffering from it. There are some similarities between misophonia and tinnitus (persistent ringing in the ears when no actual sound is present). The difference between tinnitus and misophonia is primarily in terms of where the sound is located. Misophonia is sound produced by other people while tinnitus is internally perceived sound. Neuroimaging findings may provide hypotheses on the neural basis of misophonia including linking in relevant sensory regions or an actual increase of anatomical connectivity. Pathological distortions between limbic structures and the auditory cortex could be a cause of misophonia. Misophonia may be exaggerated mechanisms already present in the general population—many of the common aversive stimuli are also deemed socially inappropriate in Western society.

Particular sounds made by other people provoke particular reactions: the worst trigger sounds tend to be chewing, pen clicking, crunching, and clock ticking. Other common trigger sounds include clicking, typing, and whistling. The person with misophonia will have a range of negative emotions, thoughts, and even physical reactions that are triggered by these sounds. Trigger sounds are felt as intrusive or disgusting and evoke anger, extreme irritation, intense anxiety, and strong feelings of being violated for the individual with misophonia. Physical symptoms include pressure on the chest, sweaty palms, tense and tightened muscles, difficulty breathing, and an increase in blood pressure and body temperature. These reactions and endless discomfort can have a serious impact on the misophone's daily life. Interactions within personal and work relationships can be affected and the potential for social isolation exists, especially if the misophone is trying to avoid problematic situations. Pharmacological agents affect misophonia. For most persons with misophonia, caffeine will intensify their reactions to the offending sound while alcohol decreases the adverse response. Self-induced trigger sounds will not evoke as much of an adverse reaction and neither will the sounds produced by animals or babies. This implies an underlying social component to misophonia.

Misophones commonly describe the onset of misophonia in childhood with responses evoked by trigger sounds modulated by context, sound source, and prior knowledge. Many times, it is the people who are the closest to the misophone or the people they are exposed to frequently who elicit the worst triggers, which can make personal relationships stressful and difficult. School settings and workplaces can also become an issue, especially if the misophone has little input in shaping that environment. Sometimes, the sound environment can make keeping a job intolerable with supervisory or teaching staff not really understanding the issue. Misophones describe themselves as being hyperfocused on background noise.

Treatment

Mimicking trigger sounds is an effective coping strategy. It appears to "overwrite" the disturbing sound and sometimes functions as a way to retaliate against the offending individual producing the sound. Some of the current treatments for misophonia are Neurofeedback (NFB), Cognitive Behavioral Therapy (CBT), psycho-therapeutic hypnotherapy, Tinnitus Retraining Therapy (TRT), and Neural Repatterning Technique/Trigger Tamer. The use of ear plugs, sound masking, and sound machines is often effective and helpful.

Carolyn Johnson Atwater

See also: Auditory Processing Disorder; Auditory System; Auditory-Tactile Synesthesia; Synesthesia

Further Reading

Cavanna, Andrea E., & Stefano Seri. (2015). Misophonia: Current perspectives. *Neuropsychiatric Disease and Treatment, 11*, 2117–2123. http://dx.doi.org/10.2147/NDT.S81438

Ro, Tony, Timothy M. Ellmore, & Michael S. Beauchamp. (2013). A neural link between feeling and hearing. *Cerebral Cortex, 23*, 1724–1730.

MOBIUS SYNDROME

Mobius syndrome is a congenital and rare neurological disorder that affects approximately 2 individuals in every 1 million births worldwide (1 individual in every 50,000 births in the United States). This disorder is characterized by facial muscle weakness/paralysis due to paralysis (palsy) of the sixth (abducens) and seventh (facial) cranial nerves. These nerves enter and exit from the back of the brain in the brainstem and are critical for the movement of facial muscles and in particular back and forth (lateral) eye movement. One of the distinguishing symptoms of Mobius syndrome is the inability to look left and right and the need to turn one's head to see to either side of the body. In some individuals the eighth (vestibulocochlear) cranial nerve is also involved. At this point, there is no known effective treatment for this disorder.

Mobius syndrome is named after Paul Julius Mobius (1853–1907), a German neurologist who fully described this syndrome in 1892. Mobius syndrome is a congenital disease and not something that an individual can develop after birth. Individuals born with Mobius syndrome have significant weakness or paralysis of the facial muscles and as a result are often unable to frown, move their eyebrows, smile, and have significant difficulty with feeding early in life due to a smaller than average mouth size and weakness in the muscles associated with sucking. These individuals also tend to have smaller than average chins (micrognathia) and smaller than normal tongues. In addition, these individuals often have difficulty with speech and exhibit significant dental problems.

There are currently four classifications/groups of Mobius syndrome. Group I individuals often exhibit simple hypoplasia or atrophy of the cranial nerve nuclei. Group II individuals will exhibit more significant lesions in the peripheral cranial nerves. Group III individuals start to show focal (localized) necrosis (death) of neuronal nuclei in the brainstem, and group IV individuals exhibit primary myopathies with no central nervous system or cranial nerve lesions.

In addition to defects seen in the face and skull, individuals with Mobius syndrome can also have general skeletal system defects. These include the presence of clubbed feet, shorter than average tibial and fibular lengths, and scoliosis. It is not uncommon to also find defects specifically of the hand including syndactyly (webbing of the fingers), absence of some fingers, and/or underdevelopment of the fingers. Lastly, some individuals may also demonstrate lack of development of the pectoral muscles of the chest. This in conjunction with scoliosis is a contributing factor to the respiratory problems that some individuals with this syndrome exhibit.

Etiology

While there is no specific known cause for Mobius syndrome, there is a growing body of evidence that the cause is most likely a combination of both environmental and genetic factors. No specific genes have been identified to date that may be the cause of this syndrome, but there is evidence that there may be changes in chromosomes 3, 10, and/or 13 in some families. There is also a growing body of evidence that this syndrome could be due in part to a disruption of blood flow to the brainstem during early fetal development, which could be a leading cause of the atrophy of the sixth and seventh cranial nerves. It is important to note that this evidence is very preliminary and much more research needs to be performed.

There is also evidence that some medications, if taken during pregnancy, could contribute to the development of this syndrome. In particular, studies completed in Brazil have shown that mothers who take misoprostol, which is a drug that is occasionally used to induce labor, or thalidomide, which was used to treat nausea during pregnancy, increase their chances of giving birth to a fetus with Mobius syndrome by a factor of 30.

Treatment

While there is no specific treatment today that can be used to prevent this syndrome, it is not uncommon to treat the secondary symptoms and difficulties that arise from this syndrome. Treatment teams often consist of neurologists, orthopedic surgeons, and plastic surgeons, to name a few. If a patient has involvement of cranial nerve VIII, an audiologist is also often part of the treatment team. Experimental surgeries that are designed to increase nervous system innervation of affected muscles as well as increase vascular supply to affected areas continue to be examined as a possible mode of treatment for this syndrome (https://www.youtube.com/watch?v=zj6om25_KX4). For individuals with significant skeletal system defects, the use of physical therapy has been shown to relieve some of the symptoms of this syndrome. Research continues to try to determine the exact cause of this syndrome and to develop more specific treatments.

Charles A. Ferguson

See also: Brain Anatomy; Brainstem; Facial Nerve; National Organization for Rare Disorders; Sacks, Oliver Wolf; Visual System

Further Reading

Bogart, Kathleen R. (2014). "People are all about appearances": A focus group of teenagers with Moebius syndrome. *Journal of Health Psychology.* http://dx.doi.org/10.1177/1359105313517277

Koren, G., & L. Schuler. (2001). Taking drugs during pregnancy. How safe are the unsafe? *Canadian Family Physician, 47,* 951–953.

National Organization for Rare Disorders (NORD). (2014). Moebius syndrome. Retrieved from http://rarediseases.org/rare-diseases/moebius-syndrome/

St. Louis Children's Hospital. (2014). Dawson's smile: Facial reanimation surgery for a child with Mobius syndrome. Retrieved from https://www.youtube.com/watch?v=zj6om25_KX4

MOSQUITO MACHINE

The Mosquito machine (or Mosquito alarm) was designed to discourage teenagers from loitering. The Mosquito machine works by emitting a high-frequency sound that can only be heard by people under 25 years of age. Younger people find the high-frequency sound annoying and will not loiter in areas with the sound. The Mosquito machine also discourages vandalism and graffiti by deterring youth from spending time in an area with the sound. Older people, on the other hand, are unable to hear the sound and are unaffected by the Mosquito machine.

History

Howard Stapleton (1966–) developed the Mosquito machine in 2005 in Wales. He released the technology to be purchased as an alarm through his company, Compound Security Solutions, in 2006. Later, Moving Sound Technologies started distributing the Mosquito machine in North America. Initially, Stapleton aimed his product at shop owners in cities with teen loitering problems. The Mosquito machine currently has customers throughout the world including school districts, shops, and transit hubs.

The Mosquito machine works by emitting high-pitched sound only audible to people under 25 years of age. The sound was selected because adults cannot hear the pitch; the sound is annoying to those who can hear it, yet exposure to the sound is not believed to damage hearing. Moving Sound Technologies, the company that markets the Mosquito machine in North America, has audio demonstrations on their website that allow people to test their hearing and determine whether they can hear the Mosquito machine pitches (Mosquito Audio Demo, 2012). Moving Sound Technologies also claims that the Mosquito machine is safe for all ages, meets all known U.S. sound regulations, and will not bother younger children or dogs (Mosquito FAQs, 2012).

Current Use

Currently, the companies marketing the Mosquito machine report successful use in many countries, but not all cities are welcoming the use of this technology. Opposition to the Mosquito machine is based on the idea that specifically targeting teenagers is discriminatory and may violate basic human and civil rights. The sound can be viewed as an invasion of personal space, and concerns have been raised that exposure to high-frequency sound could be damaging to hearing. Any action to target a specific group of people could later have discriminatory uses, particularly when the technology could be used to prevent people in a certain age range from moving around freely in public.

To address these concerns, cities may impose limits on the time and duration of use of the Mosquito machine. The city of Sheffield in South Yorkshire, England, has completely banned use of Mosquito machines. Other cities may consider limiting the duration and time of use of the Mosquito machine. For example, schools have reported a decrease in vandalism if the Mosquito machine is on during the hours when students should not be at the school. If the Mosquito machine continues to be used, in the future, cities may be challenged by human rights activists or concerned parents to limit or ban the use of Mosquito machines.

Not to be dissuaded by concerns about age discrimination, teenagers have found ways to make the Mosquito machine technology useful rather than antagonistic by creating a cellphone ringtone using the same frequencies. The ringtone, often called teen buzz, can be heard by teens and people under age 25, but not by most adults. Since many schools require ringers and alerts on cellphones to be silenced during classes, the teen buzz ringtone allows teens to communicate during class using a ringtone that most of their teachers cannot hear.

Future

Additional studies need to be conducted to verify the safety of high-pitched sounds on children's hearing. If the Mosquito machine continues to be viewed as a valid option to prevent teen loitering and the resulting vandalism, cities may be challenged to create laws surrounding the approved use of this technology.

Lisa A. Rabe

See also: Age-Related Hearing Loss; Auditory System; Tinnitus

Further Reading

Compound Security Systems. (2014). Mosquito MK4 (anti-loitering device). Retrieved from http://www.compoundsecurity.co.uk/security-equipment-mosquito-mk4-anti-loitering-device

Local teen wins campaign to ban controversial device. (2011, February 22). *Sheffield Telegraph*. Retrieved from http://www.sheffieldtelegraph.co.uk/news/local/local-teen-wins-campaign-to-ban-controversial-device-1-3104497

Mosquito Audio Demo. (2012). Retrieved from http://www.movingsoundtech.com/about-the-mosiquito/mosquito-faq

Mosquito FAQs. (2012). Retrieved from http://www.movingsoundtech.com/about-the-mosiquito/mosquito-faq

MOTION SICKNESS

Motion sickness is a multifaceted condition in which a person experiences several unpleasant symptoms during actual or sensed motion. It is a common problem that has been recognized for hundreds of years. During biblical times, it was known as "camel sickness" as that was one of the main forms of travel and often made people feel sick. When travel by sea became prevalent, it was known as seasickness. The word nausea is derived from the Greek word *naus* meaning ship.

Causes and Risk Factors

The cause of motion sickness is complex and not entirely understood. The brain senses motion using several signaling pathways. These include the inner ear, eyes, and special receptors called proprioceptors. The inner ear contains the vestibular system, which includes three semicircular canals, saccule, and utricle. The function of these organs is to sense motion, spatial orientation, and other sensory information, and they also play a role in maintaining equilibrium. Motion sickness is believed to occur when the different signaling pathways have conflicting sensory information when exposed to a motion stimulus. This creates a conflict in sensory input to the brain, which creates abnormal sensory processing.

Anyone can be affected by motion sickness, although some people are more likely to be affected than others. There is no direct way to guess who will be affected; however, there are some factors that can increase the possibility of becoming motion sick. Those more likely to be prone to motion sickness include (1) women (especially those who are pregnant); (2) children, usually between the ages of 5 and 12; (3) people who have migraines or other conditions such as ear infections or conditions that interfere with the vestibular system in the ear; and (4) athletes. Young children under the age of two are typically not affected, and the likelihood is reduced in the elderly. Other factors that can make someone more likely to experience motion sickness are lack of sleep, anxiety and stress, alcohol, smoking, and eating large meals. People react differently to motion sickness and some may be more likely to get sick from one type of activity while others will be affected more by another.

Types and Symptoms

There are many different types of motion sickness, or type of motions that can make one get motion sick. Some things or activities that can elicit symptoms include cars (carsickness), airplanes (airsickness), trains, rides (such as those at amusement parks), boats or ships (seasickness), video games, simulators, space motion sickness, and virtual reality sickness.

There are numerous signs and symptoms of motion sickness. These include a general unwell feeling, headache, nausea, vomiting, sweating, dizziness, "stomach awareness," increased salivation, burping, difficulty concentrating, fatigue, confusion, irritability, and pale skin. The most common symptom is nausea. The signs and symptoms can occur soon after experiencing the motion or it may take a while for them to develop. Symptoms will usually subside after the motion stops, but sometimes they can persist for several hours or days afterward. The severity of symptoms may vary widely, and again each person is different. Once a person experiences motion sickness, he or she is more likely to develop it again.

Diagnosis

There are no specific diagnostic tests for motion sickness. However, sometimes tests need to be performed in order to exclude other causes, such as vertigo and pregnancy. Tests performed in these situations may include a pregnancy test, computed tomography (CT) or magnetic resonance imaging (MRI), and vestibular testing. Motion sickness is not normally a cause for worry, except if the symptoms, especially vomiting, last for more than a few days. Continued vomiting can cause dehydration, electrolyte imbalances, low blood pressure, and irregular heartbeats.

Treatments

There are several ways in which to treat motion sickness including medications and behavioral modifications. Medications work best if taken before exposure to the motion stimulus occurs. It is much easier to prevent motion sickness than to treat the symptoms once they have already begun. Current motion sickness medications include anticholinergics (scopolamine), antiemetics (Zofran), antihistamines (Benadryl, Antivert, Bonine, and Dramamine), antidopaminergics (Phenergan and Zofran), and bendodiazepines (Valium). Scopolamine is probably the most effective and its effects last several days. Scopolamine usually comes as a patch, which is applied behind the ear. Many of these medications have similar side effects, which include a dry mouth, drowsiness, and blurry vision. Less common side effects include constipation, bloating, headache, and confusion. Other treatments include eating specific foods (such as crackers), getting fresh air, acupressure (at the P6 pressure point on the wrist), and eating ginger. Behavioral modifications include lying down, keeping eyes fixed on the horizon, sitting in the front seats of cars, and standing in the middle of a boat. Further research is needed to focus on the treatment of motion sickness. Medications that do not have the adverse side effects such as drowsiness and those that treat both nausea and vomiting are needed.

Shannen McNamara

See also: Dizziness; Emesis; Nausea; Vestibular System; Visual Motor System

Further Reading

Brainard, Andrew, & Chip Gresham. (2014). Prevention and treatment of motion sickness. *American Family Physician, 90*(1), 41–46. Retrieved from http://www.aafp.org/afp/2014/0701/p41.html

Lackner, James R. (2014). Motion sickness: More than nausea and vomiting. *Experimental Brain Research, 232*(8), 2493–2510.

MYASTHENIA GRAVIS

Myasthenia gravis (MG) is an autoimmune disorder that affects the neuromuscular junction (NMJ) at the postsynaptic level. Its name is derived from both Greek and Latin words meaning "grave muscular weakness." Although the cause of the disorder is unknown, the role of immune responses in its disease process is well established. The person's own immune system abnormally creates antibodies that circulate in the body and attack the nicotinic acetylcholine receptor. In normal voluntary muscle function, impulses from the brain are sent down the nerves to where the axon terminal meets the muscle fibers. A nerve action potential is created and acetylcholine (ACh) is released into the synapse. This eventually leads to muscle contraction when ACh has activated enough receptors. In myasthenia gravis, there is up to an 80 percent decrease in ACh receptors, which leads to dysfunction at the NMJ as well as produces sensory dysfunction (MGFA, 2010). Thus, the nerves cannot communicate with the muscles the way that they should.

Clinical Features

MG is not rare, with a prevalence of 50 to 125 cases per million persons (MGFA, 2010). However, this number may be much higher as MG is thought to be under-diagnosed. The incidence is age- and sex-related, generally affecting women less than 40 years old and men greater than 60 years old. The cardinal features are weakness and fatigue of skeletal muscles. The weakness tends to increase with repeated activity and improve with rest. Ptosis (drooping eyelid) and diplopia (double vision) occur early in the majority of patients. Weakness remains localized to the extraocular and eyelid muscles in about 15 percent of patients (MGFA, 2010). When the facial muscles are affected, there may be a characteristic flattened smile, "mushy" or nasal speech, and difficulty in chewing and swallowing. Generalized weakness develops in most patients. If weakness of respiration becomes severe enough to require mechanical ventilation, the patient is said to be in crisis. Some patients may have symptoms only late in the day or after physical exertion. This disorder is highly treatable so prompt recognition is crucial.

Diagnosis

Patients experiencing muscle pain that does not affect all skeletal muscles, such as arm and leg weakness with no eye muscle symptoms, are not likely to have MG. A variety of neurological conditions can mimic MG, such as botulism and amyotrophic lateral sclerosis. In addition, a large number of medications that can cause a patient to experience muscle weakness must be addressed before diagnosing the disease as MG. The list includes but is not limited to antibiotics, cardiovascular agents, and other various drugs.

The most sensitive test for MG is an ACh receptor antibody (AChR-Ab); however, not all patients with MG will present with positive antibodies. Another test to determine MG is to give the patient in question a medication—edrophonium (an acetylcholinesterase inhibitor)—and evaluate the response. This medication prevents the breakdown of ACh and therefore allows more receptors to interact with the muscle fibers. After a patient receives the drug, health care providers look for an unequivocal increase in strength. A subjective feeling of strength increase will not be enough to diagnose MG. Thus, an objective finding by the provider can be used, such as if the person's drooping eyelids improve. Clinicians can also use electrodiagnostic studies that look at nerve conduction, repetitive nerve stimulation, exercise testing, and sometimes an electromyelogram.

Treatment

Prior to 1958, the mortality rate for MG patients was very high, most had deteriorating symptoms, and very few patients improved. Since then, the mortality rate is essentially zero, and many patients lead normal functioning lives. There are four ways of treating MG: (1) acetylcholinesterase inhibitors (ACh-i), (2) thymectomy, (3) immunosuppression, and (4) plasma-exchange or immune globulin.

As discussed previously, an ACh-i will improve muscle strength in MG patients and these are popular methods of treatment. The drugs will be tailored to the patients' needs and the doses can range as well. Higher doses, however, can exacerbate muscle weakness. Since the thymus has been implicated in MG, those between puberty and age 60 should have their thymus surgically removed. The goal for any patient undergoing this procedure is remission of the disease, or at least great improvement of MG that limits the need for other medications.

Immunosuppressive therapy is indicated when the patient experiences progressive weakness despite treatment with anticholinergic drugs. Because suppressing the body's immune system puts patients at higher risk for infection and many other side effects, the decision to step up therapy is made after weighing the costs and benefits. Patients on these drugs should do their best to take care of their health like hand washing, eating well, and being vaccinated, because they will not be able to fight simple infections.

Plasmaphoresis is a technique that takes the plasma out of the patient, cleans it by taking out the ACh antibodies, and puts it back into the patient. This procedure is typically performed when an MG patient is having a crisis or if a patient is undergoing a surgical thymectomy. The effect of this treatment is seen very rapidly, but then it goes away after a few weeks, which is why this is used in emergency situations and not for long-term treatment options.

Jeremy E. Brothers

See also: Diplopia; Ptosis

Further Reading

Myasthenia Gravis Foundation of America (MGFA). (2010). *What is myasthenia gravis?* Retrieved from http://www.myasthenia.org/WhatisMG.aspx

MYOPIA

Myopia is commonly referred to as nearsightedness. In this condition, light that comes into the eye does not come directly into focus on the retina, but instead it focuses in front of the retina. This causes an object far away to be seen out of focus and an object closer to the eye to be seen in focus.

Classification

Myopia is classified in two different groups: axial and refractive. Axial myopia is due to an increase in the eye's axial length, whereas refractive myopia refers to the condition of the refractive elements of the eye. Further classifications include curvature myopia, which is excessive curvature in one or more of the refractive surfaces of the eye, mostly the cornea. Index myopia is a variation in the index of refraction of one or more ocular media. All of these classifications still result in the same basic issue, the inability of the eye to focus on objects that are far away from the lens.

Degree of Myopia

Myopia comes in different degrees depending on the person. Myopia is measured in diopters, the strength or optical power of a corrective lens that focuses distant images on the retina. Low myopia is usually −3.00 diopters or less, closer to 0.00. Medium myopia is usually between −3.00 diopters and −6.00 diopters. These individuals typically have pigment dispersion syndrome, which leads to glaucoma. High myopia is usually −6.00 diopters or more. These individuals are more likely to have retinal detachments and open angle glaucoma. Approximately 30 percent of people with myopia have high myopia. The higher the number of diopters, the worse the patient's ability to focus on objects far from the lens.

Signs and Symptoms

Myopia presents mostly with blurred vision when looking at distant objects. When examined by an ophthalmologist, the optic nerve tends to be tilted, and an area where white sclera can be seen next to a disc with a line of hyperpigmentation is separating this area from the normal retina.

Risk Factors

Genetics have been shown to be a risk factor associated with juvenile myopia, while work, higher school achievement, and less time spent doing sports activity contributed relatively little to the development of myopia in individuals. Performing close work (e.g., using a computer or microscope), however, has been implicated as a factor in the pathogenesis of myopia, as seen in the United States where the prevalence of myopia rose with family income and education level (Sperduto et al., 1983). It has been shown that persons with higher education tend to perform close work.

Prevention, Control, and Management

There is really no universally approved method of preventing myopia, although many attempts have been made. Myopia can be controlled using various methods. The most common form of control is reading glasses, contact lenses, or surgery. Pharmaceuticals such as antimuscarinic topical medications and eye drops have been shown to be effective in slowing myopia. A final form of control and management of myopia is surgery. Laser in-situ keratomileusis or laser-assisted in-situ keratomileusis (LASIK) surgery is the most common form of eye surgery, which is a procedure that includes cutting the cornea to make a corneal flap to allow a laser beam access to the exposed corneal tissue. The laser reshapes the cornea by clearing tissue to correct the misshapen lens. This results in the vision being corrected. After reshaping the cornea, the corneal flap is then flipped back over to cover the corneal tissue that was reshaped. LASIK is not painful and has a very short recovery time but has the potential for flap complications and potential loss of corneal stability. Additionally, there is sometimes a need to fine-tune the surgery to ensure 20/20 vision. Another option for correcting myopia is photo-refractive keratectomy (PRK). While very similar to LASIK in that it uses a laser to reshape the surface of the cornea, it does not remove as much tissue and no flap is formed. The reshaping happens on the surface of the cornea. This means there is a much longer healing period, but this might be a more viable option for individuals with a higher degree of myopia as there is less risk of the cornea being reduced to too small a size, as might happen with LASIK.

Renee Johnson

See also: Amblyopia; Diplopia; Hyperopia; Presbyopia; Retina; Visual Perception

Further Reading

National Eye Institute (NEI). (2010). Facts about myopia. *National Eye Institute.* Retrieved from https://nei.nih.gov/health/errors/myopia

Sivak, Jacob. (2012). The cause(s) of myopia and the efforts that have been made to prevent it. *Clinical and Experimental Optometry, 95*(6), 572–582. http://dx.doi .org/10.1111/j.1444-0938.2012.00781.x

Sperduto, Robert D., Daniel Seigel, Jean Roberts, & Michael Rowland. (1983). Prevalence of myopia in the United States. *Archives in Ophthalmology, 101*(3), 405–407. http: //dx.doi.org/10.1001/archopht.1983.01040010405011

NATIONAL ORGANIZATION FOR RARE DISORDERS

The National Organization for Rare Disorders (NORD) is not only a professional organization for basic science and clinical researchers studying rare disorders—also called orphaned diseases—but also an organization for those with rare disorders, their families, and their communities so that our society can better support them. The vision of NORD has been divided into four core areas: (1) a national awareness and recognition of the challenges endured by people living with rare diseases; (2) a culture of innovation that supports basic and translational research to create diagnostic tests and therapies for all rare diseases; (3) access for all patients to the diagnostics and therapies that will extend and improve their lives; and (4) a regulatory environment that encourages development and timely approval of safe, effective diagnostics and treatments.

The U.S. National Institutes of Health (NIH) has defined a disease as rare if there are fewer than 200,000 Americans affected by the disorder. To date, there are about 7,000 identified rare diseases with many having an effect on sensory systems. Thus, there are roughly 30 million people in the United States (or approximately 1 in every 10 persons) who are living with a rare disease. For a complete list of rare disorders, please see the following link: https://rarediseases.info.nih .gov/gard.

To promote their cause, NORD is the official U.S. sponsor of Rare Disease Day, which is always the last day of February. Rare Disease Day started in Europe in 2008 and focuses on allowing patients and their families/caregivers to promote awareness of the disease and how it challenges their everyday lives. Most recently, 65 different countries participated in Rare Disease Day.

History

Prior to the late 1970s, rare disorders were not widely studied, and thus, new and specific treatments were not being developed for patients. In 1979, patients, families, and leaders who were part of a rare disease patient organization began an Ad Hoc Coalition to bring the lack of research and treatments to the attention of the U.S. Congress. By 1983, the coalition was successful in getting the Orphan Drug Act passed, which provides financial incentives for new drugs and treatments to be developed for rare disorders. This coalition eventually became NORD.

Following is a short timeline that led to NORD and important legislation that is still in effect today.

- January 1, 1979: Dr. Marion J. Finkel, who worked for the Food and Drug Association (FDA), issued a report that focused on the lack of funding for drug development that would have limited commercial value, meaning medications for small patient populations. She is considered the leader in orphan drug development.

- January 1979–January 1980: Representative Henry Waxman (1939–) chaired the Subcommittee on Health and the Environment of the House Energy and Commerce Committee, and held hearings about the lack of orphan drugs. During this same time period, patient advocates formed the Ad Hoc Coalition to help campaign for better health care solutions for rare diseases.

- March 4, 1981: The rare diseases issue was brought to prime time on national television. Actor Jack Klugman (1922–2012) along with his brother and producer Maurice Klugman (1914–1981) made an episode of *Quincy, M.E.* (1976–1983) that highlighted problems for patients with orphaned disorders. The episode, titled "Seldom Silent, Never Heard," was about the tragic death of a teenager with Tourette's syndrome that sets Quincy to fight for orphan drug development.

- December 1982: The House and Senate passed the Orphan Drug Act. The act was originally put aside for work on other bills, but the Ad Hoc Coalition and other advocates for rare diseases mobilized support for it to be revived and become law.

- January 4, 1983: President Ronald Reagan (1911–2004) signed the Orphan Drug Act, making it a law of the United States.

- February 1, 1983: The first orphan drug (Panhematin®) was approved by the Food and Drug Administration (FDA) for acute intermittent porphyria, which can cause problems with the nervous system if porphyrin (a natural chemical needed for hemoglobin to bind red blood cells, iron, and oxygen) levels are too high.

- May 4, 1983: NORD was founded and Abbey Meyers becomes the first president of the 501(c)(3) organization, which provides support and advocacy for persons with rare disorders.

- January 1, 1984: The Orphan Drug Act Amendment was passed. This amendment included a definition of rare disorders: "any disease affecting fewer than 200,000 Americans or a disease with a higher prevalence but for which there is no reasonable expectation that a therapy would recover the cost of development."

Jennifer L. Hellier

See also: Ageusia; Anosmia; Bell's Palsy; Congenital Insensitivity to Pain; Horner Syndrome

Further Reading

Genetic and Rare Diseases Information Center (GARD). (n.d.). Diseases. National Center for Advancing Translational Sciences. Retrieved from https://rarediseases.info.nih.gov/gard

National Organization for Rare Disorders (NORD). (n.d.). Tools and resources. Retrieved from http://rarediseases.org/

NAUSEA

Nausea is the sensation of discomfort in the upper stomach that gives a person the feeling or the urge to vomit. Vomiting is the action of expelling the contents of the stomach through the mouth. Typically one feels queasy prior to vomiting; however, it is not uncommon to vomit without experiencing nausea. By itself, nausea is not debilitating unless there is a prolonged feeling of nausea.

Causes

Nausea is a nonspecific symptom and can have many causes. These causes include but are not limited to (1) food poisoning, (2) pregnancy, (3) side effects of medication, (4) anxiety, (5) stress, (6) depression, and (7) motion sickness. The two most common causes are gastrointestinal infections and food poisoning.

Food poisoning occurs when bacteria in the food one eats produces toxins, which can cause a very abrupt and sudden onset of nausea and vomiting. Nausea, or morning sickness, is commonly caused by pregnancy usually in the early stages (the first three months or trimester). Nausea from pregnancy and many other causes is usually mild and does not require treatment.

However, there are some cases of nausea that do require immediate attention, but these cases come with more often severe symptoms. These cases include but are not limited to (1) appendicitis, where the appendix becomes inflamed or infected: (2) a brain tumor; (3) a heart attack; (4) meningitis, where the meninges (protective covering that surrounds the central nervous system) becomes infectious; (5) hepatitis, an illness of the liver; and (6) carbon monoxide poisoning.

Diagnosis

The diagnosis of nausea usually begins with the patient's history. The patient is asked questions about when the nausea started, how long he or she has felt nauseated, and if it is constant. A typical diagnosis of acute onset of nausea is normally related to drugs, toxins, or infections. If nausea has been long-lasting, then it is normally related to a more chronic illness. If nausea occurs about an hour after eating, then there might be an obstruction that is proximal to the small intestine. If a patient vomits and then feels relief in the abdomen, then it is likely an obstruction is a cause and not a chronic issue like pancreatitis or gallstones (choleocystitis), both of which are not relieved by vomiting.

Physiology

The central nervous system plays a vital role in nausea suppression. Areas including the limbic system and cerebral cortex are activated by an increase in intracranial pressure, meningeal irritation, or emotional triggers. Housed in the fourth ventricle of the brain are chemoreceptor trigger zones (CTZs). CTZs are outside of the blood-brain barrier and are always exposed to substances and/or toxins circulating in the blood and cerebral spinal fluid. CTZ activation is controlled by dopamine, serotonin, and neurokinin receptors. The vestibular system is located in the inner ear and can be activated by movements that cause motion sickness and dizziness. This system is triggered via histamine and acetylcholine receptors.

These three pathways have receptors that respond to a stimulus and travel to the brainstem. This in turn activates structures including but not limited to the nucleus of the solitary tract, the dorsal motor nucleus, and the central pain generator. Continuing downstream, the body's motor response halts the muscles of the gastrointestinal tract and causes reverse propulsion of gastric contents to the mouth while abdominal contractions increase. There are autonomic effects involved that increase a sense of feeling faint, in which nausea and vomiting generally occur shortly after.

Treatment

The treatment for nausea can vary depending on the underlying cause. Treatments usually include rehydration if one is dehydrated, medication to suppress the queasiness of the stomach and bowels, acupuncture, and other alternative medications. It is recommended to seek medical care if one cannot keep any liquids down, has symptoms for more than two days, is weak, has a fever, has severe stomach pain, vomits more than two times in one day, or does not urinate for more than eight hours.

Avoiding nausea may be hard, but there are some ways to do so. The most common is eating smaller meals throughout the day, eating them slowly, and resting after eating. Avoiding certain foods that irritate one's stomach is also a good way to avoid nausea. Drinks like ginger ale are common to try when experiencing nausea as well as eating high-protein foods such as cheese or meat before standing up.

Renee Johnson

See also: Autonomic Nervous System; Chemoreception; Dizziness; Emesis; Vestibular System

Further Reading

Blake, Katie. (2015). Nausea and vomiting. *Healthline Medical Review Team*. Retrieved from http://www.healthline.com/health/nausea-and-vomiting#Prevention6

Singh, Prashant, Sonia S. Yoon, & Braden Kuo. (2016). Nausea: A review of pathophysiology and therapeutics. *Therapeutic Advances in Gastroenterology, 9*(1), 98–112. http://dx.doi.org/10.1177/1756283X15618131

NEARSIGHTEDNESS: *See* Myopia

NERVES

The nervous system derives its name from nerves—the cordlike bundles of axons that branch repeatedly to innervate tissues throughout the body. Nerves form remarkably coordinated networks that relay messages to and from the brain. These networks underlie the ability to sense stimuli and transmit signals to and from different parts of the body.

Nerve cells, or neurons, are the basic unit of the nervous system. The primary function of these cells is communication, which they do by sending electrical and chemical messages. Electric signaling is the fastest way to communicate, and nerve cells do this by sending electrical signals down their axons. Individual axons are microscopic in size and too small to see with the naked eye. Groups of axons that are bundled together outside of the brain and spinal cord form nerves. Nerves can also be too small to see. For example, the nerve that innervates taste buds on the tip of the tongue, called the chorda tympani, is about 1.7×10^{-5} inches in diameter—that is 150 times thinner than a single strand of hair. Other nerves are much larger. The widest nerve in the human body, which is also the longest nerve, is the sciatic nerve. This nerve is about three-quarters of an inch in diameter where it starts in the lower back. The sciatic nerve branches out to provide movement and feeling from the top of the leg all the way down to the foot.

Anatomy and Physiology

The function of a nerve depends on the individual axons, also called nerve fibers, that make up the nerve. Nerve fibers are broadly classified as afferent or efferent. Afferent fibers are sensory nerve fibers and constantly keep the central nervous system (CNS) informed of events that happen inside and outside of the body. This means that sensory fibers are continually sending information into the brain about what we sense in the environment, such as sights, sounds, tastes, and smells as well as details about the organs in the body. Efferent fibers are the motor nerve fibers and send information out of the brain to the many muscles and glands throughout the body. Motor fibers control both voluntary and involuntary movements. The autonomic nerve fibers are responsible for the involuntary actions of the body such as heart rate, blood pressure, muscle contractions of the digestive organs, and secretions from glands. Animals are usually unconscious of this kind of movement.

How fast electrical signals can travel down nerve fibers is determined by how thick the fiber is as well as the myelin that surrounds it. Some of the fastest nerve signals travel 400 feet in a second, which is around 144 miles per hour. Other fibers, such as those that convey pain, do not have any myelin; these nerve signals travel about three feet in a second, which is just over two miles per hour.

Nerve fibers are then bundled together to make up the peripheral nerves. Hence, nerves can also be broadly classified as sensory, motor, or mixed nerves, which contain both sensory and motor fibers. There are 12 pairs of cranial nerves that connect to the brain and 31 pairs of spinal nerves that connect to the spinal cord. Cranial nerves are numbered with Roman numerals in order of where they connect to the brain. These nerves primarily serve the sensory and motor functions of the head and neck region. Some cranial nerves are exclusively sensory nerves, such as the olfactory and optic nerves, while some are only motor nerves, such as the trochlear and abducens nerves that are involved in eye movement. The remaining cranial nerves are mixed.

Unlike the cranial nerves that serve one or a few specific functions to a broad region, the spinal nerves serve all functions to smaller segmental regions of the body. Therefore, all of the spinal nerves are mixed nerves. These nerves do not have names but are grouped and numbered according to the spinal cord level from which they stem—cervical, thoracic, lumbar, or sacral. The cervical nerves, which are numbered C1–C8, involve the shoulders, arms, neck, and hands. The thoracic nerves, T1–T12, run along the middle of the back and are involved with the chest, abdomen, and internal organs, including the heart, lungs, liver, and stomach. The lumbar nerves are L1–L5 and target muscles of the lower back, thighs, legs, and feet as well as some internal organs, such as the appendix, bladder, and reproductive organs. The sacral nerves are S1–S5 and target the hips, buttocks, thighs, and legs. The last pair of spinal nerves, simply called the coccygeal nerves, targets the skin over the back of the tailbone.

Dianna Bartel

See also: Autonomic Nervous System; Central Nervous System; Cranial Nerves; Peripheral Nervous System

Further Reading

A history of the nervous system. (n.d.). Retrieved from http://www.stanford.edu/class/history13/earlysciencelab/body/nervespages/nerves.html

Neuron basics. (n.d.). Retrieved from http://www.animatlab.com/NeuralNetworkEditor/FiringRateNeuralNet/NeuronBasics.htm

NEUROLOGICAL EXAMINATION

The neurological examination is a systematic method used by health care providers and particularly by neurologists to look for abnormalities or lesions in the nervous system. The neurological examination is not performed in isolation, but as part of a general physical examination. The following is an abbreviated neurological examination for an alert, adult patient. The neurological examination contains several broad rubrics to test the patient's (1) mental status, (2) cranial nerves, (3) reflexes and motor ability, (4) coordination and gait, and (5) sensory responses.

Mental

The mental portion of the examination is conducted informally by having a conversation with the patient. Questions are asked, such as, "Is the patient oriented?" "Confused?" "Are there alterations in short-term memory?" "In recall?" More formally, the physician may use the Folstein Mini Mental Examination, which tests for items such as orientation, registration, reading, and naming objects. These items and answers are scored on a 30-point scale.

Cranial Nerves

The cranial nerves are listed and tested as follows:

Cranial nerve I (olfactory nerve): This nerve can be tested by having the patient smell a non-noxious smell such as coffee in each nostril.

Cranial nerve II (optic nerve): Visual acuity, visual fields, and ocular fundi (the interior surface of the eye) are confirmed. Specifically, the patient's sight is tested using a handheld visual acuity card. To test the visual fields, the examiner brings his or her fingers into the visual field and has the patient indicate when he or she can see the moving fingers. The fundoscopic examination is performed using an ophthalmoscope. The physician looks for the color of the fundus, the cup to disc ratio, and the presence of spontaneous venous pulsations.

Cranial nerves II and III (oculomotor nerves): Pupillary responses are confirmed. The examiner tests to see that the pupils are of equal size and constrict in response to light, the consensual pupillary light reflex.

Cranial nerves III, IV (trochlear nerves), and VI (abducens nerve): These three nerves control eye movements and are typically tested together by having the patient follow a target, such as a pen light, and look up, look down, look side to side, and then look toward the nose to test for accommodation. One examines for the smoothness of the eye movement, conjugate eye movements, and any nystagmus.

Cranial nerve V (trigeminal nerve): The patient is asked to clench the masseter muscles, which control jaw movement. The examiner tests for asymmetry between the two sides.

Cranial nerve VII (facial nerve): The examiner looks for weakness of facial muscles during a smile and when cheeks are puffed out. Also, the examiner looks for weakness when the eyebrows are raised.

Cranial nerve VIII (vestibulocochlear nerve): The examiner rubs fingers together and has the patient report if a sound is heard. Balance is assessed during the coordination and gait exams.

Cranial nerves IX (glossopharyngeal nerve) and X (vagus nerve): The patient elevates the palate and the examiner looks for any asymmetry of movement.

Cranial nerve XI (accessory nerve): The patient shrugs the shoulders upward to test the strength of the trapezius muscles. The patient then turns the head to either side against resistance provided by the examiner to test for the strength of the sternocleidomastoid muscle of the neck.

Cranial nerve XII (hypoglossal nerve): The patient protrudes the tongue out and moves it from side to side. The examiner looks for any asymmetry of movement.

Reflexes

The deep tendon reflexes in the extremities are tested and rated on a scale of 0 to 5 or from no reflex to a presence of sustained clonus. Stroking the lateral aspect of the bottom of the foot checks the plantar response. The normal response is for the toes to move down in contraction.

Motor

One examines the muscles for any abnormalities such as fasciculation (brief, spontaneous contractions of a few muscle fibers). One tests the tone of the extremities, asking, "Are they flaccid? Spastic?" and so on. The strength of the arms and legs are tested by muscle group and then rated on a scale of 0 to 5 or from no muscle contraction present to full strength.

Coordination

Coordination is tested by examining "finger to nose to finger" testing to determine if the patient can hit the target or if there is any overshoot while attempting to hit the target. In the legs, coordination is examined by having the patient place the heel on the shin and then slide the heel up and down the shin.

Gait

One examines casual gait, then tandem gait in which one foot is placed in front of the other. The patient walks on heels and toes. This identifies any weakness in dorsi and plantar flexion of the feet.

Sensory

Pain and temperature are tested using a sharp object and the cool touch of the tuning fork. Vibration and proprioception are tested by vibration of the tuning fork and by moving a toe or finger up or down and asking the patient to identify which direction the digit is moved.

Audrey S. Yee

See also: Accommodation; Cranial Nerves; Neurologist; Nystagmus; Reflex; Touch

Further Reading

Blumenfeld, Hal. (n.d.). *Neuroanatomy through clinical cases.* Retrieved from http://www .neuroexam.com/neuroexam/content.php?p=2
Russell, Stephen, & Marc Triola. (n.d.). *The precise neurological exam.* Retrieved from http ://informatics.med.nyu.edu/modules/pub/neurosurgery/index.html

NEUROLOGIST

Neurology, the study of nerves, is a specialty within medicine. A neurologist is a physician, either a medical doctor (MD) or a doctor of osteopathy (DO), who is trained specifically in neurology and in treating the human nervous system—the central, peripheral, and autonomic nervous systems—and the blood vessels that supply them. The central nervous system includes the brain and spinal cord, while the peripheral nervous system includes the sensory and motor nerves that supply the body. The autonomic nervous system, however, has many endocrine or metabolic functions and an endocrinologist usually treats these dysfunctions. Neurology has many subspecialties including child or pediatric neurology, epileptology (the study of seizures and epilepsy), neurosurgery, movement disorders, and psychiatry (the study of mental disorders), to name a few. To become a neurologist, the physician needs to complete a residency in neurology and may need to complete a few fellowships if he or she is pursuing a subspecialty.

In general, patients will be referred to a neurologist from their primary care provider or other physicians. A neurologist will start by taking a medical history of the patient and then perform specific neurological tests to determine the person's balance, cognition (thinking and memory ability), cranial nerve functions, gait (ability to coordinate movements like walking), muscle strength, reflexes, and sensory functions (like touch, temperature, and pressure). Additional tests can be used to evaluate the health of the nervous system such as computed tomography (CT) scans, magnetic resonance imaging (MRI), and ultrasound imaging techniques (that can be used to view blood vessels to determine the location of an intercranial aneurysm). A neurophysiology test can also be performed to see brain activity (electroencephalography, EEG) and muscle and evoked potentials activity (electromyography, EMG). Finally, to determine the health of the cerebrospinal fluid, neurologists can perform a lumbar puncture. Results from the aforementioned tests can help diagnose patients with several different neurological diseases such as dementia, multiple sclerosis, Parkinson's disease, seizures, and stroke, to name a few.

Jennifer L. Hellier

See also: Autonomic Nervous System; Central Nervous System; Meniere's Disease; Neurological Examination; Peripheral Nervous System; Sacks, Oliver Wolf; Seizures; Society for Neuroscience

Further Reading

Association of American Medical Colleges. (2013). Careers in medicine: Neurology. Retrieved from https://www.aamc.org/cim/specialty/list/us/336846/neurology.html

Kandel, Eric R., James H. Schwartz, Thomas M. Jessell, Steven A. Siegelbaum, & A. J. Hudspeth (Eds.). (2012). *Principles of neural science* (5th ed.). New York, NY: McGraw-Hill.

NEUROPIL

Structurally, the neuropil is a concentrated region of synapses that consists of primarily unmyelinated axons, dendrites, and glial cells (the supportive cells of the nervous system). It is relatively devoid of neuronal cell bodies and myelinated axons, but it is a region where signals are processed. The term *neuropil* is derived from Greek meaning "nerve felt." This is because of all the integrated fibers found within the neuropil, thus making the region look like a piece of felt. The neuropil is a generic term that defines several parts of the central nervous system and is not concentrated in just one area or another. However, the largest amount of neuropil is found in the outer layer of the cerebral cortex—which is the outermost portion of the brain—and the olfactory bulb—which is responsible for the detection and discrimination of odors.

The cerebral cortex is a six-layered structure with each layer being numbered with the corresponding Roman numeral: I–VI. Although it is layered, meaning there are clear divisions of neuron layers, the majority of the cortex contains neuropil. The outermost layer is the molecular layer and is also called layer I. Alternating layers of neurons that have either a granular or pyramidal shape follow the molecular layer, thus these layers are called granular and pyramidal layers. Layer VI is polymorphic, meaning it consists of several cell types and is the deepest layer. Within layers II–V, the granular or stellate cells act as the principal interneurons (neurons between the primary neurons), and their projections do not leave the local cortex. The pyramidal cells act as the primary output neurons and typically do send projections out of the cortex. These projections frequently contact other cortical areas of the brain or subcortical areas. The neuropil can be found within and between each cortical layer. Thus the neuropil within the cerebral cortex is an amalgam of stellate cell axons projecting from one layer to another; the glial cells in the region; and the dendrites of the principal cells.

In the olfactory bulb, there are also very specific layers of neurons that are easily identifiable. Specifically, the outer surface of the olfactory bulb is made up of several circular regions called glomeruli (plural; glomerulus is the singular form). It is these glomeruli that make up some of the olfactory bulb's neuropil by the axons of the olfactory sensory neurons, the dendrites of the mitral cells, and the short dendrites and axons of the periglomerular cells. It is at this region where an odorant's perception begins to be processed by the brain.

Finally, there are other brain regions that are composed of neuropil such as the retina. The retina consists of 10 identifiable layers of neurons and both the inner and outer plexiform layers have regions of neuropil. Similar to the olfactory bulb, the neuropil regions in the retina begin the processing of vision and what is being seen or perceived.

Future

At the turn of the 21st century, neuroscientists researched the target amount of neuropil to neurons that is needed for a functioning central nervous system. They found that the volume of the tissue should contain three-fifths of neuropil for an optimally wired brain (Chklovskii et al., 2002). This information is useful for neuroscientists who are developing computer programs to better understand the brain's circuitry as well as for developing artificial intelligence.

Jennifer L. Hellier

See also: Axon; Cerebral Cortex; Nerves; Olfactory Bulb; Olfactory Sensory Neurons; Olfactory System; Retina; Visual System

Further Reading
Chklovskii, Dmitri B., Thomas Schikorski, & Charles F. Stevens. (2002). Wiring optimization in cortical circuits. *Neuron, 34*(3), 341–347.
Purves, Dale, et al. (Eds.). (2004). *Neuroscience* (3rd ed.). Sunderland, MA: Sinauer Associates.

NOCICEPTION
Nociception or pain is defined as an unpleasant sensory and emotional experience associated with actual or potential tissue damage. It is a conscious experience involving the interpretation of sensory input that signals a noxious event and is influenced by several factors. One model describes pain in terms of three hierarchical levels: a sensory-discriminative component (location, intensity, and quality), a motivational-affective component (depression and anxiety), and a cognitive-evaluative component (thoughts involving the cause and significance of the pain). This model highlights the reality that the perception of pain is determined by a combination of several components and is very complex to both understand and manage.

Classification of Pain

Acute pain warns an organism of a potentially harmful situation (like a burn) or a disease state (such as appendicitis). Acute pain serves a specific physiologic function and lasts a brief period of time. Unfortunately, if the acute pain is undertreated or severe, it can last longer than its biologic usefulness and may have many harmful effects. Acute pain caused by surgery, acute illness, or trauma is usually nociceptive (a signal from neurons that is usually due to damage to these cell types). The goal of treating acute pain is cure.

Chronic pain results when pain persists for months to years. This type of pain can be nociceptive, neuropathic/functional, or mixed. It is associated with cancer or noncancer etiologies that result in changes to the receptors and nerve fibers within the nervous system. Additionally, chronic pain is often associated with depression, insomnia, and other personal or social problems. The goal of treatment with chronic pain is not cure, but a return to functionality.

Pathophysiology of Nociceptive Pain

Nociceptive pain is "normal" pain resulting from the activation of nociceptive fibers and includes somatic and visceral pains. Sprains and strains produce mild forms of nociceptive pain, while the pain of arthritis is much more severe. Nociceptive pain is described as either somatic or visceral. Somatic pain presents as a throbbing and well-localized pain, while visceral pain presents localized to the organ from which it originates.

Nociceptive pain occurs as a result of the activation of the sensory system by persistent noxious stimuli, a process involving transduction, transmission, modulation, and perception. Transduction is the process by which noxious stimuli are converted to electrical signals in the nociceptors. Nociceptors have the ability to distinguish between noxious and innocuous stimuli and are activated and sensitized by mechanical, thermal, and chemical impulses. Noxious stimuli may result in the release of naturally occurring chemicals, such as bradykinins, hydrogen and potassium ions, prostaglandins, histamines, interleukins, tumor necrosis factor alfa, serotonin, and substance P. These chemicals sensitize or activate the nociceptors.

Pain transmission takes place in two different nerve fiber types: A delta and C-afferent fibers. A delta fibers are myelinated and have a large diameter. When stimulated, these fibers evoke a sharp, well-localized pain. C-fibers are unmyelinated and have a small diameter. When stimulated, the C-fibers produce a dull, aching, poorly localized pain. For the central nervous system to receive the pain, the signal travels from the affected area toward the brain. These afferent nociceptive fibers synapse in various layers of the spinal cord, specifically in the region where most neuronal cell bodies reside in the dorsal horn, the "gray matter of the spinal cord." This, in turn, results in the release of a variety of neurotransmitters including glutamate, substance P, and aspartate. The role of substance P in pain has been widely studied and how it aids in pain transmission to the brain. Substance P is released from C-fibers in response to tissue injury or to intense stimulation of peripheral nerves.

There are three major classes of nociceptors: thermal, mechanical, and poly-modal. Extreme temperatures activate thermal nociceptors, which have a small diameter and are myelinated, sending very rapid signals. Mechanical nociceptors are activated by intensive pressure applied to the skin. They are also thinly myeli-nated fibers that conduct signals quickly. Polymodal nociceptors are activated by high-intensity mechanical, chemical, or thermal stimuli. These nociceptors have a small diameter and are nonmyelinated, conducting signals much more slowly. The nociceptors transduce signals via specialized proteins—also known as channels—such as transient receptor potential channels or those that are activated by sodium, voltage-gated sodium channels. Depolarization of the primary afferent nerves re-sults in production of substances that are produced by tissues, inflammatory cells, and neurons. Once depolarization occurs, transmission information continues along the axon to the spinal cord and then on to higher brain centers.

Nociceptive information is transmitted from the spinal cord to the thalamus and cerebral cortex along five ascending pathways: spinothalamic, spinoreticular, spi-nomesencephalic, cervicothalamic, and spinohypothalamic tracts. The spinotha-lamic tract is the most prominent ascending nociceptive pathway in the spinal cord. These axons project into the contralateral side of the spinal cord and terminate in the thalamus. The cerebral cortex also contributes to the processing of pain. Neurons in several regions of the cerebral cortex respond selectively to nociceptive input.

At this point, pain becomes a conscious experience that takes place in higher cortical structures. The brain may take in only a limited number of pain signals, allowing cognitive and behavioral functions to modify pain sensation. Variables including relaxation, distraction, and meditation may decrease pain by limiting the number of processed pain signals. On the other hand, depression and anxiety may worsen pain.

Pain is modulated through a number of systems, including the endogenous opi-ate system. This system consists of neurotransmitters including enkephalins, dynorphins, beta endorphins, and mu, delta, and kappa receptors that are found throughout the central nervous system. The poppy plant extract, opium, binds to specialized proteins within the central nervous system. Scientists have expanded on this knowledge and have developed opioids, which are a group of chemicals that bind to one or more of the three opioid receptors in the central nervous sys-tem. Endogenous opioids, like exogenous opioids, bind to opioid receptor sites and modulate the transmission of pain impulses. Other receptors, including the N-methyl-D-aspartate (NMDA) receptors found in the dorsal horn, also influence the endogenous opiate system. Blockage of NMDA receptors may increase the mureceptors' responsiveness to opiates. In addition to this mode of modulation, the central nervous system also contains a descending system that controls pain transmission through inhibition of synaptic pain transmission at the level of the dorsal horn in the spinal cord. Neurotransmitters that play an important role in this descending system include endogenous opioids, serotonin, norepinephrine, and gamma-aminobutyric acid (GABA).

Pathophysiology of Neuropathic and Functional Pain

Neuropathic and functional pain are different from nociceptive pain in that they can become disengaged from noxious stimuli or healing and are often described in terms of chronic pain. These types of pain often present as burning, tingling, or shooting sensations. In addition, persons with chronic pain may have exaggerated painful responses to normally noxious stimuli (hyperalgesia) or painful responses to normally non-noxious stimuli (allodynia).

Neuropathic pain results from direct injury to nerves in the peripheral or central nervous system. Diabetic neuropathy and phantom limb pain are two examples of neuropathic pain. Phantom limb pain can occur after traumatic or surgical limb amputation. Functional pain syndromes include fibromyalgia, irritable bowel syndrome, tension-type headaches, and sympathetic-induced pain that results from abnormal operation of the nervous system. These types of pain syndromes are complex and can be very difficult to treat, as the pain reported is not evident by examining physical findings.

The exact mechanism of neuropathic or functional pain is complex. Overall, nerve damage or certain disease states may signal changes in inflammatory pain, ectopic excitability, enhanced sensory transmission, nerve structure reorganization, and loss of modulatory pain inhibition. Pain circuits eventually rewire themselves both anatomically and chemically, producing a mismatch between pain stimulation and inhibition. This results in an increase in the discharge of dorsal horn neurons. These changes over time help explain why this type of pain often manifests long after the actual nerve-related injury or when no actual injury is identified.

Pain Management

Successful pain management depends on a comprehensive assessment of the patient including the nature of the pain and how it is impacting the patient's life. Often, numeric rating scales are used to measure pain. Zero on the scale indicates no pain and 10 indicates the most unbearable pain. Patients should be asked frequently throughout the treatment to rate their pain in order to understand whether they are improving.

There are several classes of agents that can be used for the management of pain. These include nonsteroidal anti-inflammatory drugs (NSAIDs), opioids, anticonvulsants, and antidepressants, among others. Acute and chronic pain states are managed differently. Traditionally, acute pain is managed based on pain scores. A mild pain (score 1–3) is usually treated with a nonopioid medication like acetaminophen (Tylenol) or ibuprofen (Advil). Moderate pain (score 4–6) is treated with an immediate-release, short-acting opioid in addition to a nonopioid if needed. Severe pain (score 7–10) is usually managed with two therapy modalities, including a short-acting opioid that is rapidly titrated in addition to a nonopioid or long-acting opioid.

Danielle Stutzman

See also: Congenital Insensitivity to Pain; Nociceptors; Phantom Pain; Sensory Receptors

Further Reading

MedlinePlus. (2013). *Pain.* U.S. National Library of Medicine. Retrieved from http://www .nlm.nih.gov/medlineplus/pain.html

National Institute of Neurological Disorders and Stroke (NINDS). (2012). *NINDS chronic pain information page.* Retrieved from http://www.ninds.nih.gov/disorders/chronic _pain/chronic_pain.htm

NOCICEPTORS

Nociceptors, or pain receptors, are located across the body. They are considered "free" nerve endings; they respond to noxious or harmful stimuli such as excessive heat, excessive cold, or chemicals and send a signal to the brain of pain. Nociceptors lie in both the cutaneous and subcutaneous layers of the skin as well as the cornea and a variety of internal organs. While nociceptors provide the signal to the brain indicating pain, the two are not mutually exclusive. It is possible to feel pain without a signal from a nociceptor, and similarly it is possible to feel no pain when they are firing signals. Nociception plays an integral role in everyday life, alerting you to dangers and signaling you to avoid them. However, the body does have some control over nociceptor signals, regulating the amount of pain that is felt at specific locations.

Types and Functions

Nociceptors can be classified into a few main groups depending on the stimuli that they respond to. These groups are polymodal nociceptors, mechanical nociceptors, thermal nociceptors, and chemical nociceptors. Polymodal nociceptors is the classification that most nociceptors fall into. These nociceptors respond to mechanical, thermal, and chemical stimuli. Other nociceptors show a high degree of selectivity for their stimuli, and it is important to note that the stimuli they respond to are excessive—the stimulus is strong enough to damage tissue.

There are also two different types of axons or fibers: unmyelinated C-fibers and lightly myelinated A delta fibers. Both of these fiber types conduct signals to the brain and spinal cord relatively slowly. Nevertheless, nociception does have a fast and a slow signal. A delta fibers conduct signals fairly quickly—approximately 20 meters per second (m/s)—whereas C-fibers conduct pain signals much more slowly—closer to 2 m/s. The more selective nociceptors typically conduct their signals along A delta fibers as these stimuli tend to be more intense and dangerous, thus requiring a faster response. C-fibers tend to conduct signals from polymodal nociceptors. Recent research is finding that C-fibers also have a large selectivity for histamine and are responsible for the perception of painful itch, like a bee sting. All nociceptors have a large receptive field because it is more important for the brain to get a signal of pain than to know the exact location of that pain.

Pathway

There are two main pathways that signals from nociceptors travel down. These are the spinothalamic pathway and the trigeminal pathway. Within the spinothalamic pathway, the second-order neuron's axon crosses over immediately and travels to the brain through the spinothalamic tract. It projects through the medulla, pons, and midbrain, eventually synapsing in the thalamus. This pathway ascends contralaterally. As is indicated in the name, the trigeminal pathway mainly conveys information about painful signals from the face and head (including the cornea). The first-order neurons in the trigeminal pathway synapse on second-order neurons in the spinal trigeminal nucleus of the brainstem. Eventually the axons from the second-order neurons cross over and ascend to the thalamus through the trigeminal lemniscus. The trigeminal lemniscus conveys information about the face's orientation in space in addition to conveying information about pressure, pain, and temperature (partially through nociception).

Once the two pathways reach the thalamus, the signal is then sent to various regions of the cerebral cortex based on the location of the painful signal. This is where the signal is integrated and a potential motor reaction is created. Additionally, both pathways have many other neurons that will synapse at various levels within the brainstem and spinal cord. These synapses are important in playing a role in reflexes. Instead of your body waiting for the relatively slow signals to reach the brain, be processed, and a response to be sent back, it is more important to have a more immediate reaction. These reflexes are what tell you to pull your hand away from a hot stove before your brain registers that it is hot and that it burns. After this initial response, the brain has time to make a decision based on the information that it is receiving.

Regulation

One theory proposed in the 1960s by Melzack and Wall introduced the idea that activity in nociceptors could be reduced with the addition of vibration, pressure, or touch sensations in the same location. These signals would override the feeling of pain coming from the nociceptor, causing the individual to feel less pain. This theory is called the gate theory of pain and was used to describe why rubbing the area around a wound would often help to alleviate some of the pain.

Another form of regulation includes endogenous opioids. Opioids are natural chemicals that the body uses to reduce sensations of pain. Modern opiates (man-made chemicals) perform a similar function and are often prescribed to help alleviate pain in patients. Both endogenous and exogenous opioids will bind to several types of receptors throughout the brain. These chemicals block pain signals through nociceptors to the brain, causing the individual to feel less pain.

Riannon C. Atwater

See also: Congenital Insensitivity to Pain; Nociception

Further Reading

Dafny, Nachum. (2015). Chapter 8: Pain modulation and mechanisms. *Neuroscience Online*. John H. Byrne (Ed.). Retrieved from http://neuroscience.uth.tmc.edu/s2 /chapter08.html
Nociceptors. (2001). In D. Purves, G. J. Augustine, D. Fitzpatrick, W. C. Hall, A. LaMantia, J. O. McNamara, & S. M. Williams (Eds.), *Neuroscience* (2nd ed.). Sunderland, MA: Sinauer Associates. Retrieved from http://www.ncbi.nlm.nih.gov/books/NBK10965/

NORADRENALINE

Noradrenaline or norepinephrine is a monoamine molecule (made of one amino acid, one base unit of protein) that functions as both a hormone and a neurotransmitter. Norepinephrine is incredibly important in cognitive awareness. It is released by a presynaptic sympathetic ganglion to act on the heart as a stress molecule that increases heart rate. Not only does norepinephrine play a role in the sympathetic branch of the autonomic nervous system (ANS), it also directly affects the amygdala, which is a brain structure important in controlling attention. Norepinephrine is synthesized mainly by the adrenal medulla (a structure in the adrenals that is associated with each kidney). However, it can also be synthesized and secreted by presynaptic noradrenergic neurons in the central nervous system. Treatment of hypotension (low blood pressure) is often done by administering noradrenaline to the patient.

Synthesis and Mechanism of Action

The adrenal medulla synthesizes a large amount of norepinephrine, which is then secreted by the adrenals directly into the blood without the use of a duct. It is also synthesized by postganglionic neurons in the sympathetic nervous system (SNS) of the ANS. Additionally, a region in the brainstem called the locus coeruleus is responsible for originating most of the pathways that utilize norepinephrine as their neurotransmitter in the brain. These signals are propagated through noradrenergic neurons that are bilateral (on both sides of the brain) and that run to various locations. Some of these locations in the brain include the cerebral cortex and the limbic system. These noradrenergic neurons also run to the spinal cord. All of these pathways combined are considered a neurotransmitter system that utilizes noradrenaline. Any noradrenergic neuron is capable of synthesizing and secreting norepinephrine when trying to propagate neural signals. Norepinephrine is fairly similar in structure to epinephrine, as norepinephrine is just an oxidized version of epinephrine. Dopamine is the major precursor to norepinephrine.

Norepinephrine is fairly important in the SNS response and "fight-or-flight." The SNS is a part of the ANS that is important in responding to possible threats to the organism. When the SNS is stimulated, blood is funneled from the digestive and urinary organs to the heart, lungs, brain, and muscles. This results in the body's ability to respond properly to a threat. The effects that are felt when there is an activation of noradrenergic neurons are an increase in alertness, arousal, and positive effects on the reward system. Norepinephrine has the physiologic response of constricting the blood vessels and serum glucose levels (by stimulating glycolysis in the muscles and liver and inhibiting the production and secretion of insulin by the pancreas). The constriction of blood vessels will eventually result in an increase in blood pressure. These physiologic responses help the body have the energy, nutrients, and oxygen to respond to the threat it is encountering.

Medical Applications

Norepinephrine is extensively used to treat hypotension in patients. Hypotension is a condition in which systemic blood pressure is abnormally low. This can result in blood not circulating correctly and tissue not getting the correct amount of oxygen. Since one of the sympathetic effects of norepinephrine is the constriction of blood vessels, it can be used to treat this condition. The constriction of the blood vessels will result in higher blood pressure since the size of the vessels themselves will decrease. It is important to maintain proper levels of norepinephrine. If levels become too high, the patient might begin feeling highly stressed, anxious, and hyperactive. Low levels are linked to difficulties focusing and finding motivation along with a massive lack of focus. Additionally, there are some adverse effects of norepinephrine such as swelling of the face, lips, and tongue; uneven heart rate; alarmingly high blood pressure; blue lips and fingertips (a sign that tissues are not getting enough oxygen delivered to them); and difficulty breathing.

Riannon C. Atwater

See also: Adrenaline; Autonomic Nervous System; Carotid Body

Further Reading

Kandel, Eric R., James H. Schwartz, Thomas M. Jessell, Steven A. Siegelbaum, & A. J. Hudspeth (Eds.). (2012). *Principles of neural science* (5th ed.). New York, NY: McGraw-Hill.

Klabunde, Richard E. (2012). Norepinephrine, epinephrine and acetylcholine—Synthesis, storage, release and metabolism. In *Cardiovascular Pharmacology Concepts*. Retrieved from http://www.cvpharmacology.com/norepinephrine.htm

Purves, Dale, et al. (Eds.). (2004). *Neuroscience* (3rd ed.). Sunderland, MA: Sinauer Associates.

NOREPINEPHRINE: *See* Noradrenaline

NOSE: *See* Olfactory System

NYSTAGMUS

Nystagmus is an ophthalmic disorder that is characterized by involuntary, repetitive movements of one or both eyes. The condition presents with the eyes shifting up and down, side to side, or in a circular manner. Some even describe nystagmus as the eyes appearing to be "dancing." There are many possible etiologies of nystagmus, and removal of an identifiable cause remains the most effective form of management.

Pathophysiology

Nystagmus occurs due to a dysfunction in the areas of the brain and inner ear that regulate eye movement. When the head rotates, organs within the vestibular system of the inner ear detect the movement and send signals to the brain initiating appropriate eye adjustment. This process allows for the eyes to adapt to the motion and maintain a stable line of vision. A disruption in this signaling pathway is what leads to the inappropriate ocular muscle movements associated with nystagmus.

Based on its etiology, there are two main classifications of nystagmus: infantile nystagmus syndrome (INS) and acquired nystagmus. INS is a condition that patients are born with, typically presenting within six weeks to three months of age. The disorder is genetically inherited, and a family history will increase the likelihood of development. Conversely, acquired nystagmus occurs later in life as a result of causative factors. Several diseases and injuries in the inner ear and brain have been implicated in the development of acquired nystagmus, due to these organs' role in proper eye movement. Additionally, the presence of existing vision problems such as cataracts (cloudiness of the lens) and myopia (nearsightedness) can contribute to faster progression of nystagmus. Common medications associated with nystagmus are antiseizure drugs, such as phenytoin. Furthermore, excess use of alcohol and sedatives can lead to the condition, as a result of their effects on balance within the inner ear. Despite the multitude of implicated diseases, a cause of nystagmus cannot be identified in some patients, and this is termed idiopathic nystagmus.

Presentation

The severity of nystagmus can vary greatly between patients and from day to day, with movements of the eyes changing in speed and duration. The condition can present continuously or in intermittent episodes that occur spontaneously or are triggered by factors such as stress and fatigue. The movements associated with nystagmus can be classified as pendular, where the eyes move at the same speed in either direction, or jerk, where the eyes drift slowly in one direction and quickly in the other. Symptoms of nystagmus include oscillopsia, when objects in the visual field appear shaky. This can lead to significant vision impairment, as surroundings are viewed as blurry. Other visual defects include light sensitivity and difficulty seeing in the dark. Patients with nystagmus often feel the need to tilt their heads, as this has been known to help improve visual focus. Due to the effects on inner ear balance, patients may also experience dizziness and vertigo.

Diagnosis and Treatment

Diagnosis of nystagmus should be done with a thorough eye examination to rule out all other conditions. Tests that detect the disorder may involve the patient spinning around for several seconds, stopping, and attempting to stare at an object. When focusing on the object, the eyes will move quickly in different directions if the patient has nystagmus. Visual acuity tests can be used to determine the impact of nystagmus on a patient's vision.

When managing nystagmus, it is important to establish what is causing the disorder and treat the underlying disease. Removal of offending agents can result in spontaneous return to normal eye movement. When all etiologies have been accounted for, the only treatment options for nystagmus are to improve symptoms. Certain medications such as baclofen (a muscle relaxant) and gabapentin (a nerve-modifier) have been used in practice with variable success. Botulinum toxin injections (commercially known as Botox) have been useful in mildly paralyzing eye muscles in patients who experience severe shakiness. Prisms are corrective factors that can be added to eyeglasses to help keep the eyes in fixed positions for better visual focus. Finally, surgery is an option for severe nystagmus to alter the positions of ocular muscles, although this procedure has shown inconsistent results. Importantly, none of these therapies has demonstrated complete reversal of nystagmus, and the need for more effective treatment options remains a future area of clinical study.

Vidya Pugazhenthi

See also: Dizziness; Vestibular System; Visual System

Further Reading

American Academy of Ophthalmology. (2013). *What is nystagmus?* Retrieved from www .geteyesmart.org/eyesmart/diseases/nystagmus.cfm

Bradley, Walter G. (2004). *Neurology in clinical practice.* Philadelphia, PA: Butterworth Heinemann.

Medline Plus. (2013). *Nystagmus.* Retrieved from http://www.nlm.nih.gov/medlineplus/ency /article/003037.htm

OCCIPITAL LOBE

The occipital lobe is the primary visual processing center of the mammalian brain. It is one of the four main lobes of the brain and is located in the posterior region of the cerebral cortex. There are two occipital lobes, one each on the right and the left hemispheres of the brain. The occipital lobe is involved in visual perception and color recognition. This particular lobe is not very vulnerable to injury because of its location at the back of the brain. However, any significant trauma to the brain could cause subtle changes to the visual-perceptual system. Damage to the occipital lobe can cause blindness or a condition called cortical blindness. People with this condition have no pattern of perception and no awareness of visual information.

Anatomy and Function

The primary visual cortex (PVC) is the main region of the brain that is responsible for sight and is called Brodmann area 17. This area of the brain recognizes size, shape, color, light, motion, and dimension of objects. For example, the PVC helps a person identify the basic features of a pencil—the edges, the amount of light, and its location in space. The PVC sends signals to other cortical regions called the visual association areas, which are located in the posterior portions of the temporal and parietal lobes. It is the visual association areas that interpret the information received from the PVC and helps a person recognize an object as well as recall its name, such as goldfish, book, face, or television.

The visual cortex is made up of several neurons that will respond to a specific stimulus like light, color, or movement. The region within the occipital lobe in which a neuron will be activated is called a receptive field. The neurons contained in the receptive fields are named based on the stimulus that is needed to activate them. For example, simple cells may respond only to light. Complex cells may respond to light moving only from left to right, while hypercomplex cells may respond to a two-inch length of light moving from left to right. These receptive fields help to determine the physical features of objects that a person sees.

In addition to receptive fields, the PVC contains columns of cortical neurons that respond from input of either the left or right eye. These are called ocular dominance columns. It has been hypothesized that these columns are required for binocular vision as a person who has input from a single eye will not have well-formed columns. Other studies, however, suggest that ocular dominance columns may result from visual development and may not have a true function.

Damage to the Occipital Lobe

In rare cases, the occipital lobe may be injured from accidents such as vehicle crashes or falls. Damage to the occipital lobe can cause blindness or a condition called cortical blindness. People with this condition have no pattern of perception and no awareness of visual information. Injuries to the parietal-temporal-occipital visual association areas may cause visual defects like having (1) problems locating objects, (2) difficulty with color recognition (color agnosia), or (3) trouble with reading (alexia) and writing (agraphia).

Another common problem in the occipital lobe is occipital seizures. These seizures are often mistaken for a migraine headache due to the similar symptoms shared by the two disorders. These seizures usually begin with visual hallucinations and can often be triggered by visual stimuli, such as playing video games or staring at a television. This is because images on computer and television monitors are flickering but the brain perceives them as a constant image. Occipital lobe epilepsy accounts for about 5–10 percent of all epilepsy cases (Adcock & Panayiotopoulos, 2012). This is typically due to an unknown cause or due to a lesion in the occipital lobe. Occipital epilepsy usually begins in childhood but may occur at any age.

Renee Johnson and Jennifer L. Hellier

See also: Blindness; Brain Anatomy; Brodmann Areas; Color Perception; Ocular Dominance Columns; Optic Nerve; Visual Perception; Visual System

Further Reading

Adcock, Jane E., & Chrysostomos P. Panayiotopoulos. (2012). Occipital lobe seizures and epilepsies. *Journal of Clinical Neurophysiology*, 29(5), 397–407.

Hines, Tonya. (2011). Anatomy of the brain. *Mayfield Clinic for Brain & Spine*. Retrieved from http://www.mayfieldclinic.com/PE-AnatBrain.htm#.U_SJy0tFFfM

Kandel, Eric R., et al. (Eds.). (2012). *Principles of neural science* (5th ed.). New York, NY: McGraw-Hill.

OCULAR DOMINANCE COLUMNS

The visual system is the most well-studied sensory system of animals. From these studies it is known that processing vision within the brain is extremely complex. Part of this processing occurs within ocular dominance columns. Ocular dominance columns are groups of neurons that span several layers of the primary visual cortex. They are anatomical structures that make up the striate cortex, which is a

Dominant Eye Test

Humans do not only have a dominant hand (right or left), but also have a dominant eye. This develops during childhood and has a critical period for development. The medical term for dominant eye is ocular dominance. It means that one eye is preferred for visual input over the other eye. Ocular dominance may not be on the same side as the person's dominant hand. This is because both the left and right hemispheres of the brain control vision as well as control different halves of the visual field and of each retina (the back of the eye where objects are visually formed). Just as most humans are right-handed, most are also right-eye dominant.

Materials:

2 eyes (for one of the tests below, the person must have the ability to close one eye at a time)
2 hands, forming a triangle shape
An object in the distance (about 10 feet away)

Directions:

There are two easy ways to determine a person's dominant eye. Both tests start with having the person hold their arms out at eye level. Next have the person make the letter "L" with each hand. Specifically, have the person hold their palms outward, fingers up, and thumbs out—making the L-shape. Have the person bring their hands together and cross one over the other. This makes a triangle space: one thumb over the other and one set of fingers over the other. Next, have the person look through the triangle space made by their hands at an object with both eyes. It is preferable to have the entire object almost completely fill the space. The person will use these directions to complete both tests to determine which eye is dominant.

Test 1: Keeping the hands together, have the person bring their hands back to their face toward one eye. For example, the person will bring their triangle-shaped hands to their right eye until the base of their left thumb touches the tip of their nose. If the image stays within the open space, that is the person's dominant eye. Now have the person start over and bring their hands back to the left eye until the base of their right thumb touches their nose. The object should partially or completely disappear from the opening.

Test 2: Keeping the hands together, have the person close one eye and then the other. If the image stays within the open space, that is the person's dominant eye. The object will seem to "jump" sideways when the dominant eye is closed. To learn more about your dominant eye please see http://www.sciencemadesimple.co.uk/activities/left_or_right_eyed

Jennifer L. Hellier

portion of the primary visual cortex. Ocular dominance columns are found as a striped pattern on the surface of the striate cortex. They are perpendicular to another set of cells that make up the orientation columns. Drs. David H. Hubel (1926–2013) and Torsten N. Wiesel (1924–) discovered ocular dominance columns during their research in the primary visual cortices of cats. Since these experiments, ocular dominance columns have been found in many mammals, including humans.

Anatomy and Physiology

When an object is viewed, its image is sent to the retina of the eye and then through the optic nerve to the lateral geniculate nucleus of the thalamus. Here the image's information is sent to the primary visual cortex, where the ocular dominance columns are located. These columns are alternating bands and patches from the left and right eye preferences. Previously, it was thought that ocular dominance columns are like an orderly sensory map of the outside world that develop by activity-dependent processes. However, more recently, it has been shown that ocular dominance columns develop earlier than originally thought and that they have a predetermined specification pattern.

These columns are activated primarily from the input of one eye and not the other and they develop in utero. However, after birth there is a "critical period," which is now called the "sensitive period," for ocular dominance columns. Visual input from both eyes is required for developing vision. However, after a baby is born, it is crucial that both of the baby's eyes have visual input, as the columns undergo activity-dependent plasticity. This means the ocular dominance columns can degrade during the sensitive period. Hubel and Wiesel found that blocking vision in one eye during the critical period resulted in the unaffected eye developing ocular columns in regions of the striate cortex that would normally be developed by the blocked eye.

Originally, ocular dominance columns were hypothesized to be important for binocular vision. However, these columns are not as distinct or well developed in all animals with binocular vision, such as rats and squirrel monkeys. Now, scientists are wondering if ocular dominance columns are more a result of development, particularly from synaptic plasticity or Hebbian learning. These functions can occur from the spontaneous activity of the retina of the developing fetus or from the lateral geniculate nucleus of the thalamus that projects to the striate cortex. Other studies, however, suggest that ocular dominance columns may be just a result from visual development and may not have a true function.

Jennifer L. Hellier

See also: Blindness; Hubel, David H.; Optic Nerve; Visual Fields; Visual Perception; Visual System; Wiesel, Torsten N.

Further Reading

Adams, Daniel L., Lawrence C. Sincich, & Jonathan C. Horton. (2007). Complete pattern of ocular dominance columns in human primary visual cortex. *Journal of Neuroscience, 27*, 10391–10403.

Purves, Dale, et al. (2008). *Neuroscience* (4th ed.). Sunderland, MA: Sinauer Associates.

Tomita, Koichi, Max Sperling, Sidney B. Cambridge, Tobias Bonhoeffer, & Mark Hübener. (2013). A molecular correlate of ocular dominance columns in the developing mammalian visual cortex. *Cerebral Cortex, 23*(11), 2531–2541. http://dx.doi.org/10.1093/cercor/bhs232. Retrieved from http://cercor.oxfordjournals.org/content/23/11/2531.long

ODOR INTENSITY SCALE

Neuroscientists have identified four dimensions of an odor including odor concentration (an odor's pervasiveness), hedonic tone (the odor is ranked from extremely unpleasant to extremely pleasant), character (description of the odor to distinguish it from another), and odor intensity. How strongly an odor is perceived through the nose and interpreted by the brain is the odor's intensity. An odor's intensity is a property of the olfactory system that helps animals locate an odor's source. It is also essential for determining if an odor is a nuisance and to warn the animal of potential danger (e.g., spoiled food or a gas leak). Odor intensity is analogous to the perception of temperature sensation in humans, such as identifying whether an object is warm or cold. However, individuals can perceive an odor differently. Just as in the children's story "Goldilocks and the Three Bears," an odor may be too strong for one person, barely detectable by another individual, and just right for a third person. Thus, the field of psychophysics was developed to quantify the relationship between a physical stimulus (like an odor) and the perception and sensation it affects in humans.

Psychophysics and Odor Intensity

German physician Ernst Heinrich Weber (1795–1878) was the first person to quantify a human response to a physical stimulus. Using 5-pound dumbbells and slightly changing the weight by half a pound (0.5 pound), he asked individuals if they could detect the difference (if it was heavier). From these experiments, he developed Weber's law, which states that the just-noticeable difference between two stimuli is proportional to the magnitude of the stimuli and the person's sensitivity. This means if a person can detect the difference of 0.5 pound on a 5-pound dumbbell, the person should also be able to detect the difference of 1 pound on a 10-pound dumbbell. Weber's student Gustav Theodor Fechner (1801–1887), who was a German physicist and experimental psychologist, added to Weber's law to develop a psychophysical scale. This scale described the relationship between the physical magnitude of a stimulus (such as odor, sound, or light intensity) and the perceived intensity by the subject. Fechner's scale states that subjective sensation is proportional to the logarithm of the stimulus intensity. This scale is now often called the Weber-Fechner law.

In psychophysics, an odor's intensity is related to its physical concentration and strength and can be measured by the Weber-Fechner law: $I = a \times \log(c) + b$, where I is the perceived psychological intensity at the dilution step on the butanol scale, a is the Weber-Fechner coefficient, C is the chemical concentration, and b is the intercept constant (0.5 by definition; Jiang et al., 2006).

Not everyone can quickly calculate the Weber-Fechner law to determine an odor's intensity, thus neuroscientists have produced a verbal odor intensity scale to describe the odor's sensation. This numbered scale ranges from 0 to 6 with specific words to describe an odor's intensity. A score of 0 represents no odor. A score of 1 is a very weak odor and when an odor is first detected, an odor's threshold. A score of 2 represents a weak odor. A score of 3 is a distinct odor, generally when a person can quickly identify the name or character of the smell. A score of 4 represents a strong odor. A score of 5 means a very strong odor, which for some people can be distracting. Finally, a score of 6 denotes the odor is intolerable, meaning for most individuals it is a very annoying or bothersome smell. Today, this descriptive odor intensity scale is used in the laboratory by highly and suitably trained observers, who can quickly and easily determine the nuances of the scale to identify an odor's intensity.

Patricia A. Bloomquist and Jennifer L. Hellier

See also: Odor Threshold; Olfactory Mucosa; Olfactory Reference Syndrome; Olfactory Sensory Neurons; Olfactory System; Primary Odors

Further Reading

Alobid, Isam, Santiago Nogue, Adriana Izquierdo-Dominguez, Silvia Centellas, Manuel Bernal-Sprekelsen, & Joaquim Mullol. (2014). Multiple chemical sensitivity worsens quality of life and cognitive and sensorial features of sense of smell. *European Archives of Oto-rhino-laryngology, 271*(12), 3203–3208. http://dx.doi.org/10.1007/s00405-014-3015-5

Jiang, John, Patrick Coffey, & Brendan Toohey. (2006). Improvement of odor intensity measurement using dynamic olfactometry. *Journal of Air and Waste Management, 56*, 675–683. http://dx.doi.org/10.1038/17383

Wojcik, Pawel T., & Yevgeniy B. Sirotin. (2014). Single scale for odor intensity in rat olfaction. *Current Biology, 24*(5), 568–573. http://dx.doi.org/10.1016/j.cub.2014.01.059

ODOR THRESHOLD

Neuroscientists have identified four dimensions of an odor including odor concentration (an odor's pervasiveness), hedonic tone (the odor is ranked from extremely unpleasant to extremely pleasant), character (description of the odor to distinguish it from another), and odor intensity (how strongly an odor is perceived). Odor threshold is the lowest concentration of an odorant that can be first detected by the human nose in either air or a liquid, such as water or oil. Thus, the resulting minimal concentration of the odor is the odor threshold value (OTV), which is generally expressed as a concentration in air or as a concentration in liquid (for example, 0.1 percent in mineral oil).

Testing Odor Threshold in Research

Mice are often used in research as their olfaction abilities can easily be tested with an olfactometer. An olfactometer is a specialized machine that presents a subject (a mouse in this case) with an odorant at different concentrations. The olfactometer can be used in a simple go-no-go behavioral task that the mouse learns and is rewarded with water. In these types of experiments, "go" is the positive stimulus (S+) that rewards with water and "no-go" is the negative stimulus (S–) that provides no reward. Thus, a go-no-go behavioral task requires mice to learn to lick on a water-rewarded stimulus (for example, 1 percent isoamyl acetate—a banana-like smell—in mineral oil; S+) and not to lick on an unrewarded stimulus (mineral oil alone—the control; S-). After completion of three consecutive blocks with greater than 85 percent accuracy, it is determined that a mouse has learned the go-no-go task. The olfactometer can be used for additional behavioral experiments, such as Maximum Likelihood Parameter ESTimation (MLPEST, Clevenger & Restrepo, 2006). This method is reliable and accurately assesses olfactory detection threshold within a single day. As MLPEST is a difficult behavioral task, mice are first trained on the go-no-go behavioral task before being tested in MLPEST to determine their ability to identify an odor's threshold.

Odor Threshold and Neurological Diseases or Disorders

Changes in a person's sense of smell can be associated with neurological disease such as Alzheimer's disease and schizophrenia or neurodegenerative disorders like Parkinson's disease. Because it is an easy and noninvasive way to quickly determine a person's olfactory dysfunction, neurologists will test a patient's sense of smell. Generally, odor threshold (T) is often tested along with odor discrimination (D) and odor identity (I). Patients are presented with a series of 16 "sniffing sticks" using a three-alternative forced-choice task and a staircase paradigm. Each stick has a specific concentration of an odorant, which is usually a rose-like odor (phenylethyl alcohol). Patients are given the lowest concentration stick along with two blank sticks (for controls). They sniff each stick independently and are asked if they can smell anything. If not, they are given the next concentration stick with two blank sticks and repeat the sniffing sequence. Two successive correct identifications or one incorrect identification, respectively, triggers a reversal of the staircase. Odor threshold is then represented by the mean of the last four out of seven staircase reversals. In general, most patients with Parkinson's disease will need a higher concentration of odorant for them to be able to detect the odor's threshold compared to control adults.

Jennifer L. Hellier

See also: Anosmia; Odor Intensity Scale; Olfactory Mucosa; Olfactory Reference Syndrome; Olfactory Sensory Neurons; Olfactory System; Primary Odors

Further Reading

Alobid, Isam, Santiago Nogue, Adriana Izquierdo-Dominguez, Silvia Centellas, Manuel Bernal-Sprekelsen, & Joaquim Mullol. (2014). Multiple chemical sensitivity worsens quality of life and cognitive and sensorial features of sense of smell. *European Archives of Oto-rhino-laryngology, 271*(12), 3203–3208. http://dx.doi.org/10.1007/s00405-014 -3015-5

Clevenger, Amy C., & Diego Restrepo. (2006). Evaluation of the validity of a maximum likelihood adaptive staircase procedure for measurement of olfactory detection threshold in mice. *Chemical Senses, 31*, 9–26.

Lotsch, Jorn, Heinz Reichmann, & Thomas Hummel. (2007). Different odor tests contribute differently to the evaluation of olfactory loss. *Chemical Senses, 33*(1), 17–21. Retrieved from http://chemse.oxfordjournals.org/content/33/1/17.full

OLFACTORY BULB

The olfactory system plays an important role in an organism's ability to grasp its environment. One of the most important regions of the brain responsible for olfaction is the olfactory bulb. The olfactory bulb processes molecular information from specific chemoreceptors called olfactory receptors and interprets it as a scent. This organ is responsible for an organism's ability to identify smell, also known as the olfactory sense. In addition to being an important sensory system for survival for many organisms, the sense of smell is thought to be most associated with memory due to the olfactory bulb's location in the brain.

History and Function

Richard Axel (1946–) and Linda Buck (1947–) were awarded the 2004 Nobel Prize in Medicine for their work with olfactory receptors (Keeley, 2004). During their study, they discovered the genes responsible for olfactory receptors. They also found that olfactory receptors have high specificity to vaporizable molecules, also known as aromatics.

These receptors have axons that extend all the way to the olfactory bulb. Because these receptors are highly specific to their binding agent, they can be classified into families. Each family of receptors converge to a single point, creating a bundle of nerve endings called a glomerulus. The main olfactory bulb is home to these glomeruli, and it is where scents are identified and interpreted.

An activated glomerulus enables the olfactory bulb to decipher the scent specific to those receptors. Because each glomerulus is associated with a single type of molecule, scientists have mapped the main olfactory bulb to locate where different odors are deciphered within it.

The accessory olfactory bulb is part of the olfactory bulb and has been attributed to mating and social behaviors in organisms. It responds to pheromones in addition to ordinary aromatics. Although the existence of this structure has been largely identified in mice and rodents, it is thought to be absent in adult humans. Scientists found an accessory olfactory bulb in human embryo, but later stages show the structure simplifies and eventually disappears as the embryo develops (Shepherd, 2010).

Anatomy and Physiology

The olfactory bulb is located on the inferior part of the forebrain. Olfactory receptors bind to specific molecules in the air. Correct molecules will trigger a cascade of action potentials, serving as a signal that is then relayed to the specific glomerulus of the receptors. This information is then relayed to other parts of the brain, such as the hippocampus and amygdala. The hippocampus is responsible for memory formation whereas the amygdala is the primary processor of emotions. The olfactory bulb is directly linked to both of these structures. This is thought to be the reason for the strong correlation between scents and memories.

The vomeronasal system is a part of the auxiliary olfactory system that is largely governed by the accessory olfactory bulb. Although adult humans largely lose the accessory olfactory bulb during development, it plays a huge role in other mammals in choosing partners (Shepherd, 2010). Pheromones are airborne hormones detectable by the vomeronasal system, which contributes to the chemistry of attraction during mating season in many animals. The accessory olfactory bulb is located in the nasal passage and is directly connected to the amygdala. Due to the absence of this structure in adult humans, it is unclear whether or not the vomeronasal system exists outside of animals.

Disease and Disorders

Disease and disorders in the olfactory bulb cause an inability to distinguish scents. The degree of the defect depends on the severity. Many mechanisms can cause a defect, including facial trauma and neurodegeneration (Attems et al., 2014). Due to the location of the olfactory bulb, facial trauma can cause damage to the receptors as well as the bulb itself. Neurodegenerative diseases such as Parkinson's and Alzheimer's are also known to affect the olfactory bulb as the disease progresses. Any damage to the olfactory bulb and its associated receptors will cause a deficit in the organism's ability to process scents from its surrounding. This may affect appetite as well because the smell of food is known to contribute to gustation, or sense of taste.

Melissa Tjandra

See also: Anosmia; Axel, Richard; Bowman's Glands; Buck, Linda; Olfactory System

Further Reading

Attems, Johannes, Lauren Walker, & Kurt A. Jellinger. (2014). Olfactory bulb involvement in neurodegenerative diseases. *Acta Neuropathologica*, *127*(4), 459–475. Retrieved from http://www.ncbi.nlm.nih.gov/pubmed/24554308

Keeley, Jim. (2004). Richard Axel and Linda Buck awarded 2004 Nobel Prize in Physiology or Medicine. Howard Hughes Medical Institution. Retrieved from http://www.hhmi .org/news/richard-axel-and-linda-buck-awarded-2004-nobel-prize-physiology-or -medicine

Shepherd, Gordon M. (2010). New perspectives on olfactory processing. In A. Menini (Ed.), *The Neurobiology of Olfaction* (Chap. 16). Boca Raton, FL: CRC Press/Taylor & Francis. Retrieved from http://www.ncbi.nlm.nih.gov/books/NBK55977/

OLFACTORY MUCOSA

The sense of smell begins with an odorant binding to olfactory sensory neurons that reside in the olfactory mucosa of the nasal cavity. These olfactory sensory neurons face the external environment, which is unique to just the sense of smell. Because of the exposure to the environment, olfactory sensory neurons are much more vulnerable to infections and changes in the airway surface liquid or mucus. Thus, the olfactory mucosa is designed to protect these sensory neurons and undergo repair if necessary.

The olfactory system is also unusual compared to other sensory systems, as its sensory receptors are true neurons that project directly to the central nervous system. This is a potential route to transport bacteria or other infectious agents from the external environment to the central nervous system. This is why olfactory sensory neurons can be damaged easily. Recent studies have shown, however, that the olfactory system can repair itself particularly better than other sensory systems. This ability allows the olfactory system to maintain its sensory function.

Anatomy and Physiology

The nasal cavity is found between the ethmoid bone superiorly and the palate inferiorly. It is divided into two sections by the nasal septum. The nasal cavity is essential for conditioning the air that passes into the lungs as well as acting as a resonance chamber to enhance a person's speech. Within the nasal cavity lie the nasal and olfactory epithelia. This entry will focus on the olfactory mucosa and epithelium.

The olfactory mucosa contains the olfactory epithelium (also called the neuroepithelium to describe the olfactory sensory neurons within it) and the lamina propria, which lies just below the olfactory epithelium. The olfactory mucosa is located in the posterior and dorsal portion of the nasal cavity. The cell bodies within the olfactory epithelium are aligned, making the tissue appear stratified. There are four main cell types within the epithelium: (1) sustentacular cells (located near the apical surface), (2) mature olfactory sensory neurons (which have cilia that project into the external environment of the nasal cavity), (3) globose basal cells, and (4) horizontal basal cells (which are closest to the basal lamina). Sustentacular cells are support cells that express proteins associated with detoxifying mechanisms. This suggests that sustentacular cells assist in protecting olfactory sensory neurons from toxins and other foreign bodies. Mature olfactory sensory neurons are bipolar in shape with a ciliated dendrite that extends to the apical portion of the epithelium. These cilia contain receptors that bind specific odorants, converting the chemical signal to an electrical impulse (action potential), which begins the process of odor perception. The axons of the olfactory sensory neurons leave the epithelium through the basal layer and project to the olfactory bulb, carrying the action potential. There is a ratio of immature to mature olfactory sensory neurons within the epithelium, which allows a constant and/or continual replacement of neurons that become damaged. Immature sensory neurons have been shown to mature in about a week, including reinnervating the olfactory bulb. Lastly, the globose and horizontal basal cells proliferate at different rates, globose at a higher rate than horizontal cells, which maintains the normal function of the epithelium.

Within the lamina propria of the olfactory mucosa are the Bowman's glands. These are specialized cells that protrude through the olfactory epithelium so that its duct can release fluid onto the apical surface, allowing the cilia of the olfactory sensory neurons to be bathed in a protective discharge. Secretions from Bowman's glands, including lysozyme (an enzyme that damages bacterial cell walls to fight infection), amylase (an enzyme that breaks up starches), and immunoglobulin A (an antibody that is necessary for mucosal immunity), help moisten the epithelium in the nasal passages.

Regenerating the Olfactory Mucosa

There are two general types of injuries to the olfactory system: (1) direct damage to the olfactory epithelium via exposure to toxic chemicals that damage several different cell types, and (2) damage to the axons of the olfactory sensory neuron, which prevents the electrical signal from reaching the olfactory bulb. In cases where the epithelium is damaged, the toxin may not spread evenly throughout the nasal cavity, resulting in several regions of the olfactory mucosa being spared. The damaged area will have some recovery, but it may be incomplete. Severely damaged regions can recover but generally become respiratory epithelium instead of olfactory. In cases where the olfactory nerve is damaged, this signals an increase in maturing of immature olfactory sensory neurons so that the olfactory bulb can be reinnervated. Full recovery may or may not occur depending on the severity of the original lesion.

Jennifer L. Hellier

See also: Anosmia; Bowman's Glands; Dysosmia; Olfactory Bulb; Olfactory Sensory Neurons; Olfactory System

Further Reading

Farbman, Albert I. (1992). *Cell biology of olfaction.* New York, NY: Cambridge University Press.

Schwob, James E. (2002). Neural regeneration and the peripheral olfactory system. *Anatomical Record, 269*(1), 33–49.

OLFACTORY NERVE

The sense of smell is mediated via the olfactory nerve, which is one of the 12 pairs of cranial nerves. The olfactory nerve is purely sensory and has no motor component. It is the first cranial nerve and is also known as cranial nerve I. The olfactory nerve enters the brain and synapses (terminates) within the glomerular layer of the olfactory bulb. This is where an odor is first detected, filtered, and identified. The meaning or perception of the odor is determined in other regions of the brain in association with olfactory cortices. Collectively, structures involved in olfaction are part of the rhinencephalon, which translates from Latin as "nose brain."

General Functional Component

The olfactory nerve has one component, special sensory (special afferent). Its function is the sensation of olfaction, or the sense of smell. The inability to smell is called anosmia, which can be a congenital (present at birth) defect or associated with degenerative neurological diseases such as Parkinson's and Alzheimer's diseases.

Anatomy

Neurons that make up the olfactory nerve are found in the olfactory epithelium within the nasal passageway, specifically in the roof of the nasal cavity, the superior nasal conchae, and the nasal septum. These are special sensory neurons as they include the sensory receptor (a specialized protein) on the anterior end and the posterior end (axon) makes up the nerve. These neurons are called olfactory sensory neurons, which are activated when a specific chemical component of an odor binds to the receptor. When an odor enters the nostril, olfactory gland secretions dissolve the scent. These secretions also keep the olfactory epithelium moist.

Roughly 20 axons bundle together making several small branches of the olfactory nerve. These branches pass through the numerous foramina (holes) of the cribiform plate of the ethmoid bone. The axons then terminate on the secondary sensory neurons (mitral and tufted cells) of the olfactory bulb. Here the odor is filtered and identified before its signal is relayed to other brain regions, such as the limbic system that includes the amygdala and entorhinal cortex. The olfactory system is unique as it is the only sensory system that bypasses the thalamus, which is a deep structure in the brain that modulates neuronal signals (or alters the perception of the sense). Instead, the olfactory message directly enters the limbic system, which is associated with memories. This is why a specific smell, like a perfume, can instantly bring back memories of a certain place (for example, Grandma's house) or feelings.

Physiology

The olfactory system is also associated with the autonomic nervous system, particularly for visceral responses. The smell of food cooking will induce salivation if it is a pleasant odor, while unpleasant odors induce nausea. This is due to the complex medial forebrain bundle, the stria medullaris thalami, and stria terminals pathways.

Most animals have a very strong sense of smell, as it is important for finding food and potential mates as well as to determine nearby predators. Thus, nonhuman mammals and reptiles have two systems: the main olfactory system to detect volatile odors and an accessory olfactory system to detect fluid-phase stimuli. Fluid-phase stimuli are commonly known as pheromones, and it is important to note that some pheromones can be detected via the main olfactory system. The accessory olfactory system has a special organ to sense the fluid-phase stimuli. This structure is a bone that separates the left and right nasal cavities (between the nose and the mouth) and is called the vomeronasal organ. Mammals curl back their upper lip (flehmen) to stimulate the vomeronasal organ, while snakes stick out their tongue while touching the vomeronasal organ to detect prey.

Clinical Symptoms

Injury to cranial nerve I may occur during a fall or injury to the head especially if the cribiform plate breaks. This is because the nerve passes through the foramina of the cribiform plate and is easily severed. Tumors in the base of the anterior skull can also damage the olfactory nerve. The major symptom of a damaged nerve is the inability to smell in one (unilateral) or both (bilateral) nostrils. Anosmia may improve over time as the nerve regenerates. Persons with anosmia generally have a loss of appetite because they can no longer smell and their food lacks flavor.

Jennifer L. Hellier

See also: Anosmia; Cranial Nerves; Olfactory Bulb; Olfactory Sensory Neurons; Olfactory System; Sensory Receptors

Further Reading

Liang, Barbara. (2012). *The 12 cranial nerves.* Retrieved from http://www.wisc-online.com/objects/ViewObject.aspx?ID=AP11504

Wilson-Pauwels, Linda, E. J. Akesson, & Patricia A. Stewart. (1988). *Cranial nerves. Anatomy and clinical comments.* Philadelphia, PA: B. C. Decker.

OLFACTORY REFERENCE SYNDROME

Olfactory reference syndrome (ORS) is a psychiatric disorder. The term was first created in 1971 by neurologist William Pryse-Phillips. There have been many reported cases of ORS around the world, and several cases were reported in the literature between 1891 and 1966. People who have this disorder have an irrational and extreme fear, believing that they are producing a foul, unpleasant, and offensive odor. People with ORS believe that others around them can smell the odor and sometimes they may think that they themselves can smell the odor too. They may believe that they smell natural body smells, such as anal, vaginal, or overall body odor or a nonbody odor, such as a chemical odor. Patients feel ashamed and embarrassed, which can cause a great amount of distress and behavioral change. ORS can significantly impair a person's life. Many times people affected with ORS will stop working and will not be involved in social situations, because they wish to avoid the embarrassment they think they will experience. ORS can also have an effect on a person's academic life and relationships. A recent study showed that of patients with ORS who experienced symptoms, 74 percent avoided social circumstances and 47 percent avoided job-related, academic, or other significant activities (Feusner et al., 2010). People with ORS may also become depressed and may have suicidal feelings and/or actions. Furthermore, a study by Pryse-Phillips that included 26 patients reported that 43 percent experienced suicidal thoughts or actions. During their follow-up period, which is believed to have been approximately one to two years, 5.6 percent of the patients committed suicide (Feusner et al., 2010). People with ORS many times will construe others' actions as a reaction to their alleged body odor. Actions such as scratching the face, sneezing, turning away, or making comments can be misunderstood. Patients with ORS will usually perform certain characteristic repetitive behaviors. These include smelling/checking themselves; taking many unneeded showers; attempting to disguise the smell; changing their clothes often; using an excessive amount of deodorant, cologne, or perfumes; asking others around them for reassurance that they do not smell; avoiding public locations; and going to the doctor multiple times about their odor.

Classification and Diagnosis

ORS has not been defined as its own category in the *Diagnostic and Statistical Manual of Mental Disorders* (DSM). There are several different psychological disorders that ORS can resemble. These psychological disorders include social anxiety disorder (SAD), avoidant personality disorder (APD), Taijin Kyofusho (TKS), body dysmorphic disorder (BDD), hypochondriasis, obsessive compulsive disorder (OCD), major depression and social withdrawal, and psychotic disorders such as schizophrenia or delusional disorder. There are also general medical conditions such as skin conditions and infections that could be causing the odor. These medical conditions must be ruled out before making an ORS diagnosis. It is believed that ORS and BDD are closely related and that BDD would probably come closest to an ORS diagnosis. BDD is the condition of imagining one's body is somehow deformed in appearance. However, there are data demonstrating that individuals with BDD also have obsessions regarding odor. The diagnosis of ORS can be difficult. This is mostly because ORS does not have its own classification, and there are no specific diagnostic criteria. Many people with ORS are never properly diagnosed. Often, they will receive no diagnosis or will receive an incorrect diagnosis.

Treatment

The treatment for ORS uses many of the same techniques and treatments that are used to treat other related disorders such as OCD. Most treatments focus on cognitive behavioral intervention, using cognitive behavioral therapy (CBT) methods. Types of CBT methods include exposure and response prevention (ERP), imaginal exposure, cognitive restructuring, and mindfulness-based cognitive behavioral therapy. Cognitive restructuring can lessen the frequency and extent of the obsession. In exposure and response prevention, patients are exposed to situations they would normally avoid, while not being allowed to use their normal behaviors related to their perceived odor such as checking the odor or trying to get rid of it. In imaginal exposure, prerecorded videos are used to allow the patients to be exposed to experiences and situations that they are fearful of and imagine. In mindfulness-based CBT, the aim is to get the patient to be more willing to experience the fears, feelings, and urges without using any obsessive repetitive behaviors such as asking for reassurance. Some medications can also be used to treat ORS. These include antidepressants, specifically a type known as selective serotonin reuptake inhibitors (SSRIs), and antipsychotic drugs.

There are limited data and research regarding ORS, thus further research is warranted. Research should focus on developing specific diagnostic criteria and also deciding if ORS should have its own classification or if it should be classified under another disorder.

Shannen McNamara

See also: Dysosmia; Odor Intensity Scale; Odor Threshold; Olfactory System

Further Reading

Feusner, Jamie D., Katharine A. Phillips, & Dan J. Stein. (2010). Olfactory reference syndrome: Issues for DSM-V. *Depression and Anxiety*, 27(6), 592–599. Retrieved from http://www.dsm5.org/Research/Documents/Feusner_ORS.pdf

Houston OCD Program. (2016). *Olfactory reference syndrome*. Retrieved from http://houstonocdprogram.org/olfactory-reference-syndrome/

Lochner, Christine, & Dan J. Stein. (2003). Olfactory reference syndrome: Diagnostic criteria and differential diagnosis. *Journal of Post-Graduate Medicine*, 49(4), 328–331.

OLFACTORY SENSORY NEURONS

An olfactory sensory neuron (OSN) is a component within the olfactory system used to detect airborne chemicals that are inhaled, which gives rise to the sense of olfaction or smell. Olfactory sensory neurons are transduction cells that total about six million in humans (Moran et al., 1982). Transduction cells convert chemical signals into electrical signals that travel to the brain, so smells can be perceived. OSNs are classified as bipolar neurons due to having two processes that emerge from the cell body. These neurons are arranged with dendrites positioned in the inferior space of the nasal cavity and an axon that projects through the cribriform plate to the olfactory nerve, and subsequently the olfactory bulb. OSNs are located in the olfactory epithelium in the nose, where its cell bodies are distributed among all three of its stratified layers.

The olfactory epithelium has a thin layer of mucus covering its surface. There are many cilia that project into this mucus layer from the olfactory sensory neuron's dendrites. The surface of these hair-like cilia is blanketed with olfactory receptors. These olfactory receptors are a type of G protein–coupled receptor, which means the receptors are inherently metabotropic. This means the receptor is indirectly activated when ions enter an ion channel, which is done by the secondary messenger, G protein molecules.

Biochemistry

In this activation process, an odorant molecule will dissolve into the mucous membrane of the olfactory epithelium and subsequently bind to an olfactory receptor. This ligand-receptor binding is variable. Each receptor can bind to a variety of odorants with differing affinities. The varying strength of these intermolecular interactions gives rise to variability in activating neurons and results in the detection of unique smells (Bieri et al., 2004). Olfactory receptors on different OSNs can detect new odors from background environmental odors. Activated olfactory receptors then activate intracellular G protein, guanine nucleotide binding protein (GNAL), adenylate cyclase, and the production of cyclic adenosine monophosphate (cAMP). Molecules of cAMP cause ion channels within the cell membrane to open, which ultimately results in depolarization of the neuron and the generation of an action potential, due to an influx of sodium and calcium and an efflux of chloride ions.

Desensitization

The olfactory sensory neuron is equipped with a rapid negative feedback mechanism upon depolarization. During the depolarization event, when cAMP binds to the cyclic nucleotide-gated (CNG) ion channels, sodium and calcium diffuse into the cell. When calcium diffuses into the cell, a series of events occur. Initially, calcium binds to calmodulin to form CaM. Then, CaM molecules will do a couple of things. For one, they will find CNG channels and close them, halting the influx of sodium and calcium. CaM will also activate calmodulin-dependent protein kinase II (CaMKII). CaMKII will reduce cAMP levels by both deactivating adenyl cyclase and by activating phosphodiesterase, which hydrolyzes cAMP (Wei et al., 1998). This negative feedback response inhibits the OSNs from being activated again when other odor molecules are introduced. The feedback system allows vertebrates to adapt to a stimulus.

Olfactory System

Each OSN singly expresses only one type of olfactory receptor, which is a phenomenon that has been called the "one neuron, one receptor" rule. Olfactory receptors are the largest gene family. It is estimated that there are 1,000 different genes that code for olfactory receptors. That being said, there are many separate OSNs that express olfactory receptors, which bind to the same set of odors. The axons of these OSNs that express the same olfactory receptors come together to form glomeruli in the olfactory bulb. These axons touch the dendrites of mitral cells inside the glomerulus. Mitral cells innervate the following brain areas: the medial amygdala, anterior olfactory nucleus, entorhinal cortex, olfactory tubercle, and piriform cortex.

The medial amygdala is associated with social functions like mating and recognizing others. The entorhinal cortex is involved with memory such as pairing odors with memories. The piriform cortex is an area involved with identifying odors. Individual odors are characterized by patterns of activated neurons in an olfactory region. These functions of the central nervous system are still being researched and are debatable (Scott et al., 1980).

Drake E. Sisneros

See also: Anosmia; Dysosmia; G Proteins; Odor Threshold; Olfactory Bulb; Olfactory Mucosa; Olfactory Nerve; Olfactory System; Phantosmia; Pregnancy and Sense of Smell

Further Reading

Bieri, Stephan, Katherine Monastyrskaia, & Boris Schilling. (2004). Olfactory receptor neuron profiling using sandalwood odorants. *Chemical Senses, 29*(6), 483–487.
Moran, David T., J. Carter Rowley III, Bruce W. Jafek, & Mark A. Lovell. (1982). The fine structure of the olfactory mucosa in man. *Journal of Neurocytology, 11*(5), 721–746.

Scott, John W., Russell L. McBride, & Stephen P. Schneider. (1980). The organization of projections from the olfactory bulb to the piriform cortex and olfactory tubercle in the rat. *Journal of Comparative Neurology, 194*(3), 519–534.

Wei, Jia, et al. (1998). Phosphorylation and inhibition of olfactory adenyl cyclase by CaM kinase II in neurons: A mechanism for attenuation of olfactory signals. *Neuron, 21*(3), 495–504.

OLFACTORY SYSTEM

The olfactory system is responsible for the sense of smell, also known as olfaction. The act of smelling is deceptively simple. With a single sniff, the average human is capable of discriminating between millions of different odors with little or no training, and with little regard for the chemical or physical properties of odor molecules. Olfaction is considered to be one of the oldest senses, and it can be traced back through the genetic record as one of the earliest sensory systems used by an organism to interact with its environment. For example, smells can help identify potential mates or competitors, find prey and other food sources, and identify places to live. Mammals also use their sense of smell as an advanced warning system to detect environmental hazards, such as spoiled food, smoke, leaking natural gas, airborne pollutants, or the presence of predators. Notably, mammals, and particularly humans, use their sense of smell to determine the flavor of foods and beverages. This is why it is very difficult or almost impossible to taste anything when a person has a cold (other than the sweet, salty, bitter, or sour information relayed by the tongue). Any deviation in the ability to smell can adversely impact one's quality of life, influence what and how much one eats, whom one talks to, and where one may go.

Anatomical Organization

Across species, animals use very similar cellular and molecular strategies to detect odors. In both invertebrate and vertebrate animals, the primary sensory cells responsible for detecting odorants are bipolar neurons with cilia or microvilli on one end and a typically unbranched axon at the other end. These sensory neurons are wired into the nervous system in a remarkably similar fashion: each sensory cell sends an axon to a spherical structure in the olfactory bulb called a glomerulus. At the molecular level, the proteins used to detect odorants belong to the odorant receptor family, which are all G protein–coupled receptors. These proteins have seven transmembrane domains and activate G protein–based signaling cascades, which can amplify the molecular signal. Mammals and reptiles often split their olfactory systems into two parallel systems: the main olfactory system and the accessory olfactory system. The main olfactory system detects airborne volatile chemicals, while the accessory olfactory system can detect both volatile chemicals and nonvolatile proteins or hydrocarbons.

Jelly Belly® Experiment

Before a person takes a bite of pizza, Hawaiian-style with ham and pineapple, they smell the rich aroma and their nose can distinguish the different notes of the foods that make up the pizza. This perception of odors enters the nose during sniffing, also called orthonasal olfaction. Taking that first bite, a person tastes the sweetness of the pineapple, the saltiness of the meat, and the savoriness of the cheese. A person will also perceive the food's odorants through chewing and eating, which is retronasal olfaction where odors enter the nose via the pharynx. Together these tastants stimulate the gustatory system and the odorants stimulate the olfactory system. Thus, the chemical senses of both the taste and olfactory systems are necessary for the ability to perceive flavors of foods and beverages.

The sense of smell is the most important chemical sense for flavor to be distinguished. This is why food does not taste as flavorful when a person has a stuffy or runny nose from a head cold, flu, or sinusitis. Anosmia is the inability to smell, whether the instance is acute (temporary) or chronic (permanent). Any deviation in a person's ability to smell can adversely impact their quality of life and influence what and how much they eat. However, it is important to note that the sense of taste is still intact, and a person with a cold or anosmia can still sense sweet, salty, bitter, umami, or sour information that is relayed by the tongue.

Jelly Belly® candies have significant amounts of odorants trapped within them, which makes the flavor of the bean more intense compared to other candies. However, other foods can be used for this experiment.

Materials:

A variety of flavors of Jelly Belly® jelly beans or other highly flavored candies

Directions:

For best results, make sure your nasal passage is clear and that you can take a deep breath. With one hand, plug your nose. Place the Jelly Belly® (or other food) in your mouth and chew about 5–10 times with your nose still plugged. You should only be able to taste if the food is bitter, salty, sour, and/or sweet. Unplug your nose, as this will allow retronasal olfaction to take place. Instantly, you should be able to identify the flavor of the Jelly Belly® bean.

Jennifer L. Hellier

Main Olfactory System

In the vertebrate main olfactory system, the primary sensory neurons (called olfactory sensory neurons, OSNs) are found in specialized tissue called the main olfactory epithelium (MOE), which lines a portion of the nasal passage. OSNs have a long dendrite capped by a tuft of tiny hair-like cilia, which protrude directly into the mucosal lining that covers the olfactory epithelium and are directly exposed to ambient air. Odor molecules enter the nasal passage and bind to proteins that are bound in the cilia membrane. These proteins then activate the signal transduction machinery responsible for creating a signal that indicates that an odor has been detected. The brain tissue responsible for the initial processing of this odor signal is called the main olfactory bulb (MOB). Several distinct layers make up the MOB. The outermost layer contains the olfactory nerve, which is the first cranial nerve pair (cranial nerve I). Beneath this outer nerve layer is the inner nerve layer, then the glomerular layer, the external plexiform layer, the mitral cell layer, the internal plexiform layer, and finally the granule cell layer. The granule cell layer is the innermost layer found at the center of the olfactory bulb.

From the MOE, the OSN cell body extends a single axon through the bone between the eyes and into the surface of the MOB. This axon synapses directly onto mitral cells and tufted cells in a spherical tangle of axons and dendrites called a glomerulus. In coronal sections of the olfactory bulb, these circular glomeruli can be found just inside the perimeter of the tissue cross-section. Each glomerulus represents a massive convergence of olfactory information as axons from tens of thousands of OSNs synapse onto only 25 mitral cells in a given glomerulus. Moreover, only axons from OSNs that express the same odorant receptor type converge on the same glomerulus. Each OSN responds to a limited number of odor features, which is determined by its odorant receptor type. For example, the smell of "apple" actually contains thousands of different odor features and will activate millions of different OSNs. OSNs that have the same odorant receptor type will respond to just one of these odor features and will synapse in the same glomerulus in the MOB. Similarly, a different odor feature in the apple smell will activate a different population of OSNs that will target a different glomerulus. Thus, the collective OSN response to the apple smell will activate a specific pattern of glomeruli across the surface of the MOB. This signal is then integrated and modulated by the large number of interneurons found in the different layers of the MOB, including periglomerular cells and granule cells. This signal is then relayed via the mitral cells to the regions of the brain where the apple smell will be perceived.

Mitral cell axons are the main output of the MOB and leave via the lateral olfactory tract (LOT). The LOT targets five distinct regions of the brain: the anterior olfactory nucleus, olfactory tubercle, amygdala, piriform cortex, and entorhinal cortex. Most of these targets are part of the limbic system, which are the memory and emotional centers of the brain. These direct connections into the limbic system are the reasons why smells rarely are neutral, meaning odors tend to be either attractive or repellent to a person or animal. It is also why certain smells are often associated with strong memories; for example, the smell of a rose or violets might bring back memories of a grandmother. Interestingly, the MOB receives more inputs from the rest of the brain than the number of outputs that leave the bulb. Although these inputs coming from the cerebrum are thought to modulate olfactory behavior, their anatomical and functional significance remains unclear.

Odorant Receptors

Mammalian odorant receptors (OR) are proteins that specialize in detecting and responding to specific chemical signals known as odorants. An easily recognizable odor, such as "apple," is actually a complex mixture of many different odorants at varying concentrations. A given OR type (defined by its genetic code) will often respond to just a small subset of the different odorants that make up the "apple" smell, and a distinct OR (one with a slightly different protein sequence) will respond to a different subset of the odorants.

OR proteins can be found bound to the cell membrane in the cilia of the OSN. Each OR protein is made from a gene that belongs to a relatively large family of similar genes (gene family), and each OR gene codes for a slightly different OR protein that is sensitive to only a limited number of odorants. The mammalian OR gene family is the largest gene family found in any species. In fact, it represents 1–5 percent of the entire mammalian genome. For example, humans have nearly 500 genes devoted to detecting odor molecules. Since there are only about 30,000 genes in the human genome, nearly 1 in every 50 genes is devoted to a person's sense of smell.

ORs belong to a family of specialized receptors that are known as G protein–coupled receptors. Each OR can be likened to a tiny molecular lock that can be opened by a small, specific number of odorants. The binding of an odorant by an OR initiates a signal transduction cascade by changing the shape of the receptor protein. This conformational change releases a coupled G protein, specifically G_{olf}, which then binds to adenylase cyclase. This cascade causes multiple biochemical reactions in the cilia that ultimately produces an action potential, which is relayed to the glomerulus in the MOB.

Only one OR gene from the entire OR gene family is expressed in any given OSN, so the entire neuron responds only to the odorants detected by the expressed OR in that cell, such as a few of the chemicals that make up the "apple" smell. OSNs expressing the same odorant gene all send signals from their axons to the same glomerulus in the MOB. This means that each glomerulus receives axons from neurons that have the same OR and are sensitive to the same set of odorants. In this way, each glomerulus integrates axonal activity from OSNs that all respond to the same odor signal. As such, each glomerulus functions as an independent processing unit in a complex topographical map of OSN activation found on the surface of the MOB. This map is known as an odor map, and different odors generate different odor maps.

The Accessory Olfactory System

An accessory olfactory system (AOS) can be found in many animals, excluding humans. This system is designed to detect nonvolatile chemical cues, often including pheromones, and requires direct contact with the odor source. In this system, the primary sensory neurons are contained within a vomeronasal organ (VNO). The VNO extends its axons to the accessory olfactory bulb. The VNO contains a vascular pump that delivers stimuli through a thin duct into the lumen within the VNO that houses the sensory neurons. The AOS differs in the types of receptor proteins and components of the signal transduction cascade that it uses to detect and respond to odor stimuli. The VNO is typically used to detect important social and sexual information, and it plays an important role in sexual reproduction and social interactions.

Ernesto Salcedo

See also: Anosmia; Buck, Linda; Dysosmia; G Proteins; Interrelatedness of Taste and Smell; Limbic System; Olfactory Bulb; Olfactory Mucosa; Olfactory Nerve; Olfactory Reference Syndrome; Olfactory Sensory Neurons; Phantosmia; Pheromones

Further Reading

Buck, Linda, & Richard Axel. (1991). A novel multigene family may encode odorant receptors: A molecular basis for odor recognition. *Cell, 65*(1), 175–187.
Finger, Thomas E., Wayne L. Silver, & Diego Restrepo. (2000). *The neurobiology of taste and smell.* New York, NY: Wiley-Liss.
Mombaerts, Peter. (2001). How smell develops. *Nature Neuroscience, 4,* 1192–1198.

OPTIC NERVE

The optic nerve is the pathway that directly connects the eye to the brain. It is a sensory nerve that is responsible for the transmission of all visual information. It is the second of the 12 paired cranial nerves and, therefore, is also known as cranial nerve II.

Anatomy

There are approximately 1.2 million nerve cell axons in each optic nerve. The optic nerve acts like a cable connecting the eye to the brain. The diameter of the optic nerve varies from about two to four millimeters. The optic nerve is mainly composed of axons from the ganglion cells of the retina, making it a pure white matter tract. This means it is actually more like brain tissue than nerve tissue, and therefore, its development and functions are similar to other typical central nervous system brain cells. Thus, oligodendrocytes cover the axons with a myelin sheath, astrocytes give biochemical and homeostatic support to the optic nerve, and finally, microglia, a type of resident macrophage used for immune protection of the brain, scavenge the nerve for extracellular components and infectious agents. The optic nerve is also covered with all three layers of the specialized brain coverings called the meninges: dura, arachnoid, and pia maters.

The optic nerve can be broken down into three parts: the optic nerve, optic chiasma (or chiasm), and optic tract. The nerve fibers of the retina exit the eye through the optic nerve, and there is no retinal tissue over the head of the optic nerve. The optic nerve head or optic disc is oval shaped and is around 1.5 to 1.75 millimeters in circumference. It leaves the back of the eye socket through the optic canal. It is approximately 30 millimeters in length from the retina to the optic canal. The nerve then runs 5 to 12 millimeters through the canal. Once it enters the cranium, the length varies from 8 to 19 millimeters as it runs posterior and medial to the optic chiasma.

The optic chiasma is an "X-shaped" intersection of both left and right optic nerves and is located directly below the hypothalamus and directly above the pituitary gland. As the two optic nerves meet, around half of the nerve fibers cross over and continue on the opposite side. For example, the nerves that originate on the nose or nasal half of the left retina cross over at the chiasma and will proceed onto the right side of the brain. On the other hand, the nerve fibers that originate on the lateral or temporal side of the left retina will proceed onto the left side of the brain. This causes a partial crossing of the fibers from the visual fields of both eyes. In other words, visual information from the nasal part of each eye ultimately reaches the visual centers of the opposite side of the brain.

Anatomically, the optic nerve ends at the chiasma, but the retinal ganglion cell axons continue on to make up the optic tract. As the nerve ends leave the chiasma, the optic tract moves posterior and laterally toward its terminations. The optic nerve has four main terminations within the brain: the lateral geniculate nucleus (LGN), the pretectal nucleus and pulvinar, the superior colliculus, and the hypothalamus.

Physiology

The main function of the optic nerve is to carry visual information from the retina to various parts of the brain. Approximately 90 percent of all optic nerve fibers terminate at the LGN of the thalamus, as its main role is to regulate the flow of visual information to the primary visual cortex. Other functions are (1) to aid in the pupillary response, (2) to help coordinate head and eye movements based on visual information sent to the superior colliculus, and (3) to aid circadian control of sleep-wake cycles, temperature, and other systematic functions.

Diseases

In a healthy optic nerve, all of the nerve fibers that receive light signals from the outside world pass the signals to the brain, meaning that the entire field of vision should be seen. In any disease or disorder, functioning nerve fibers decrease at a rate much faster than would occur through the normal aging process. This decrease may be due to increased intraocular pressure, lack of blood flow, some other mechanism, or a combination of mechanisms. When these nerve fibers die, they leave an empty space where they used to be. When enough nerve fibers die, an empty space on the optic disc becomes visible through examination. These traumas to the optic nerve may cause severe or even permanent loss of vision. Since each eye has a left and right visual hemifield, the particular loss to these visual fields mainly depends on which parts of the optic nerve are damaged.

The most common injuries to the optic nerve are from glaucoma, optic neuritis, and anterior ischemic optic neuropathy. Glaucoma is not just a single disease but a group of eye conditions. It results in optic nerve damage, which may ultimately cause loss of vision. Abnormally high pressure inside the eye is the usual cause of this damage. Glaucoma cannot be cured and neither can damage caused to the optic nerve, but treatment may prevent vision loss in early glaucoma. The main way to treat glaucoma is to lower pressure in the eye. This may be done by directly lowering the eye pressure, increasing drainage of fluid in the eye, or lowering the amount of fluid produced by the eye.

Optic neuritis is inflammation of the optic nerve. It is mainly found in those younger than 50 years of age. It is most commonly associated with diseases that involve demyelination, such as multiple sclerosis. Other causes of optic neuritis include infection, autoimmune disorders, inflammatory bowel disease, and diabetes. An ophthalmologist will treat optic neuritis by prescribing eye drops containing antibiotics and/or steroids to stop the infection and inflammation. Anterior ischemic optic neuropathy is a condition involving damage to the optic nerve from insufficient blood supply and usually affects patients that are over the age of 50. The most common congenital optic nerve damage is optic nerve hypoplasia, which is the underdevelopment of the optic nerve causing little to no vision. This hypoplasia occurs during fetal development and has no cure.

Mario J. Perez

See also: Circadian Rhythm; Cranial Nerves; Optic Nerve Hypoplasia; Retina; Thalamus; Visual System

Further Reading

Kolb, Helga, Ralph Nelson, Eduardo Fernandez, & Bryan Jones (Eds.). (2011). *Webvision: The organization of the retina and visual system.* Retrieved from http://webvision.med.utah.edu/book/

Machemer, Robert, & Georg Michelson. (2012). *The atlas of ophthalmology: Online multimedia database*. Retrieved from http://www.atlasophthalmology.com/atlas/frontpage.jsf

OPTIC NERVE HYPOPLASIA

Optic nerve hypoplasia (ONH) is the most common type of congenital blindness. Persons with ONH have small, underdeveloped optic nerves (cranial nerve II) as well as small optic discs known to affect one or both eyes. This condition can occur alone or in occurrence with additional physiological abnormalities, such as a dysfunctional pituitary gland. Depending on the severity of the abnormalities, ONH has been associated with septo-optic dysplasia or de Morsier's disease. However, recent findings have shown that septo-optic dysplasia is a different disease and is not ONH (Garcia-Filion & Borchert, 2013).

ONH is a congenital defect in children, but can become an event in adults. The main characteristic of ONH is the abnormal color and shape of the optic nerve, which looks similar to a doughnut with a pink rim and white depression when viewed through an ophthalmoscope. Abnormal characteristics of the optic nerve are an indication of unusual function. A normal functioning optic disc should look orange-pink when viewed through an ophthalmoscope.

In the event of ONH occurring, the affected optic nerve seizes function and becomes white in color. Some common causes of optic nerve fiber failure result from inflammation, increased pressures (as in glaucoma), and/or reduced blood flow to the tissue. In cases of ONH associated with glaucoma, ophthalmologists and optometrists use a measurement called the cup-to-disc ratio to determine the progression of the disease. This is a measurement of the optic disc's (the area where the optic nerve and associated blood vessels enter the retina, creating an anatomical "blind spot") flatness to its natural cupping formation. The normal cup-to-disc ratio should not exceed 0.5 in diameter. However, if the cup-to-disc ratio measures greater than 0.5, this is an indication that the optic nerve is most likely pathological in nature. These characteristics are a result of a patient likely experiencing glaucoma. Furthermore, an abnormal optic disc will display a shade of white, as the dead nerve fibers are replaced by a pale appearance.

History

The first documented case of ONH was in 1915, but previous ONH cases could have occurred at a much earlier time. In 1915, German physician O. Schwarz produced the first drawing of a postmortem patient with ONH, which contained an illustration of the eye's optic disc. Since then and in the past 30 years, ONH has been recognized as an epidemic cause of congenital blindness, but current research in endocrinology has developed treatments to improve this syndrome.

Eye Function and Brain Function

A person's eyes take in outside light and send pictures through the optic nerves to the brain. In normal eye function, more than 1 million nerve fibers make up a single optic nerve that connects the brain to the eye. However, an individual who has ONH will have smaller or absent optic nerves traveling from the brain to the eye. Therefore, individuals with this condition have a reduced connection between the brain and the affected eye(s). In some cases, people with ONH have normal vision in only one eye, others experience reduced vision in each eye, and some people are nearly or completely blind.

Treatment

A patient's vision will need to be monitored on a semiannual or annual basis. Children who have been diagnosed with ONH by an optometrist or ophthalmologist should be referred to an endocrinologist who specializes in hormone treatment. This is to determine if any other physiological functions are being impaired or if their pituitary gland is functionally normally. For adults with an event of ONH, an ophthalmologist should monitor them regularly, particularly if glaucoma is suspected.

Outcomes

Treatment for OHN is provided to patients with the outcome of having increased vision. Patching therapy—where a patient wears a patch over the good eye during the daytime—has been used as an old method of treatment. In severe cases, this old style of treatment may result in developmental and learning setbacks in pediatric patients. Physiological and/or endocrine conditions that are correlated with ONH can be treated with daily medications. However, even with proper medical care, the lack of endocrine deficiencies can have adverse affects in certain patients, and thus they will need to be monitored very closely.

Michael Freer

See also: Blindness; Optic Nerve; Visual Perception; Visual System

Further Reading

Borchert, Mark, & Pamela Garcia-Filion. (2008). The syndrome of optic nerve hypoplasia. *Current Neurology and Neuroscience Reports, 8*, 395–403. Retrieved from http://www.chla.org/sites/default/files/migrated/ONH_Review_Article.pdf

Garcia-Filion, Pamela, & Mark Borchert. (2013). Optic nerve hypoplasia syndrome: A review of the epidemiology and clinical associations. *Current Treatment Options in Neurology, 15*(1), 78–89. http://dx.doi.org/10.1007/s11940-012-0209-2. Retrieved from http://www.ncbi.nlm.nih.gov/pmc/articles/PMC3576022/#R1

Kaufman, Francine, et al. (n.d.). Optic nerve hypoplasia: A guide for parents. One Small Voice Foundation. Retrieved from http://www.onesmallvoicefoundation.org/pdf/ONH%20pamphlet_sm.pdf

ORTHOSTATIC HYPOTENSION

A delicate balance between heart rate, blood volume, and arterial diameter maintains normal blood pressure within the human body. In the typical adult, blood pressure is considered to be normal when the systolic pressure is less than 120 mm Hg and the diastolic pressure is less than 80 mm Hg; however, there is significant variation in these numbers depending on the person's position when blood pressure is measured. It is common for a person's blood pressure, particularly systolic pressure, to momentarily drop 8–10 mm Hg when standing up from a sitting or lying position. This is due in part to the effects of gravity and blood pooling lower in the body. Under normal conditions, a number of events take place in our bodies to reestablish a normal functioning blood pressure. When a person's blood pressure drops more than 20 mm Hg upon standing, this is defined as orthostatic hypotension.

Normal Control of Blood Pressure

To maintain a normal or mean arterial blood pressure, the body must create a balance between cardiac output (how much blood the heart is pumping per contraction), total peripheral resistance (how dilated the vessels are), and blood volume (how many liters of blood exist in the body). The primary structure that orchestrates all of this is called the baroreceptor (pressure sensor), which is found in the aortic arch of the vascular system. Under normal conditions, the baroreceptors fire action potentials through the autonomic nervous system to the heart and vessels, regulating heart rate and how dilated or constricted the vessels should be. If blood pressure drops, the baroreceptors will increase the number of action potentials being fired, which results in an increase in heart rate and a constriction of the great vessels of the body, both of which result in an increase in blood pressure. The converse is true if blood pressure becomes too high.

Orthostatic Hypotension

Orthostatic hypotension (OT) is defined as a drop of greater than 20 mm Hg in systolic blood pressure or a drop in diastolic blood pressure of greater than 10 mm Hg over three minutes of standing (https://www.youtube.com/watch?v=QZj0EmFV2to). There are two general categories of OT: (1) initial orthostatic hypotension, which develops within the first five minutes of standing erect, and (2) delayed orthostatic hypotension, which develops later, often 15–45 minutes after standing. There are multiple potential causes for OT. Some predisposing factors for development of OT include dehydration (decreased volume in the vascular system), deconditioning (inability of the heart to increase heart rate quickly enough to respond to a drop in pressure), nutritional factors, and aging. There are also a number of medications that can increase the incidence of OT including (1) tricyclic antidepressants, (2) antihypertensives and diuretics, (3) general vasodilators, and (4) tizanidine (Zanaflex, which is a short-acting muscle relaxant).

In addition to pharmacological agents there are a number of other pathologies/conditions that can lead to OT including (1) autonomic neuropathies, (2) Parkinson's disease, (3) dementia, (4) dopamine β hydroxylase deficiency, (5) brainstem lesions/injuries, and (6) spinal cord injuries.

Treatment

Treatment for OT is varied depending on the specific symptoms and the potential causative agent. Often, OT is a secondary symptom of some other disease process and in treating the primary disease process, the OT issue is lessened. However, there are some general behavioral changes that can be made to help individuals with benign OT. These include (1) staying well hydrated so that blood volume remains high, (2) decreasing alcohol consumption (which can cause dehydration), (3) when getting up from bed, coming to a sitting position first, and slowly allowing the body to respond to the changes in pressure, (4) wearing compression stockings, which apply pressure to the legs and prevent blood from pooling in the lower legs, (5) raising the head of the bed when sleeping, and (6) avoiding prolonged standing during the day.

Orthostatic hypotension is a significant issue within the geriatric population and often requires more treatment. Orthostatic hypotension occurs in about 20–25 percent of the elderly, and the incidence increases with the presence of coexisting disease processes. This often results in increased numbers of falls, which could lead to head injuries and fractures, particularly of the shoulder and hip. It is thought that as we age, baroreceptor sensitivity and response times become more delayed, which results in a decreased response in heart rate and peripheral resistance. Significant care must be taken to help older patients develop safe habits to prevent further injury as a result of OT.

Charles A. Ferguson

See also: Baroreceptors

Further Reading
Beitzkea, Markus, Peter Pfistera, Jürgen Fortinb, & Falko Skrabal. (2002). Autonomic dysfunction and hemodynamics in vitamin B12 deficiency. *Autonomic Neuroscience, 97*(1), 45–54.
Cleveland Clinic. (2013). Diseases & conditions: Orthostatic hypotension. Retrieved from https://my.clevelandclinic.org/health/diseases_conditions/hic_orthostatic_hypotension

Logan, Ian C., & Miles D. Witham. (2012). Efficacy of treatments for orthostatic hypotension: A systematic review. *Age and Ageing, 41*(5), 587–594.

Robertson, David. (2008). The pathophysiology and diagnosis of orthostatic hypotension. *Clinical Autonomic Research, 18*(1), 2–7.

OTOACOUSTIC EMISSIONS

The ability to hear is essential for social interactions, cognition, and understanding emotions. Thus, infants and young children need to have their hearing checked as soon as possible to determine if they have any type of hearing loss. Even a mild hearing loss can lead to the child's inability to learn how to speak clearly or to understand language. If caught early, hearing loss can be treated. Thus, hearing should be evaluated before a newborn leaves the hospital.

Causes of hearing loss include but are not limited to premature birth, complications at birth, frequent ear infections, and being exposed to very loud sounds even if it is for a brief time. Hearing loss comes in two different forms: (1) conductive hearing loss, which is caused by interference in the transmission of sound to the inner ear, and (2) sensorineural hearing loss, which is caused by malformation, dysfunction, or damage to the inner ear. Thus, tests have been developed to determine the function of hearing. These physiologic tests include auditory brainstem response, auditory steady state response, tympanometry, middle ear muscle reflex, and otoacoustic emissions.

Auditory brainstem response predicts how well a baby's inner ear and lower part of the auditory system (brainstem) is functioning. Auditory steady state response is performed under sedation and a computer is used to pick up the brain's response to a sound and establish hearing level. Tympanometry is actually a procedure to show how well the eardrum moves when a soft sound and air pressure are introduced into the ear canal. Middle ear muscle reflex tests how well the ear responds to loud sounds, which in a healthy ear causes the middle ear to contract. Finally, otoacoustic emissions test how healthy the outer hair cells are and if they are functioning properly. Otoacoustic emissions tests are of clinical importance because they are a simple, noninvasive test for hearing defects in newborns as well as in children who are too young to cooperate with conventional hearing tests.

Otoacoustic emissions are sounds originating from the cochlea in the ear. A microphone that is fitted into the ear canal records these sounds. When sound stimulates the cochlea, the outer hair cells vibrate, producing a nearly inaudible sound that echoes back to the middle ear. A person with normal hearing can produce otoacoustic emissions, but if an individual has hearing loss that is greater than 25 to 30 decibels (dB), he or she will not produce otoacoustic emissions. In the United States, an otoacoustic emissions test is typically performed as part of the newborn hearing screening program and can detect blockages of the outer ear canal and the presence of middle ear fluid or damage to the outer hair cells.

Types of Otoacoustic Emissions

There are two types of otoacoustic emissions: spontaneous and evoked. Spontaneous otoacoustic emissions are emitted from the ear without any sort of stimulation and can be measured with a microphone fitted into the ear canal. About 35 to 50 percent of the population can detect at least one spontaneous otoacoustic emission. Most people are completely unaware of spontaneous otoacoustic emissions and about 10 percent of people perceive them as a very irritating tinnitus, or the hearing of a sound when one is not actually present.

Evoked otoacoustic emissions are currently evoked with three different processes: stimulus frequency, transient-evoked, and distortion product. Stimulus frequency–evoked otoacoustic emissions are detected by the difference between a stimulus wavelength and the recorded wavelength the individual hears. Transient-evoked otoacoustic emissions are evoked via a clicking or tone burst (pure tone) stimulus. Response from the clicking can cover a frequency ranging up to around 4 kilohertz (kHz), but a tone burst will only produce a response that has the same frequency as the pure tone. Lastly, distortion product otoacoustic emissions are evoked with a pair of primary tones with particular intensities and ratios. These tones are presented at the same time to the cochlea; the response determines the intermodulation distortion and the other determines the reflection by the cochlea.

Renee Johnson

See also: Age-Related Hearing Loss; Auditory Hallucinations; Auditory Processing Disorder; Brainstem Auditory Evoked Potentials; Cochlea; Deafness; Tinnitus

Further Reading

Akron Children's Hospital. (2012). Hearing evaluation in children. Reviewed by Thierry Morlet. Retrieved from https://www.akronchildrens.org/cms/procedures_tests/Otoacoustic_Emissions_Test/

Kemp, David T. (2002). Otoacoustic emissions, their origin in cochlear function, and use. *British Medical Bulletin, 63*(1), 223–241. Retrieved from http://bmb.oxfordjournals.org/content/63/1/223.full

Shahid, Ramzan, Michaela Vigilante, Heidi Deyro, Irma Reyes, Beverly Gonzalez, & Stephanie Kliethermes. (2015). Risk factors for failed newborn otoacoustic emissions hearing screen. *Clinical Pediatrics (Philadelphia).* http://dx.doi.org/10.1177/0009922815615826

OTOLITHS

The human ear is composed of both the auditory system that we use for hearing, and the vestibular system that is found within the inner ear and plays a significant role in maintaining balance, helping us with spatial orientation, and maintaining a sense of where we are within a three-dimensional space (proprioception). The vestibular system is composed of two primary components that include the semicircular canal system, which provides information about rotational movements of our heads, and the otoliths, which are small stones of calcium carbonate within the semicircular canals and also play a role in providing information about rotation as well as linear acceleration. The vestibular system is also integrated very closely with the muscles that control eye movement and the general body muscles that help us maintain an upright position.

Anatomy and Physiology of the Otolithic System

The vestibular system is composed of several structures including three semicircular canals, which are filled with a viscous fluid that moves within the canals as our heads move. These three semicircular canals known as the horizontal, anterior, and posterior canals connect with two other structures critical to balance known as the utricle and the saccule. In humans, the utricle is oriented in a horizontal direction and detects motion in a horizontal plane, while the saccule is oriented in a vertical direction and detects motion in a vertical plane. Both of these structures contain special "hairs" whose tips are embedded in the otolithic membrane of the inner ear. In addition to these hairs or "stereocilia," there are small stones made of calcium carbonate called otoliths that are embedded in the membrane of the utricle and saccule. As individuals move their heads from one position to another, the otoliths move in response to positional change and/or acceleration and in doing so, create a sheering force across the stereocilia, stimulating the vestibular system. This information is sent to the brain via the vestibulocochlear nerve for further integration with information from the eyes and muscles of the neck.

Otolith Reflexes

There are a number of reflexes in the body that are associated with the vestibular system and otoliths in particular. These include, first, the otolith-ocular reflexes, which include (1) linear nystagmus, (2) a condition known as ocular counter-roll where the eyes rotate around a specific line of sight in the opposite direction when the head is tilted to the side, and (3) off-vertical axis nystagmus, which is induced when the head is moved in a lateral direction. Second, the otolith-body reflexes include the righting reflex, which allows us to respond to temporary loss of balance and maintain an upright position; and third are the otolith-canal interactions.

Pathologies of the Vestibular System

There are a number of different pathologies associated with the vestibular system that involve the various structures within this system. Virtually all of them are capable of producing vertigo (defined as a sensation of motion in which the individual's surroundings seem to move even when the person is not moving), difficulty maintaining balance, and significant nausea and vomiting. The three most common diseases of the vestibular system include labyrinthitis, an infection of the inner ear, Meniere's disease, and benign paroxysmal positional vertigo or BPPV. Benign paroxysmal positional vertigo is most likely caused by the abnormal movement or dislodging of the otoliths within the utricle and saccule of the inner ear. It is thought that as these stones become dislodged or break into smaller pieces, some of those pieces migrate over time into the semicircular canals and disrupt the normal flow of fluid within the canals. This creates a sense of vertigo that patients often describe. The most common location where these stones collect is within the posterior canal. Vertigo can be brought on by rapid movement of the head such as looking up or down, rolling over in bed, or rapidly tilting the head from side to side. BPPV is most commonly treated using a number of different repositioning maneuvers such as the Epley maneuver, the Semont maneuver, or the Brandt-Daroff exercises. The most common of these is the Epley maneuver, which uses deliberate movement of the head and gravity to reposition the otoliths within the utricle and saccule. In addition to these procedures, BPPV can be treated with more traditional medications such as antihistamines to reduce the fluid within the ear, and anticholinergic drugs such as meclizine or scopolamine, which help reduce the sense of dizziness and nausea. There are some surgical procedures that can be done to treat BPPV, but they are reserved as a last-choice option and not frequently performed.

Charles A. Ferguson

See also: Saccule; Semicircular Canals; Utricle; Vestibular System; Vestibulocochlear Nerve

Further Reading

Hain, Timothy C. (2010). Otoliths. Retrieved from http://www.dizziness-and-balance.com/disorders/bppv/otoliths.html

Ivanenk, Y.P., R. Grasso, I. Israel, & A. Berthoz. (1997). The contribution of otoliths and semicircular canals to the perception of two-dimensional passive whole-body motion in humans. *Journal of Physiology, 502*(1), 223–233.

Sheykholeslami, Kianoush, & Kimitaka Kaga. (2002). The otolithic organ as a receptor of vestibular hearing revealed by vestibular-evoked myogenic potentials in patients with inner ear anomalies. *Hearing Research, 165*(1–2), 62–67.

PACINIAN CORPUSCLES

Named for Italian anatomist Filippo Pacini (1812–1883), Pacinian corpuscles, also known as lamellar corpuscles, are one of the four major types of mechanoreceptors (touch receptors) found in the skin. They consist of free nerve endings within the skin that are responsible for sensitivity to vibration and pressure. These nerve endings respond to deformation by pressure or the removal of this pressure as might occur during vibrations. The sensitivity of the Pacinian corpuscles to pressure helps us to determine if a specific surface is smooth or rough. Pacinian corpuscles can also be found within the gut lining and joint capsules and play a role in proprioception, which is the ability to sense where joints and limbs are with respect to the rest of the body and in space. Pacinian corpuscles are especially sensitive to vibrations and are the primary skin receptor for vibration, specifically vibrations around 200 to 300 hertz (Hz).

Structure

Pacinian corpuscles look like tiny onions in the deeper layer of the skin, within the subcutaneous adipose tissue. They can also be found in joint capsules helping the brain sense and determine where the limbs are in relation to the rest of the body. Finally, Pacinian corpuscles are also located within the gut and help with visceral sensation. They are larger in size but fewer in number than Merkel cells and Ruffini corpuscles, other types of mechanoreceptors. They are approximately one millimeter in length and are encased in connective tissue. Pacinian corpuscles are modified Schwann cells (glial cells in the peripheral nervous system that produce myelin) and are very thin and flat. In the center of the corpuscles, there is a fluid-filled cavity with a single primary afferent (travels and sends a signal to the central nervous system), unmyelinated nerve ending. The primary afferent neuron is coated in layers of laminar cells, fluid-filled epithelial cells. Inside the corpuscle is a conduction structure called the first node of Ranvier, with a nerve sheath contained within. This nerve sheath is made of an electrically insulating myelin sheath. It is the deformation of these fluid-filled epithelial cells that initiates the electrical signal that transmits to the central nervous system.

Function

When a Pacinian corpuscle is deformed by pressure, the membrane allows sodium ions to "leak" out of the neuron. This causes a graded potential at the membrane, which is based on the strength of the stimulus creating the leakage. Every time pressure changes occur, a new graded potential is generated. These graded potentials reduce over time. If the sum of the graded potentials is high enough to reach membrane threshold, an action potential will be generated. This action potential is an all or nothing electrical signal. It is initiated in the nerve ending at the first node of Ranvier. The impulse from this action potential travels down the axon by causing sodium ion channels to open along the axon's length. A sodium/potassium ion pump along with potassium ion channels will reset the membrane of the axon behind the action potential. The signal from the Pacinian corpuscle will travel along this primary afferent neuron to the spinal cord and then to the brain for processing.

Pacinian corpuscles have a large receptor field, meaning that they are capable of picking up sensations from a very large amount of area on the surface of the skin. Additionally, they are rapidly adapting, meaning that while they will quickly respond to a stimulus, that response does not last very long even if the stimulus persists. Once the pressure stimulus is removed, these corpuscles will send out another response.

Defects and Treatment

Although rare, a Pacinian corpuscle may develop a neuroma (tumor), as it is a free nerve ending. Other abnormal features are Pacinian corpuscle hyperplasia, which can be the precursor to a neuroma. In both cases, the patient will have extreme pain wherever the neuroma or hyperplasia is located. To date, the best treatment is surgery to remove the neuroma and then, in general, all symptoms are resolved.

Riannon C. Atwater and Renee Johnson

See also: Discriminative Touch; Mechanoreceptors; Meissner's Corpuscles; Merkel Cell; Reflex; Sensory Receptors

Further Reading

Narayanamurthy, V. B., A. Thomas Winston, & Amit Gupta. (2005). A rare case of Pacinian corpuscle neuroma. *Canadian Journal of Plastic Surgery, 13*(1), 43–45. Retrieved from http://www.ncbi.nlm.nih.gov/pmc/articles/PMC3822480/

Purves, Dale, et al. (Eds.). (2001). Mechanoreceptors specialized to receive tactile information. In *Neuroscience* (2nd ed.). Sunderland, MA: Sinauer Associates. Retrieved from http://www.ncbi.nlm.nih.gov/books/NBK10895/

PAIN: *See* Nociception

PALLESTHESIA: *See* Vibration Sensation

PARESTHESIA

Paresthesia is a term that describes a burning or prickling—"pins and needles"—sensation in the body. Paresthesia has also been described as tingling, numbness, the sensation of crawling skin, or an itching sensation. This is most common in the hands, arms, legs, and feet, although paresthesia can be felt in other parts of the body as well. The sensation can occur at any time without a warning and is generally not painful.

Types and Causes of Paresthesia

There are two types of paresthesia: (1) acute or temporary, and (2) chronic. In temporary paresthesia, the most common form is from an acutely compressed nerve. Falling asleep with an arm draped over the back of a chair may result in a condition known as "Saturday night palsy," which is caused by continual nerve compression by the prolonged pressure of the chair. When the person wakes, the muscles in the arm may be weakened, painful, and experience "pins and needles" as the compression begins to heal. Another possible nontraumatic injury may occur when a patient wakens from a surgical procedure to find the table edges or surfaces produced a slight compression injury known as "intraoperative positioning injuries." In fact, the feeling of numbness and tingling when a person falls asleep on his or her arm, or sits with legs crossed for too long, are some of the early symptoms of acute nerve compression. In the majority of cases, as soon as the pressure is relieved from the compressed nerve, the sensation begins to go away.

In chronic paresthesia, there is usually an underlying disease that is the cause or traumatic damage to a nerve, such as a severe compression injury. Chronic paresthesia can be associated with nerve damage occurring over a period of time. Compression of a nerve may be the direct result of a physical condition, such as being bed-bound for an extended period of time, or it may be the result of a disease or disorder. Included within this category are conditions such as (1) degenerative disc disease affecting the spinal cord; (2) carpal tunnel syndrome (compression of the nerves of the wrist), radial tunnel syndrome (compression of the radial nerve in the arm that serves the muscles on the side of the thumb), and cubital tunnel syndrome (compression of the ulnar nerve in the arm, also called the "funny bone"), all of which affect the upper extremities; (3) "cyclist's palsy," a condition frequently experienced by cyclists affecting their hands from constant pressure on the handlebars; (4) pressure exerted on the nerves by the presence of inflammation or a growth such as a tumor; (5) multiple sclerosis; and (6) stroke or transient ischemic attacks (mini-strokes).

Chronic paresthesia may result in a condition known as peripheral neuropathy. Peripheral nerves relay sensory information to the central nervous system such as a feeling of burn on touching a hot pan, pain when one receives a paper cut, or pressure when pushing open a door, for example. Any form of damage to the peripheral nerves in the peripheral nervous system will have detrimental effects on these crucial connections. Similar to a bad telephone line or poor Internet connection, the presence of peripheral neuropathy may alter, interrupt, or impede the messages passed between the peripheral and central nervous systems.

Because every peripheral nerve in different regions of the body possesses a highly specialized function that is specific to its location, peripheral neuropathy may produce an enormous array of varying symptoms. Patients may experience a variety of sensations ranging from mild to severe, which include temporary numbness, tingling, pricking, sensitivity to touch, muscle weakness, or outright discomfort. Some of the more extreme symptoms include burning pain (especially at night), muscle wasting, paralysis, or organ or gland dysfunction. People may be unable to digest food easily, maintain safe levels of blood pressure, sweat normally, or experience normal sexual function. In the most extreme cases, breathing may become difficult or organ failure may occur.

Treatments

For acute or temporary paresthesia, if the source of pressure is relieved, the blood will return to the region and the sensation will begin to dissipate. Nerves will begin to heal, provided the cell bodies are not completely destroyed, scarred, or damaged too severely, and functionality will return. The blood–nerve barrier will be restored and the symptoms of the compression injury will subside. In chronic paresthesia, treating the underlying cause needs to be addressed for best results.

Jennifer L. Hellier

See also: Central Nervous System; Free Nerve Endings; Nerves; Nociception

Further Reading

National Institute of Neurological Disorders and Stroke (NINDS). (2015). *NINDS paresthesia information page.* Retrieved from http://www.ninds.nih.gov/disorders/paresthesia/paresthesia.htm

National Institute of Neurological Disorders and Stroke (NINDS). (2016). *NINDS peripheral neuropathy information page.* Retrieved from http://www.ninds.nih.gov/disorders/peripheralneuropathy/peripheralneuropathy.htm

PARIETAL LOBE

The cerebrum is divided into four major divisions with the parietal lobe being located posterior to the frontal lobe, anterior to the occipital lobe, and superior to the temporal lobe. The parietal lobe is generally associated with integrating sensory information as well as spatial orientation. It has also been shown to be important for processing language and spirituality. Because there are two hemispheres of the brain, there are two parietal lobes present, both with the same functions.

Brain Cut-Out Hat Activity

The brain consists of the cerebral cortex and deep structures, such as the thalamus, hypothalamus, insula, and hippocampus. The main functions of the brain are to integrate and modulate both sensory and motor information as well as to produce cognition, higher reasoning, and thinking. The cerebral cortex is divided into two hemispheres with each containing the same lobes and deep structures. The four lobes and their general function are the frontal lobe, which produces higher reasoning and motor activities; the parietal lobe containing the somatosensory cortex—senses from the body, mainly touch, language processing, visual association cortices; the occipital lobe, which processes vision; and the temporal lobe, which stores memories, is the seat of many emotions, and is essential for language comprehension. The function of the thalamus is to modulate all sensory and motor function except for olfaction (the sense of smell). The hypothalamus is important for maintaining body temperature, while the insula plays a role in consciousness, emotion, maintaining homeostasis, perception, and self-awareness. Lastly, the hippocampus is necessary for building and storing memories.

Materials:

Scissors, white glue, tape, paper clips, card stock (preferably two different colors to represent the left and right hemispheres), and pencil or pen

Directions:

Print out the left brain hemisphere (see Appendix in this book) hat pattern on one color of the card stock, and repeat with the right brain hemisphere pattern on the other color of card stock. With a writing instrument, label the functions of each lobe and draw pictures pertaining to those functions. Note that the left hemisphere, in most humans, contains Broca's area (forming sentences) and Wernicke's area (understanding language), both necessary for language. When ready, cut out each hemisphere's pattern. Then cut all of the solid lines that form the Vs along the edges of the brain. Pull the cut edge to the back side of the paper, making a flap to the dashed line. Glue these in place using the paper clips to hold them together until they dry. Next, place one hemisphere about an eighth of an inch or less underneath the other and tape together. Place on head, making sure the frontal lobe is in the front. Enjoy!

Riannon C. Atwater and Jennifer L. Hellier

Anatomical Divisions

The parietal lobe has three distinct anatomical boundaries. First, the central sulcus separates the parietal lobe anteriorly from the frontal lobe. The central sulcus is a prominent landmark in the mammalian brain as it is the longest, uninterrupted, "straight" groove on the lateral aspect of the cerebral hemisphere. Second, the parieto-occipital sulcus divides the posterior portion of the parietal lobe from the anterior portion of the occipital lobe. Lastly, the lateral or Sylvian fissure separates the ventral region of the parietal lobe from the dorsal region of the temporal lobe.

The parietal lobe is divided into anterior and posterior portions. The posterior parietal lobe can be further divided into the superior parietal lobule and the inferior parietal lobule. Within these regions, specific gyri have specific functions. Within the anterior parietal lobe, the narrow strip of brain tissue found just posterior to the central sulcus is called the postcentral gyrus and is the primary somatosensory cortex. Thus, the somatosensory cortex is the most anterior portion of the parietal lobe. Moving toward the occipital lobe, the somatosensory cortex and the posterior parietal lobe are separated by the postcentral sulcus. Lastly, the intraparietal sulcus divides the superior parietal lobule and the inferior parietal lobule.

Function

The postcentral gyrus is the somatosensory cortex with the function of integrating and processing all sensory information from the body's surface and the underlying viscera. It is also important for the perception of the senses, particularly of touch, pain, and temperature. The somatosensory cortex is often referred to as Brodmann areas 3, 1, and 2. The number order for the somatosensory cortex may seem strange to the reader. This is because when German anatomist Korbinian Brodmann (1868–1918) first sectioned the brain, he did so at an oblique angle. The first area he studied was named Brodmann area 1. As he continued his research, he continued to number the regions based on the order in which he studied them.

The superior parietal lobule is a sensory association cortex, meaning it is used to integrate and process additional sensory information such as vision. Its integration of visual signals is used in spatial orientation of where the body is in space as well as compared to other items. This region is also known as Brodmann areas 5 and 7. The main function of Brodmann area 5 is being an association cortex to the somatosensory cortex, while the primary function of Brodmann area 7 is involved with spatial awareness. Most neuroanatomists consider this region as the dorsal stream of vision (the vision of "where" something is), while the ventral stream of vision (the vision of "what" or "how") projects to the temporal lobe.

The inferior parietal lobule is a sensory association cortex that processes auditory information as well as language. It is also known as Brodmann areas 39 and 40. In most humans, the function of language is dispersed along the left hemisphere. Thus, the inferior parietal lobule, just around the posterior end of the lateral fissure, is called Wernicke's area. This region is not only involved with understanding language but also the ability to read.

In addition to being association cortices, recent studies have shown that both the left and right parietal lobes (particularly the inferior parietal lobule) may be involved with a person's understanding of spirituality or self-transcendence. Specifically, an imaging study revealed that the fronto-parieto-temporal network was activated when the person was describing spiritual experiences. This study suggests that there is a neurobiological basis for religious attitudes and behaviors in humans (Urgesi et al., 2010).

Diseases and Disorders

Damage to the parietal lobe can cause devastating consequences. Specifically, lesions to the right parietal lobe result in the loss of imagery, problems understanding visual relationships, and spatial neglect of the left side of the body. It is often caused by stroke and is characterized by the inability to attend to or interact with people or objects on the opposite side of the affected area. In severe cases, the person may act as if the left side of his or her body never existed. Damage to the left parietal lobe causes problems in understanding symbols—both written letters and mathematics—and language.

Jennifer L. Hellier

See also: Brain Anatomy; Brodmann Areas; Somatosensory Cortex; Somatosensory System; Visual System

Further Reading

Urgesi, Cosimo, Salvatore M. Aglioti, Miran Skrap, & Franco Fabbro. (2010). The spiritual brain: Selective cortical lesions modulate human self-transcendence. *Neuron, 65*(3), 309–319.

Van Vleet, Thomas M., & Joseph M. DeGutis. (2013). The nonspatial side of spatial neglect and related approaches to treatment. *Progress in Brain Research, 207,* 327–349.

PERCEPTION

Have you ever wondered why one person sees images in a painting differently from another person, or how an individual can appreciate the nuances of a musical piece when another person cannot tell the differences in horns being played? This slight variance in how one person perceives the same sensory information differently from another is perception. Specifically, perception is the organization, identification, and interpretation of sensory stimuli (information) produced by neuronal signals within the brain so that an individual can understand the surrounding environment. The sensory organs will receive the stimulus, such as light or sound, and transmit that information to the brain where it is interpreted. However, perception of the sensory information is modulated in the brain by a person's ability to learn, previous memories, expectations, and how attentive the person was at the time of the stimulus. Because perception is a very integrated process, this is why eyewitnesses to a car accident may not remember specific details the same way.

Perception has two processes for integrating sensory information. The first is processing initial low-level sensory stimuli into higher-level information that the brain understands or can identify. An example is seeing a ball and identifying its shape (large, round) and color (orange), or object recognition. The second step in perception processing is connecting the person's expectation (knowledge) and concepts with sensory stimuli. This is influenced by how attentive the person is at the time during the first part of perception processing. Continuing the example, the brain will process the use of the ball and the complex goals of the games associated with the ball. Here the goal of a large orange ball is to be bounced, passed, and shot through a high basket to score two or three points. This additional information (complex rules and strategy for playing basketball) is instantly linked to the object. As a person has more experience with a basketball, his or her understanding and perception will be different from that of someone just learning.

Sensory stimuli, whether it is light, sound, and so on, is not always persistent and is often incomplete or rapidly changing. The brain, however, helps us to feel that our external environment is stable by modulating the sensory information when it is received. For some types of sensory information the brain has developed sensory maps, which connect external stimuli to specific locations across the surface of the brain. These maps are also interconnected and often will influence each other.

Visual Perception

The visual system is a sensory system that is responsible for the sense of sight or vision. Visual perception, however, consists of the psychological process of how an animal or person sees a visual image. Thus, visual perception takes the information from visual processing and attempts to "make sense" of the object. Additionally, visual perception is important for the perception of movement, the perception of depth, and perception of color. These three types of visual perception are based in Gestalt psychology, which tries to understand how the human eye sees objects first as a whole and then as a sum of its individual parts. It also looks at how the entire object is anticipated even when the parts are not integrated, such as filling in the "blind spots" of the visual field to complete the entire image.

Perception of Movement

To perceive movement, the neurons located in region V5 are activated when the speed and direction of an object are seen. In humans, the vestibular system is also necessary for understanding motion perception. This is because it compares the speed of the person against the speed of the object to determine the motion.

Perception of Depth

Seeing the world in three dimensions (3D) and seeing how far an object is from a person is called depth perception. This perception is best with binocular vision as well as utilizing depth cues such as stereopsis (viewing a 3D scene with both eyes), parallax (looking at an object along two different lines of sight and measuring it against the angle made by the two lines), and convergence of the eyes (looking toward the center or "crossing your eyes").

Color Perception

As light hits an object, the color an individual perceives is actually the color of light being reflected by the object's surface. Ratios of S-, M-, and L-cones located in the retina are activated based on the amount and wavelengths of light that enter the eye. As more cones are activated, the eye is able to differentiate more hues and vibrancy of a color. Additionally, color perception requires visual experience so that the brain can interpret what the person is seeing. This is called visual-experience-dependent neural plasticity.

Jennifer L. Hellier

See also: Color Perception; Visual Perception

Further Reading

Bear, Mark F., Barry W. Connors, & Michael A. Paradiso. (2007). *Neuroscience exploring the brain* (3rd ed.). Baltimore, MD: Lippincott Williams & Wilkins.
Kandel, Eric R., James H. Schwartz, Thomas M. Jessell, Steven A. Siegelbaum, & A. J. Hudspeth (Eds.). (2012). *Principles of neural science* (5th ed.). New York, NY: McGraw-Hill.

PERIPHERAL NERVOUS SYSTEM

The peripheral nervous system (PNS) is made up of both nerves and ganglia, and its primary role is to connect the central nervous system (CNS) to the organs, limbs, and skin. The nerves of the PNS extend from the CNS to these outermost areas of the body. Axons that originate from neurons located in the CNS make up the PNS and are responsible for delivering signals to the most distant parts of the body. The PNS, unlike the CNS, is not protected by bone or the blood–brain barrier. This makes it vulnerable to toxins and mechanical injury.

Anatomy and Physiology

The PNS consists of 31 pairs of spinal nerves that originate in the spinal cord and 12 pairs of cranial nerves that originate in the brain. There are two important types of cells within the PNS: glial cells and neurons. Glial cells of the PNS include

Schwann cells that surround nerve fibers and perineuronal satellite cells that surround the cell body. Both types of cells produce myelin sheaths around axons and some cell bodies of ganglia. Myelin is essential for fast communication between neurons. Schwann cells also have the ability to become phagocytes in response to nerve injury and inflammation. Neurons specialize in rapid nerve impulse conduction, allowing for the exchange of signals with other neurons. The body of the neuron, or soma, is located in the CNS while the axon projects and terminates in the skin, organs, or muscles, allowing for rapid communication between the CNS and PNS.

Somatic and Autonomic Nervous Systems

The PNS is divided into two parts: the somatic and autonomic nervous systems. The somatic nervous system conveys and processes conscious and unconscious sensory information including vision, pain, and touch. Additionally, this system is responsible for motor control of voluntary muscles, allowing for coordinated muscle activity that can be adjusted based on an animal's environment. This system contains two major types of neurons: sensory neurons that carry information from the nerves to the CNS and motor neurons that carry information away from the CNS toward muscle fibers throughout the body.

In addition to controlling voluntary movements, the somatic nervous system is associated with involuntary movements. These involuntary movements are known as reflex arcs, during which muscles move involuntarily without input from the brain and a nerve pathway connects directly to the spinal cord. Placing one's hand on a hot stove and pulling it away quickly is an example of a reflex arc. A sensory receptor responds to an environmental stimulus (hot stove) and afferent fibers (A delta and C pain fibers) convey this signal through peripheral nerves to the gray matter of the spinal cord. The afferent root enters the spinal cord and synapses with an interneuron, which synapses with alpha motoneurons. Alpha-motoneurons transmit an impulse to voluntary muscles, allowing the person to pull his or her hand away.

The autonomic nervous system conveys and processes sensory input from visceral organs in addition to motor control of the involuntary and cardiac musculature. It is responsible for control of involuntary or visceral bodily functions including cardiovascular, respiratory, digestive, urinary, and reproductive systems. Examples of these body functions include heartbeat, digestion, and breathing. Additionally, it plays a key role in the way the body handles stress and recovers from stressful situations.

Sympathetic and Parasympathetic Nervous Systems

The autonomic nervous system is further divided into the sympathetic and parasympathetic nervous systems. The sympathetic nervous system regulates the "fight-or-flight" response, allowing the body to function under stress. A sympathetic response dilates pupils, inhibits salivation, relaxes the bronchi (to ease breathing), decreases digestive activity, and stimulates secretion of epinephrine and norepinephrine from the kidney. Additionally, stimulation increases blood flow to skeletal muscles, increases chronotropic and inotropic effects of the heart, and releases glucose stores from the liver. All of these reactions enable a person to respond immediately to an emergent, stressful situation such as avoiding a car accident while driving.

Based on the organization of the sympathetic nervous system, it is also referred to as the thoracolumbar or adrenergic system. All preganglionic fibers within the sympathetic nervous system emerge from the thoracic and upper two lumbar levels of the spinal cord. Norepinephrine and epinephrine are the primary neurotransmitters released by postganglionic fibers within this system and are responsible for many effects seen in the fight-or-flight response. The sympathetic system is designed to exert its effects over widespread body regions for a sustained period of time.

The parasympathetic nervous system regulates the "rest and digest" response, returning the body to normal function in order to conserve physical resources. A parasympathetic response constricts pupils, stimulates salivation, reduces heart rate, constricts bronchi, stimulates digestive activity, and contracts the bladder. All of these responses allow a person to conserve energy during times of relaxation, preparing the person for more stressful situations. The vagus nerve (the 10th pair of the 12 cranial nerves) is the main regulator of automatic functions within the parasympathetic nervous system.

The parasympathetic nervous system is also referred to as the craniosacral or cholinergic system. Preganglionic fibers within the parasympathetic nervous system emerge with several cranial nerve pairs (III—oculomotor, VII—facial, IX—glossopharyngeal, and X—vagus) and at the sacral division (S2–S4) of the spinal cord. Acetylcholine is the neurotransmitter released by postganglionic fibers within the parasympathetic nervous system and is responsible for many effects of rest and digest. The parasympathetic nervous system is organized to respond transiently to a stimulus in a localized region of the body.

Danielle Stutzman

See also: Afferent Tracts; Autonomic Nervous System; Central Nervous System; Cranial Nerves; Nociception

Further Reading

Kandel, Eric R., James H. Schwartz, Thomas M. Jessell, Steven A. Siegelbaum, & A. J. Hudspeth. (2013). *Principles of neural science* (5th ed.).New York, NY: McGraw-Hill.

Kiernan, John A. (2009). *Barr's the human nervous system: An anatomical viewpoint* (9th ed.). Baltimore, MD: Lippincott Williams & Wilkins.

Noback, Charles R., Norman L. Strominger, Robert J. Demarest, & David A. Ruggiero. (2005). *The human nervous system structure and function* (6th ed.). Totowa, NJ: Humana Press.

PERIPHERAL NEUROPATHY

The term peripheral neuropathy, or just neuropathy, is a universal expression to describe myriad syndromes that cause disease or damage to the peripheral nerves. The nerves that could be affected by peripheral neuropathy are the sensory nerves that receive sensations of heat, pain, or touch; the motor nerves that control voluntary motor movements; and the autonomic nerves that control blood pressure, heart rate, digestion, and bladder function. Depending on the severity of the disorder and/or which nerve is damaged, it can affect sensation, movement, or gland/organ function. This damage results in the nerve's decreased ability to transmit and/or receive its signals to and from the central nervous system. In mild cases of neuropathy, a person may feel a tingling sensation, numbness, or paresthesia when using a certain body part for movement. A person with severe neuropathy, however, may experience muscle wasting (hypotrophy), paralysis, or organ dysfunction, such as having problems digesting food.

Types

Neuropathies are classified as acute, chronic, or idiopathic. Cases of acute peripheral neuropathies have a sudden onset and progress quickly. In these cases, an urgent diagnosis and treatment must be made to ensure that the neuropathy can resolve. In chronic neuropathies, the condition is long term and symptoms progress slowly and may be subtle. In fact, a person may not even realize that he or she is experiencing any signs until it is more severe. Some patients will have bouts of relief, but the symptoms usually return. In other cases, some persons will have a progression of symptoms that eventually plateau. Chronic neuropathies are usually the cause of another disorder such as diabetes. Lastly, idiopathic neuropathies are named as such because the cause is unknown.

Single Nerve Damage

If a single nerve is damaged, it results in a condition called mononeuropathy. This is usually caused by localized nerve compression or trauma to a region supplied by a single nerve. Physical compression of the nerve is the most common cause of mononeuropathy, like carpal tunnel syndrome where the median nerve is compressed as it travels through the wrist; or when a person is sitting with his or her leg crossed for an extended period of time resulting in the foot "falling asleep." This is a temporary condition and the pins and needles sensation is caused by a compression mononeuropathy. By moving around and adjusting to a better position, a person can be easily relieved from this condition.

An example of damage to a single nerve is seen in Bell's palsy. This condition is characterized by unilateral temporary weakness or total paralysis of the facial nerve, which is responsible for controlling the muscles of facial expression and for the sense of taste from the anterior two-thirds of the tongue. It also provides innervation to lacrimal glands, salivary glands, and the stapes.

Multiple Nerve Damage

It is most common for more than one nerve to be affected. This condition, called polyneuropathy, generally affects more than one limb or several regions of a body. Polyneuropathy is a serious condition because of the large regions it affects as well as the fact that it usually produces symmetrical symptoms on both sides of the body. These may include muscle weakness; tingling and/or burning sensations covering large areas; the loss of fine touch like the inability to distinguish between textures; problems feeling temperatures; and difficulty in balance when standing or walking. Most of these symptoms tend to appear first in nerves that are long such as those that supply the feet and hands, and over time progress toward the trunk. Common causes of polyneuropathies are diabetes, Lyme disease, blood disorders, and neurotoxins.

Three types of polyneuropathy include distal axonopathy, demyelinating polyneuropathies, and neuronopathy. In distal axonopathy, the axons are damaged while the cell bodies are normal. This is seen most often in patients with diabetes with a very distinct pattern of progression. The farthest part of the axon is damaged first and the cell death slowly progresses toward the trunk as the disease advances. Thus, a person first loses sensation in the toes and the soles of the feet, then the lower leg, and eventually the entire leg. Next, the hands are affected starting with the fingers, the palms, and then the entire arm. Ultimately, the trunk of the body can be affected.

In demyelinating polyneuropathies, the protective covering of the axon is affected. This results in decreased ability to conduct nerve impulses along the length of the axon. Persons with this type of disease often have muscle weakness and decreased sensation because the nerve impulse is weakened in both motor and sensory nerves. The most common cause of this type of polyneuropathy is multiple sclerosis.

Finally, neuronopathy, a rare polyneuropathy, is the opposite of distal axonopathy. Here the cell body of the neuron is damaged and the axon is relatively fine. Usually only one type of neuron is affected, like the motor neurons, which are located in the spinal cord; their axons are the peripheral nerves. This would produce a syndrome called motor neuron disease with most sensory function being normal. If the sensory neurons are damaged, then it can disturb pain, temperature, touch sensation and its ability to be perceived by the brain, but motor function may be unchanged.

Patricia A. Bloomquist

See also: Bell's Palsy; Nerves; Nociception; Paresthesia

Further Reading

Donofrio, Peter D. (Ed.). (2012). *Textbook of peripheral neuropathy.* New York, NY: Demos Medical Publishing.

National Institute of Neurological Disorders and Stroke (NINDS). (2012). *Peripheral neuropathy fact sheet.* Retrieved from http://www.ninds.nih.gov/disorders/peripheralneuropathy/detail_peripheralneuropathy.htm

PHANTOM PAIN

Phantom pain is the pain and sensations that are felt at the location of a missing limb or organ as though that missing body part could still experience sensations. Most of the time, these sensations are felt in an amputated limb or portion of a limb. It is sometimes associated with feelings that the amputated limb is still a part of the body. Phantom pain can also occur in individuals who were born without limbs. Sensations caused by phantom pain are not limited only to pain; other common sensations are pressure, touch, tingling, burning, and movement, to name a few.

Risk Factors and Symptoms

There are some risk factors associated with phantom pain, especially in amputees. If an individual experiences preamputation pain, he or she is more likely to feel pain in the amputated limb after the procedure. In part, this could be due to the nervous system "remembering" the pain and continuing to send pain signals. Stump pain caused by neuromas (abnormal outgrowths of nerve endings resulting in nerve pain) can also have phantom pain or sensations associated with it. An ill-fitting prosthetic replacement can create phantom pain in the amputated limb as well. Individuals who have bilateral limb amputations, lower limb amputations, or other pain are at risk for phantom pain.

Phantom pain can happen anywhere from a few days after amputation up to a few weeks after amputation. It is a neuropathic pain, caused by malfunctioning of the nervous system rather than a real injury. This is because the limb in which the pain is felt is no longer connected to the patient's body. Paresthesias are often associated with phantom pain. Patients with phantom pain rarely have persistent pain; rather they feel pain in their phantom limb intermittently. Approximately 50 to 80 percent of amputees experience phantom pain at some point after amputation (Virtual Medical Center, 2009). Persistent pain in the phantom limb only occurs in approximately 5 percent of amputees (Virtual Medical Center, 2009). In most amputees, phantom pain disappears after two years postamputation.

Pathophysiology

The mechanisms behind phantom pain are still not well known, but it is currently being studied. One known cause of phantom pain is a neurological condition called neuromas. There are two different types of neuromas that are linked to phantom pain: tumor and traumatic. Since the amputation damages the nerve fibers, abnormal nerve growth occurs to try to compensate for the missing portions. This causes extreme pain in patients. Other theories on possible causes of phantom pain are based on neurological pathways and mechanisms.

Management

Since the causes of phantom limb pain are still not completely understood, it is difficult to treat phantom pain. Additionally, each individual reacts differently to the pain and to the various treatments available, so there is no cure-all for phantom pain. Multiple types of treatments can be used to manage phantom pain, including medicine, surgical therapies, and alternative therapies. Analgesics, a broad class of painkiller that works with the peripheral and central nervous systems, can be used to treat this disorder, but they do not ease pain in most patients. Anticonvulsants and tricyclic antidepressants have been proven to work more effectively at treating phantom pain and neuropathic pain in general.

Chronic phantom pain can be treated by surgical placement of a deep-brain stimulator. In deep-brain stimulation, the location of the misfiring neurons involved with phantom pain within the brain is determined using positron emission tomography scans and magnetic resonance imaging. Once the location has been determined, surgeons open the skull and stimulate this region on the brain with electrodes until the patient feels the most relief from the pain. The electrode is then left in the brain and secured so that the patient continues to get relief while going about his or her life. A pulse-generator is connected to continue the stimulation and is implanted below the skin above the collarbone.

Alternative therapies to treat phantom limb pain include mirror-box therapy and acupuncture. Mirror-box therapy is one of the most well-known alternative treatments for phantom limb pain. In mirror-box therapy, the stump from the amputated limb and the intact limb are placed in a box with a mirror that reflects the intact limb as though it is the phantom limb. The patient then undergoes various exercises while watching the mirrored image. This can trick the brain into believing that the phantom limb is clenching, unclenching, or doing a variety of other things.

Lastly, acupuncture can be provided, where very small, fine, sterilized needles are stuck into the skin at certain locations. Acupuncture is thought to stimulate the central nervous system to release endorphins, which often act as natural pain relievers. This relief of endorphins helps to counteract the pain felt at the amputated limb.

Riannon C. Atwater

See also: Central Nervous System; Homunculus; Nociception; Sensory Receptors; Somatosensory Cortex; Somatosensory System

Further Reading

Mayo Clinic. (2011). *Diseases and conditions: Phantom pain.* Retrieved from http://www .mayoclinic.org/diseases-conditions/phantom-pain/basics/symptoms/con-20023268

Virtual Medical Center. (2009). *Phantom limb pain.* Retrieved from http://www.myvmc. com/diseases/phantom-limb-pain/#Symptoms

PHANTOSMIA

Phantosmia, from the Greek *phant-* meaning phantom and *osme* meaning smell, is an olfactory hallucination. The disorder is frequently associated with neurological and psychological conditions. Some of these conditions include migraines, epilepsy, Parkinson's disease, neuroblastoma (cancer of neural tissue), and schizophrenia. Causes of the disorder vary, and the smells patients experience can be anywhere on a scale of pleasant to disgusting. Phantosmia can be classified into three main categories: unirhinal (from one nostril), episodic, and recurrent. Since the causes of phantosmia are varied and some are psychological rather than physiological, there is no defined treatment. For serious cases, surgery can be performed to remove the olfactory bulb. This results in anosmia, or the complete lack of sense of smell, which would also affect the flavor of food. Thus, the surgical option is not highly valued.

Causes and Diagnosis

There are a wide variety of causes of phantosmia including both neurological and psychological causes. These include less severe causes such as smoking, dental problems, nasal infection (the phantosmia typically disappears after the infection has cleared in this case), migraines (especially migraines with auras where the smell can occur before or during the migraine), nasal polyps (abnormal growths within the nasal cavity that can be either malignant—a precursor to cancer, or benign—a relatively harmless growth), and exposure to some chemicals (this includes insecticides and solvents). More severe causes of phantosmia include: schizophrenia, Alzheimer's disease, Parkinson's disease, cancer, stroke, and head injury. Additionally, the cause in some afflicted individuals can be purely psychological. One very well-documented cause of phantosmia is epilepsy involving seizures within the temporal lobe. Following seizure some patients reported phantom smells right before the seizure. Patients who do not experience seizures but have tumors growing within the temporal lobe also have a higher risk of phantosmia. In these neurological causes the issue can be that nerves are misfiring, sending the incorrect information to the brain, or the problem could be within the brain itself and how it processes these signals.

In order to diagnose phantosmia the physician needs to distinguish the condition from a gustatory issue (since the two systems are so interconnected) and from other olfactory conditions such as anosmia and parosmia (where the smell is coming from an object within the environment but this smell is becoming distorted). Both of these are typically due to damage of the olfactory system. During diagnosis, the physician will also attempt to discover the cause for the phantosmia. Techniques include nasal endoscopy (using a small flexible camera to examine the nasal cavity), a full medical history (especially looking for signs of head trauma and upper and lower respiratory infections), and imaging techniques (to look for seizures and cancers that could be the cause).

Symptoms and Treatment

The primary defining symptom of phantosmia is the perception of a smell when there is no odorant present. Phantosmia is typically worse in one nostril than the other, typically the nostril with the lower ability for smell. Scientists distinguish the terms *phantosmia* and *olfactory hallucinations* based on how long the symptoms persist. Olfactory hallucinations are the perception of a smell without an odorant present that lasts for only a few seconds. As such, phantosmia is the perception without odorant stimulus that persists for longer than a few seconds. Often, patients also report the feeling of the phantosmia about to happen. This feeling persists even after treatment to remove the smell. In this situation, patients still report the same feeling of the phantosmia about to occur but it never does.

One of the biggest ways to treat phantosmia is to treat the underlying cause of the disorder. For example, if epilepsy and seizures of the temporal lobe are what is causing the phantosmia, the reduction of seizures should help alleviate phantosmia for the patient. Sometimes the symptoms of phantosmia will reduce and eventually disappear with time, so one possible treatment for patients who can handle the smells is to wait it out and continue to monitor for a more serious neurological condition that could be the root cause. Some drugs that are used to treat depression and epilepsy have also been shown to be effective treatments in some cases. Finally, surgical treatment is an option. This can include removal of the olfactory epithelium (which has been shown to be fairly effective in a majority of cases) or removal of the olfactory bulb. One side effect of the removal of the olfactory bulb is that it can often lead to anosmia.

Riannon C. Atwater

See also: Anosmia; Dysosmia; Olfactory System

Further Reading

Leopold, Donald. (2002). Distortion of olfactory perception: Diagnosis and treatment. *Chemical Senses, 27*(7), 611–615. Retrieved from http://chemse.oxfordjournals.org/content/27/7/611.full

NHS Choices. (2014). Phantosmia (smelling odours that aren't there). Retrieved from http://www.nhs.uk/conditions/phantosmia/Pages/Introduction.aspx

PHEROMONES

Pheromones (from the Greek *pherein* meaning to transport and *hormone* meaning to stimulate) are small chemicals that are released by the body that signal a message to other individuals of the same species. They have been well documented as a communication method between many species of insects and even within prokaryotic organisms. The subject of whether humans use pheromones as a method of communication is of large interest to the scientific community and is currently being researched. Some evidence points to this being true—some pheromones are used and can alter human physiology. The vomernasal organ (VNO), thought to be a vestigial organ (an organ that remains but no longer plays a role in the species as it evolves), has been associated with the reception of pheromones. One point of evidence in favor of pheromones being a mode of communication among humans is the synchronization of female menstrual cycles.

Types of Pheromones

Many species use pheromones as a form of communication between individuals of that species. As such, these pheromones can convey a multitude of information based on their chemical composition. Pheromones are classified by the signal that they provide and their chemical composition. These include two main categories of pheromones: releaser pheromones and primer pheromones. Releaser pheromones are responsible for an immediate response in the organism that is receiving the signal. There are three main types of releaser pheromones: sex pheromones, alarm pheromones, and recruitment pheromones. On the other hand, primer pheromones create a physiological change that will then result in a behavioral response. One example of this is the release of gonadotropin-releasing hormone that will elicit mating behaviors in female rats called lordosis (this helps to attract male rats in order to mate).

Sex pheromones are one of the most widely known pheromones. These chemicals typically indicate that a specific individual is ready for breeding, especially females. In many species, the female is only prepared to copulate when she is ovulating. Pheromones help to identify those ovulating females so that males of that species can fertilize offspring. Additionally, males will release sex pheromones particularly to convey information about their genotypes so that females can select a mate. Some sex pheromones will suppress reproductive behavior of the same sex so as to create a monopoly on resources (the other sex of the species). These pheromones are also the mostly widely studied in humans with varied conclusions. Overall, it appears that far too many things are going into the human olfactory system to concretely state that pheromones play a definitive role in human sex behaviors.

Alarm pheromones play a role in a synchronized response to predators. These pheromones are volatile compounds that typically trigger either aggression or fear in members of the same species. This helps to preserve the species as other members are aware of the danger. Aggregation pheromones are responsible for driving the species to one physical location. Typically, the males of the species are the ones that release this pheromone, which is attractive to both males and females of the species. This form of pheromone is beneficial for the species as it helps with the synchronization of attack by the same species. It also plays a role in reproduction by attracting many potential mates to the same location.

Pheromones and the Menstrual Cycle

One of the first and largest studies in favor of pheromones being utilized by humans is a study performed demonstrating the effects of male and female pheromones (male and female sex-specific hormone precursors) on the female menstrual cycle. It is well documented that the menstrual cycles of women who spend a large amount of time together become synchronized. This is sometimes referred to as the McClintock effect. It is suggested that female pheromones influence other females to lengthen or shorten parts of the menstrual cycle until synchronization is achieved. Male hormones have also been demonstrated to alter female cycles by decreasing fertility issues as well as regulating the menstrual cycle by altering the length of each portion of the cycle. Unfortunately, this evidence is not entirely convincing as there are many other factors affecting the female cycle including sleep, stress, and other behavioral patterns.

Vomeronasal Organ

Within most species that utilize pheromones to communicate, the vomeronasal organ is the sensory organ responsible for the detection of pheromones. It plays a large role in reproductive behaviors and other social behaviors in part by the responses generated to pheromones. In humans it is largely regarded as a vestigial organ, or an organ that is "extra" and does not serve an obvious purpose. However, this is not completely accepted and some research is demonstrating that it might play a role in human pheromone reception, integration, and response.

Riannon C. Atwater

See also: Olfactory System; Vomeronasal Organ

Further Resources

Doty, Richard L. (2014). Chapter 19: Human pheromones. In C. Mucignat-Caretta (Ed.), *Neurobiology of chemical communication*. Boca Raton, FL: CRC Press/Taylor & Francis. Retrieved from http://www.ncbi.nlm.nih.gov/books/NBK200980/

Human pheromones. Retrieved from http://www.macalester.edu/academics/psychology/whathap/ubnrp/pheromone10/human%20pheromones.html

PHOTORECEPTORS: *See* Cones; Rods

PREGNANCY AND SENSE OF SMELL

Women have often reported that their sense of smell increases during pregnancy and that they are more sensitive to scent, particularly food and cooking odors. In fact, some women claim that this heightened sense of smell was their first indication that they were pregnant. Are there any scientific data to back up this anecdotal claim?

The Sense of Smell

The sense of smell, or olfaction, allows humans to differentiate between one trillion different odorants (Bushdid et al., 2014). Scent enters the nose and travels to the top of the nasal cavity where molecules enter the olfactory cleft. Receptors in the olfactory cleft send signals along nerve fibers to the olfactory bulb located in the brain. The olfactory bulb then relays signals to other parts of the brain, explaining why the sense of smell can be closely linked to emotion, memory, and learning.

Significance of Sense of Smell in Pregnancy

During pregnancy many women complain of increased sense of smell, sometimes called hyperosmia. This enhanced sense of smell could function to keep women away from "danger." This danger could take many forms. Perhaps a woman's heightened sense of smell will stop her from eating food that smells different due to bacterial or fungal contamination. Other sources of danger for the embryo could be in the form of chemicals or air pollution. Even body odor could alert a pregnant woman that a person is ill and therefore a potential danger to herself and her developing embryo.

Conflicting Evidence for Increased Sense of Smell During Pregnancy

Many studies report increases in women's perceived sense of smell during pregnancy. A few studies, conversely, report that women rate their sense of smell as lower when pregnant. Self-reporting leads to inclusive and conflicting data because of the subjectivity of these reports and the variability of the questions asked and rating scales used. To address these inconsistencies, researchers have measured pregnant women's ability to detect certain odors and compared these data to control groups consisting of women who were not pregnant and men. Again, the results vary depending on the odor tested.

Perhaps each woman becomes sensitive to different smells during pregnancy. Due to hormonal changes during pregnancy, a woman may become more easily conditioned to associate a smell with nausea and vomiting, making some odors seem stronger or more unpleasant. The close association between sense of smell and emotions and memory might protect humans from repeat experiences with foods that cause illness. Yet linking the memory of scents with nausea and vomiting could lead to increased nausea and vomiting when a woman is exposed to common scents. Linking the memory of a scent with the memory of nausea would certainly make a woman more aware of scents in her environment. Each woman is exposed to a different group of odors on a daily basis, which could explain the different sensitivities women demonstrate in different studies and the seemingly conflicting data revealed by many studies.

Estrogen, a hormone that fluctuates during a woman's monthly cycle and then rises throughout pregnancy, has been hypothesized to cause increased sensitivity to smell. While estrogen does rise during pregnancy, sensitivity to smells seems to decrease after the first trimester of pregnancy. Estrogen may be working in combination with a variety of other hormones to alter a woman's sense of smell during pregnancy, particularly during the first trimester when nausea and vomiting also seem to peak.

Future Research

Understanding the changes in the sense of smell during pregnancy will help us learn how the sense of smell works. If odor perception has measurable changes during pregnancy, further investigation could be undertaken to answer whether this change contributes to nausea and vomiting experienced during pregnancy. For some women, nausea and vomiting can become severe. Further research could determine whether aromatherapy or other alternative therapies could be effective in treating nausea and vomiting in pregnancy. Burning candles and sniffing lemons or herbs are common cures recommended to help with morning sickness; these cures may have a basis in fact due to the increased sense of smell experienced by some during pregnancy.

Lisa A. Rabe

See also: Anosmia; Dysosmia; Odor Intensity Scale; Olfactory Bulb; Olfactory Sensory Neurons; Perception

Further Reading

Bushdid, C., Marcelo O. Magnasco, Leslie B. Vosshall, & Andreas Keller. (2014). Humans can discriminate more than 1 trillion olfactory stimuli. *Science, 343*(6177), 1370–1372. http://dx.doi.org/10.1126/science.1249168

Cameron, E. Leslie. (2014). Pregnancy and olfaction: A review. *Frontiers in Psychology, 5*, 67. Retrieved from http://www.ncbi.nlm.nih.gov/pmc/articles/PMC3915141/

Gilbert, Avery N., & Charles J. Wysocki. (1991). Quantitative assessment of olfactory experience during pregnancy. *Psychosomatic Medicine, 53*, 693–700.

PRESBYCUSIS: *See* Age-Related Hearing Loss

PRESBYOPIA

Often referred to as "old man's eyes" or the "aging eye condition," presbyopia is the gradual loss of a person's eyes' ability to focus on nearby objects. It is a very natural result of aging and usually becomes noticeable in early to mid-40-year-olds and continues to worsen until about age 65. A basic eye exam can confirm presbyopia and it can be corrected with glasses, contact lenses, or surgery.

Anatomy and Physiology

The eyes are organs necessary for vision and use light to focus an image on the retinas, which are the photosensitive layers at the back of the eyes. At the front of the eye are the cornea, pupil, lens, and ciliary muscles. For vision to be clear, the eye must rely on the cornea and lens to focus light onto the retina. The lens can change shape with the help of contracting ciliary muscles that flank it. This process is called accommodation, which changes the optical power of the lens and maintains a clear image on the retina. Accommodation allows a person to see from a far distance and then up close (within centimeters from the face) without losing focus. Accommodation occurs very rapidly, particularly in young persons, within hundreds of milliseconds; however, the ability to accommodate decreases in older adults. This is because the lens in the eye is very prone to aging. Lenses do not have the ability to turn over proteins within their centers (nuclei). This results in a thickening or scar tissue (sclerosis) buildup within the nucleus of the lens. Thus, the elasticity of the lens reduces over time and its ability to change shape is decreased.

Research was performed to determine the stiffness of different regions of human lenses as a function of age and to correlate the biophysical measurements in the lens center with nuclear water content. A custom-made probe was designed to fit a dynamic mechanical analyzer that was used to measure stiffness values at 1-millimeter increments across humans'? lenses. The results showed there was a pronounced increase in the nucleus of the lens as well as stiffness over the age range from 14 to 78 years old. Thus, the thickness of the lens nucleus was shown to be a major contributing factor to presbyopia.

Signs and Symptoms

The primary sign and symptom of presbyopia is blurred vision at normal reading distances. This is most notable when a person is trying to read a menu and needs to hold the menu farther away to make the words clear. Additionally, persons with presbyopia may develop headaches after reading or doing close work. These symptoms can worsen when tired, drinking alcohol, or in dimly lit or dark rooms.

Treatment

A person should visit an eye doctor (optometrist) if blurry close-up vision is keeping him or her from reading, doing close work, or doing other normal activities. Current treatments for presbyopia include prescription glasses, prescription contact lens, or surgery.

If the patient does not require corrective lenses for distance vision, then the best treatment is an optical aid for near vision. These can include prescription glasses or over-the-counter magnifying/reading glasses purchased at a pharmacy or grocery store.

For patients who are diagnosed with myopia (nearsightedness, which requires corrective lenses for their distance vision), it is best if they take off their glasses to read up close. Most people with myopia can read without their corrective lenses well past the age of 40. However, if an adult patient is considering refractive surgery like LASIK (laser in-situ keratomileusis or laser-assisted in-situ keratomileusis), the ophthalmologist will advise that correcting the nearsightedness will not slow down the natural aging process of presbyopia. Thus, the patient may need reading glasses when he or she is older.

Some myopic patients may also have astigmatism. As these persons age, they may have better up-close vision without their corrective lens. However, if their astigmatism is severe, their optometrist may prescribe two different contact lenses. One eye would be the "reading eye" and the other the "distance eye." This is called monovision. If the patient likes monovision produced by contact lenses, then he or she has the option to make it permanent by a surgical technique that reshapes the corneas. Monovision is not suggested for glasses, as the wearer may not always look through the center of the lens, which would result in double images.

Persons with hyperopia (farsightedness) may need a prescription that corrects both distance and near vision with bifocal lenses.

Renee Johnson and Jennifer L. Hellier

See also: Accommodation; Amblyopia; Astigmatism; Diplopia; Myopia; Visual System

Further Reading

Ai Hong Chen, Daniel J. O'Leary, & Edwin R. Howell. (2000). Near visual function in young children. *Ophthalmology, Physiology, and Optometry, 20*, 185–198.

Heys, Karl R., Sandra L. Cram, & Roger J. W. Truscott. (2004). Massive increase in the stiffness of the human lens nucleus with age: The basis for presbyopia? *Molecular Vision, 10*, 956–963. Retrieved from http://www.molvis.org/molvis/v10/a114/

National Eye Institute (NEI). (2010). Facts about presbyopia. Retrieved from https://nei.nih.gov/health/errors/presbyopia

PRIMARY ODORS

Smells and scents are terms used for odorants (or aroma compounds) that can be either pleasant or unpleasant. Other terms for odorants tend to have more specific meanings. For example, enjoyable smells are also called fragrances, perfumes, and aromas, whereas disagreeable smells are termed stench, stink, and reek. Nonetheless, all smells are odorants, which are the chemical stimuli of the olfactory system. Today, scientists have grouped odorants into seven primary odor types: (1) camphoraceous, (2) ethereal, (3) floral, (4) musky, (5) pepperminty, (6) pungent, and (7) putrid. These seven categories of odors, however, may not be complete as science continues to study the sense of smell in humans and animals.

Anatomy and Physiology

The sense of smell is mediated by a volatilized odorant (either in air or liquid) that binds to olfactory sensory neurons (also called olfactory receptor neurons). These neurons are located in the olfactory epithelium in the posterior portion of the nasal cavity. Scientific studies have shown that there are millions of olfactory receptor neurons in the olfactory epithelium. Each neuron has cilia that protrude from the olfactory epithelium into the airway of the nasal cavity. This direct contact with air allows the volatized odorants to bind on to the receptors located in the ends of the cilia. Once a neuron binds its specific odorant, an action potential is generated and travels through the neuron's axon to the brain for perception and identification. The axons of the olfactory sensory neurons make up the first cranial nerve (CN I) or the olfactory nerve.

Aroma Compounds

Aroma compounds are chemical compounds that have a smell or scent that can be volatilized so as to enter the posterior portion of the nasal cavity. This means that most aroma compounds have a molecular weight that is less than 300 and are generally classified by chemical structure, such as alcohols, aldehydes, amines, aromatic, esters, ketones, lactones, linear- and cyclic-terpenes, and thiols.

Camphoraceous Smells

Camphoraceous smells are often found in mothballs, medicated ointments (e.g., Vicks® VapoRub™), and rosemary leaves. Camphor is the main ingredient in the above items and it is found in the camphor laurel (a large evergreen tree), which is native to Asia. Camphor is a terpenoid (similar to cyclic-terpenes) and is a waxy, flammable solid. Because of its strong smell, most insects stay away from items with camphor, making it a successful bug repellent.

Ethereal Smells

Ether-like or cleaning fluid smells are called ethereal. These smells are often found in essential oils (e.g., lavender, eucalyptus, and sandalwood) as well as dry-cleaning solution. Most of these kinds of smells are types of ethers.

Floral Smells

Floral smells are those scents from flowers, such as roses, lilies, and lilacs. Some floral odorants may have a sweet smell. Many perfumes in cosmetics and laundry powders use a commercial compound, Lilial, which has a floral scent. Lilial is a synthetic aldehyde and in rare cases can develop as an allergen for some people.

Musky Smells

Musky smells are scents derived from glandular secretions from animals, particularly the musk deer, and plants that emit similar smells. Musky odorants have been used for the base notes of perfumes and colognes since ancient Greek times. Today, a synthetic form of musk is used called muscone, which is a ketone.

Pepperminty Smells

Pepperminty smells are scents derived from mint plants, such as watermint, spearmint, and peppermint (which is a hybrid plant, *Mentha* x *piperita*). Peppermints are used in many gums and candies as the scent has been shown to freshen breath. Peppermint is a terpenoid (similar to terpenes) and its oil has been used topically for muscle pain.

Pungent Smells

Pungent smells are those that are strong and sharp, such as vinegar. In food science, pungency is a reference for spiciness from mild to hot. Capsaicin and other spices such as piperine mediate a spicy sensation by stimulating the free nerve endings of the trigeminal nerve.

Putrid Smells

Putrid smells are those that are associated with decomposition of proteins. Usually it is the smell of a decomposing body of a dead animal or rotten eggs. It is a very strong and unpleasant smell that can cause some people to vomit.

Jennifer L. Hellier

See also: Anosmia; Olfactory System; Pregnancy and Sense of Smell

Further Reading

Agapakis, Christina. (2011). What does this smell like? Wine snobbery made easy. *Scientific American*. Retrieved from http://blogs.scientificamerican.com/oscillator/what-does-this-smell-like-wine-snobbery-made-easy/

Gilbert, Avery N. (2014). *What the nose knows: The science of scent in everyday life*. New York, NY: Crown Publishing Group.

Schoenfeld, Thomas A., & Thomas A. Clenland. (2005). The anatomical logic of smell. *Trends in Neurosciences, 28*(11), 620–627.

PROPRIOCEPTION

Proprioception, from Latin *proprius* (one's own) and *capere* (to take or grasp), is the sense of your own body in space, in time. The vestibular system, mainly responsible for the body's sense of balance, plays a huge role in conveying information about equilibrium and the body's orientation in space to the proprioceptive system. Kinesthesia is monitored by mechanoreceptors, neural receptors triggered by a mechanical deformation, and provides information about the body's motion in space. Together the vestibular and kinesthetic systems make up proprioception. Additionally, proprioception can be divided into two subcategories: interoception—or the sense of the body's internal physiology; and exteroception—the sense of the body's external physiology. Proprioception plays a large role in everyday life as it is what provides motor control to the body and allows you to move without directly looking at each of your limbs as they create the motion.

Joint Receptors and Joint Position Sense

Joint Receptors

Receptors within the joint have historically been associated with proprioception and with providing information to the brain about where the joint is in relation to the body, as well as the joint's angle relative to itself. Research is moving away from this idea that joint receptors are the main receptor for joint position sense and proprioception. Part of the reason for this is that joint receptors are not as specific as was once thought and cannot provide information about the exact degree of bend. However, they do play a larger role in joint position sense in certain joints over others. Joint position sense is thought to be one of the main ways the brain is able to determine the location of body parts relative to space and itself. Research will continue to refine what is accepted as the main receptors of joint position sense.

Muscle Spindles

Research is pointing more and more in the direction of spindle fibers and their associated neurons as the main sensory receptors for joint position sense. Muscle spindles are enclosed in a capsule and innervated by three neurons: alpha motor neurons (α-MN), gamma motor neurons (γ-MN), and muscle spindle afferent neurons. These capsules are found throughout the muscle body and are partly responsible for maintaining muscle tone. The motor neurons co-activate each other in a process called alpha-gamma co-activation. This stimulus causes the muscle fiber to contract in order to maintain a specific spindle length to allow the muscle spindle afferents to remain responsive. When the spindle lengthens during muscle movement, it is the muscle spindle afferent that is triggered, sending a response to the brain about movement in that muscle. Spindle fibers mainly help to relay information about muscle length and relative velocity to the brain.

Golgi Tendon Organs

Golgi tendon organs are another large category of receptors for joint position sense. However, rather than being located within the muscle body itself, as spindle fibers are, Golgi tendon organs are located within muscle tendons. These organs are innervated by neurons called Golgi tendon afferents. These neurons are activated when the tendon is stretched through muscle contraction. This then produces a signal relaying muscle tension to the brain. Overall, Golgi tendon organs relay a sense of force on the muscle and are responsible for the sensation of "heaviness" that can occur within the muscle.

Loss of Proprioception

Proprioception loss is associated with a variety of causes. These include muscle fatigue, sudden gain or loss of weight (especially muscle weight), overstimulation of the parietal cortex due to migraines and epilepsy, and loss of limb as in phantom limb pain. Some common neurological diseases are also associated with proprioception errors. One example of this is multiple sclerosis (MS). These errors in MS occur mainly because of the loss of myelination of nerves that is caused by and characteristic of the disease. The alpha motor neurons are specifically damaged as MS progresses, leading to proprioceptive ataxia (or loss of proprioception). Damage to the spinal cord can also result in a loss of proprioception by preventing neurons from being able to relay their information to the brain.

One main disorder of the proprioceptive system is proprioception deficit disorder (PDD) also known as Sacks's syndrome or Descartes's disease. PDD is associated with the complete loss of proprioception resulting in the feeling of being disembodied. Individuals with PDD have limited control of their bodies and often do not realize that the body part they feel touching them is indeed their own, as they cannot feel their limb in space at that location. Overall the partial loss or complete loss of proprioception can cause difficulties for afflicted individuals as they cannot move properly without an extreme amount of visual focus on the body part.

Further Research

Proprioception is a huge area of research, as it is still not well understood. Some research has proposed that proprioception also includes a large amount of anticipation of where your limbs will be in space before moving them. Joint position sense cannot entirely explain this phenomenon. Additionally, while it is known that proprioception is processed partially in the cortex, exact processes have not been described.

Riannon C. Atwater

See also: Golgi Tendon Organs; Proprioception Deficit Disorders

Further Reading

Proske, Uwe, & Simon C. Gandevia. (2012). The proprioceptive senses: Their roles in signaling body shape, body position and movement, and muscle force. *Physiological Reviews, 92*(4), 1651–1697. Retrieved from http://physrev.physiology.org/content/92/4/1651

PROPRIOCEPTION DEFICIT DISORDERS

A major component of proprioception is joint position sense, which is a measurement of the accuracy of joint-angle replication from what was initiated from the brain. This can be conducted actively or passively as well as in an open or closed chain environment. Proprioception is the sense of relative position of neighboring parts of the body and strength of effort being employed during movement. Proprioceptors in striated muscles (skeletal muscles), tendons, and joints provide proprioception in humans.

History

Originally described by Julius Caesar Scaliger (1484–1558) as a "sense of locomotion" and later described as a "muscle sense" by Charles Bell (1774–1842), proprioception was one of the first descriptions of physiologic feedback mechanisms. Charles Scott Sherrington (1857–1952) introduced the terms *proprioception, interoception*, and *exteroception*, which all provide information as to where information originates. Joint position sense tests involve the ability of an individual to perceive the position of a joint without the aid of vision. Experimental evidence shows there is no strong relationship between these two aspects.

Applications and Impairment

Many applications of proprioception are used in things including but not limited to field sobriety tests, diagnosis, learning new skills, training, and joint-position matching. Being asked to touch your finger to your nose with your eyes closed is a common field sobriety test. Those with no deficits can do this with little to no error. Those with deficits, or alcohol intoxication, will fail this test because they cannot locate their limbs in space in relation to their nose. A very similar test is also done to diagnose neurological disorders. Proprioception is what allows a person to learn how to walk in complete darkness without losing balance.

Proprioception can be impaired in individuals with diseases or injuries including but not limited to (1) just being tired, (2) seizures and epilepsy, (3) vitamin B_6 overdose, (4) Ehlers-Danlos syndrome (an inherited disease that affects the connective tissues, particularly of the spine and cranioverbral junction), and (5) a spectrum of autism disorders like Asperger's syndrome, to name just a few.

Research

In 2013, Elke Heremans and colleagues wrote a review of current research about freezing of gait in Parkinson's disease. They defined freezing of gait "as a brief, episodic absence or marked reduction of forward progression of feet despite the intention to walk." Additionally, freezing of gait is one of the most debilitating motor symptoms that patients with Parkinson's disease exhibit and is the leading cause of falls in these patients. Heremans and colleagues found that freezing of gait consists of both motor deficits and cognitive deficits, and that the main cause of freezing of gait is an abnormal gait pattern generation.

Another study by Toby Smith and colleagues (2013) addressed joint proprioception in people with benign joint hypermobility syndrome (BJHS). This research focused on determining whether people with BJHS exhibit reduced joint proprioception and if they do, if it is evident in all age groups. BJHS is one of the most common heritable connective tissue disorders and is associated with joint laxity, instability, and pain. It typically manifests with symptoms including but not limited to decreased stiffness and stability from tendons, ligaments, and join capsules. Their study mostly consisted of database searches in MEDLINE, Embase, CINAHL, AMED, PubMed, and PEDro using keywords including but not limited to position sense, proprioception, postural balance, and instability. They initially found 116 individuals from the search but only 18 were potentially eligible for the study. However, the number decreased to five individuals being eligible after full text review. Following the analysis of the data Smith and colleagues collected, they concluded that people with BJHS demonstrate poorer lower limb joint position sense and threshold detection to movement with statistically different results from those without joint hypermobility. Very few studies Smith et al. looked at addressed upper limbs, so results were not significant in their study as this sample size was too small to make any conclusions.

Renee Johnson

See also: Exteroception; Interoception; Proprioception

Further Reading
Heremans, Elke, Alice Nieuwboer, & Sarah Vercruysse. (2013). Freezing of gait in Parkinson's disease: Where are we now? *Current Neurology and Neuroscience Reports, 13*(6), 350.

Scheper, Mark C., Janneke E. de Vries, Jeanine Verbunt, & Raoul H. Engelbert. (2015). Chronic pain in hypermobility syndrome and Ehlers-Danlos syndrome (hypermobility type): It is a challenge. *Journal of Pain Research, 8,* 591–601.

Smith, Toby O., Emma Jerman, Victoria Easton, Holly Bacon, Kate Armon, Fiona Poland, & Alex J. Macgregor. (2013). Do people with benign joint hypermobility syndrome (BJHS) have reduced joint proprioception? A systematic review and meta-analysis. *Rheumatology International, 33*(11), 2709–2716. Retrieved from http://link.springer.com/article/10.1007/s00296-013-2790-4#/page-2

PTOSIS

When the upper or lower eyelid is drooping, the medical term used to describe this condition is ptosis. It is derived from a Greek word meaning "to fall" and the "p" in "ptosis" is silent. Thus, the word is pronounced / ˈtōsəs/. Ptosis occurs when the muscles of the eyelid (the levator palpebrae superioris and the superior tarsal) are weakened or paralyzed and are unable to raise the eyelid. Over the course of the day, the weakened muscles can become tired and the drooping is usually worse in the evening compared to the morning.

Signs and Symptoms

Ptosis can affect one or both eyes. With ptosis, the drooping upper eyelid reduces a person's field of vision. Depending on how much the eyelid droops will determine how much of the visual field is affected. Thus, individuals with ptosis will compensate for their reduced vision by arching their eyebrow to raise the affected eyelid. If the ptosis is severe, a person may have to physically lift the eyelid with the fingers to be able to see. Additionally, if severe ptosis is left untreated, it can produce other eye conditions such as amblyopia ("lazy eye") or astigmatism (blurry vision from a misshapen cornea).

Causes

Ptosis may occur at any age but it is predominantly seen in the elderly as the eye muscles weaken with age, as does the skin of the upper eyelid. Specifically, the tendon that supports the levator palpebrae superioris muscle becomes stretched over time. Thus, the tendon cannot hold the eyelid open as well, making it the most common cause of ptosis. The tendon and/or muscle can also be stretched during eye surgery, such as cataract removal or LASIK (laser-assisted in-situ keratomileusis). Excess baggy skin of the upper eyelid can add to the severity of the ptosis.

If an infant is born with ptosis, it is an inherited condition called congenital ptosis and its cause is currently unknown. If ptosis is diagnosed in a young child, it must be corrected quickly to avoid permanent damage to the child's eyesight. Ptosis can also be caused by damage to the superior cervical sympathetic ganglion (part of the autonomic nervous system) or to the cranial nerve supplying the eyelid muscles, which is the oculomotor nerve (cranial nerve III). Damage to this nerve is usually a sign of an underlying disease or disorder such as a brain tumor, diabetes, drug abuse, myasthenia gravis, or stroke, to name a few. Persons who abuse (take multiple and/or high doses) opioid drugs (either illegal or prescription) may have a side effect of ptosis. The most common opioid drugs that can produce ptosis are heroin, hydrocodone (Vicodin), morphine, oxycodone (Oxycotin), or pregabalin (Lyrica).

Treatment

To date, the best way to treat ptosis is by surgery. An ophthalmologist who has experience in cosmetic and reconstructive facial surgery and who specializes in the eyelids will need to tighten the tendon of the levator palpebrae superioris muscle or may have to tighten the muscle itself. In some cases, if the muscle is too stretched or weakened, then a "sling" may need to be made. In this operation the forehead muscle will be used to hold the eyelid up. The main goal for a successful surgery is providing a complete field of vision for the eye as well as symmetry with the unaffected eye's upper lid.

Jennifer L. Hellier

See also: Amblyopia; Astigmatism; Cranial Nerves; Diplopia; Hyperopia; Myopia; Visual Fields; Visual System

Further Reading

American Society of Ophthalmic Plastic & Reconstructive Surgery. (2015). Ptosis (droopy upper eyelid). Retrieved from https://www.asoprs.org/i4a/pages/index.cfm?pageid =3669

Bagheri, Abbas, Mehdi Tavakoli, Hadi Najmi, Reza Erfanian Salim, & Shahin Yazdani. (2016). Comparison between eyelid indices of ptotic eye and normal fellow eye in patients with unilateral congenital ptosis. *Journal of Plastic, Reconstructive & Aesthetic Surgery, 69*(1), e5–e9. http://dx.doi.org/10.1016/j.bjps.2015.10.004

Finsterer, Josef. (2003). Ptosis: Causes, presentation, and management. *Aesthetic Plastic Surgery, 27*(3), 193–204.

R

RAMÓN Y CAJAL, SANTIAGO

Often referred to as Ramón y Cajal or just Cajal, Santiago Ramón y Cajal (1852–1934) was a Spanish histologist, neuroscientist, and pathologist, who investigated the morphology (shape) of brain cells by using a simple light microscope. He is most famous for his remarkable detailed drawings of these microscopic structures, particularly of their delicate arborizations (fine-branching structures of dendrites and/or axons) and their connections in the central nervous system. Although he used just a light microscope, his artistic drawings and anatomical analyses have proven correct in many brain regions. For his research and histological findings, Ramón y Cajal is considered to be the father of neuroscience. In fact, Ramón y Cajal's detailed drawings are still used today to teach neuroscience and neuro-anatomy to students.

Ramón y Cajal was born in Navarre, Spain, and was the son of Justo Ramón, a physician and anatomy professor, and Antonia Cajal. His last name contains both of his parents' last names: Ramón y Cajal. Santiago was kicked out of many schools because of his rebellious behavior and disagreement with authority. In fact, at the age of 11 he was imprisoned for demolishing a neighbor's gate with a homemade cannon. He was a natural artist and painter, but his father did not encourage Ramón y Cajal to develop these skills. Instead, his father made Ramón y Cajal an apprentice to a cobbler and a barber.

Eventually, Ramón y Cajal attended the University of Zaragoza School of Medicine, where his father taught. Ramón y Cajal graduated in 1873 and became a medical officer for the Spanish army where he completed a tour in Cuba from 1874 to 1875. Ramón y Cajal returned to school and received his PhD in medicine in 1877. Ultimately, he became an anatomy professor at the University of Valencia in 1883 and then at the University of Barcelona in 1887. Ramón y Cajal's neuroscience research began while at the University of Barcelona where he learned of Camillo Golgi's (1843–1926) silver nitrate histological technique. Here he used his natural artistic skills with Golgi's stain and began his neuroanatomy research. Specifically, Ramón y Cajal studied and drew the central nervous systems of many animal species. During this time he identified dendritic spines as well as the axonal growth cone, which is the terminal end of an axon that seeks its synaptic target. Additionally, Ramón y Cajal was the pioneer in showing evidence for the neuron doctrine, which is the foundation of today's neuroscience. One fundamental concept of the neuron doctrine states that the central nervous system is made up of individual cells and is not a continuous mass. Ramón y Cajal was able to draw these distinct cells and show how they connect to each other, meaning that the central nervous system is a contiguous system. For his findings and contribution to neuroscience, Ramón y Cajal received the Nobel Prize in Physiology or Medicine in 1906.

Jennifer L. Hellier

See also: Brain Anatomy; Neuropil; Olfactory Sensory Neurons

Further Reading

Ramón y Cajal, Santiago. (1999) [1897]. *Advice for a young investigator* (Neely Swanson and Larry W. Swanson, Trans.). Cambridge, MA: MIT Press.

REFLEX

From a surface level, reflexes do not appear very complicated. Most people have been to a doctor's office and had their knee hit with a rubber tool in hopes that the leg will slightly kick. This action is called a reflex. Yet how does that slight force applied to the knee cause a kick without a conscious command from the brain? The topic of reflexes becomes even more complicated when examining cranial nerve, human infant, and post–spinal cord injury reflexes.

Simply defined, a reflex movement is an involuntary, rapid response to a given stimulus. The purpose of these quick, automatic movements is to avoid pain or injury. In the example of the knee-jerk reflex, a sensory nerve quickly transmits information about the force on the patellar ligament to the spinal cord. Nerves within the spinal cord relay a "contract now" motor signal to the quadriceps. The resulting "kick" is a way to relieve tension on the patellar tendon and prevent injury of the connected muscles or knee structure.

Anatomy and Physiology

It is useful to separate reflexes into monosynaptic and polysynaptic categories. The monosynaptic category is most commonly discussed through the lens of the knee-jerk reflex. Others in this category include the biceps, triceps, brachioradialis, and Achilles reflexes. To recap, a stretch sensation is detected by a sensory neuron in the muscle body. This signal is relayed to the spinal cord and a single synapse exists between the sensory fibers and the motor unit neurons. From this point, a signal to contract is relayed to a muscle in the hopes of reducing the stretch.

Several important concepts exist in this monosynaptic model. First, how does the sensory neuron "detect" stretch? The answer can be found by examining the neuronal plasma membrane. Once there is an actual physical stretch, special chemical channels are opened in the neuronal cell membrane and the action

Reflex Test

The neurological examination is a systematic method used by health care providers and particularly by neurologists to look for abnormalities or lesions in the nervous system. The neurological examination contains several broad rubrics: (1) the mental status examination, (2) the cranial nerve examination, (3) the reflex and motor examination, (4) the coordination and gait examination, and (5) the sensory examination. This examination provides a robust method to test for nervous system function. This sidebar focuses on why a health care provider tests a patient's reflexes.

Simply defined, a reflex movement is an involuntary, rapid response to a given stimulus. The purpose of these quick, automatic movements is to avoid pain or injury. In the example of the knee-jerk reflex, a sensory nerve quickly transmits information about the force on the patellar ligament (a ligament attached to the kneecap) to the spinal cord. Nerves within the spinal cord relay a "contract now" motor signal to the quadriceps. The resulting "kick" is a way to relieve tension on the patellar tendon and prevent injury to the connected muscles or knee structure.

Materials:

Reflex hammer (can be purchased at Amazon.com) to test all four extremities
Volunteer
Something to sit on that will allow the person's legs to dangle

Directions:

Patellar reflex (knee-jerk reflex): Have the person sit on the edge of a table or desk so that their legs are dangling. Using the rubber end of the reflex hammer, gently tap the right quadriceps tendon that is located just below the right kneecap. The person's right leg should automatically jerk and then swing back and forth one or two times. If there is no reaction, tap just to the left or right of the first tap. If no reflex response is observed, the person might be focused on the knee so that no reflex takes place. Ask the person to interlock their hands and focus on pulling them apart while the rubber hammer lightly hits the knee. Repeat this test with the left leg and compare the responses.

Babinski reflex (plantar reflex): Have the person remove their shoes and socks, and then sit on the edge of a table or desk so that their legs are dangling. Using the rubber end of the reflex hammer, drag the hammer from the person's heel to the toes. The normal response is for the toes to move down in contraction. The great toe moving up is an abnormal response called the Babinski sign.

Biceps-jerk reflex: Ask the person to relax their arm and hold their elbow at a 90-degree angle. Gently tap the biceps tendon (front of the upper arm). Repeat this test with the other arm and compare the responses.

Nicholas Breitnauer and Audrey S. Yee

potential signal of "stretch" is relayed to the spinal cord by traveling the length of the neuron's axon. Second, how does this reflex occur so quickly? This is because sensory and motor neurons are not all created equally. The fastest conducting neurons (Ia sensory and α-motor neurons) are utilized in these circuits in order to reduce the chance of injury from excessive muscle stretch. Lastly, how does the reflex reduce the muscle tone of opposing muscle groups, like the hamstrings in the leg? Each monosynaptic sensory signal not only activates specific motor neurons, but also simultaneously antagonizes/relaxes other motor neurons. This allows for a specific action based on a single sensory input.

With an understanding of the monosynaptic reflex concept, polysynaptic reflexes accomplish an end result, such as movement, just with more intermediate neuronal synapses. The central pattern generator (CPG) is one example. A conscious decision is made to walk, at which point the CPG is initiated. Parts of the complex reflex exist in the various areas of the brain that are involved in motion as well as in the spinal cord. All work in symphony in order to coordinate the various movements involved in walking so a person can resume thinking of other matters.

Another example of a polysynaptic reflex is called the "flexor withdrawal." Imagine touching a hot stove or stepping on a sharp tack. Almost without thinking, the hand is quickly withdrawn and the foot is lifted up. Pain fibers (Ic) sense these types of noxious stimuli—though not as fast as stretch receptors—and synapse with interneurons in the spinal cord. These neurons amplify or mute pain before they synapse onto a motor fiber. Interestingly, the story gets a little more complicated than simply flexing to withdraw a hand or foot. The other limb simultaneously receives a signal from the contralateral spinal cord neurons to extend certain muscle groups. This is important, for example, to maintain balance if one foot is lifted up into the air.

Any discussion of reflexes would be incomplete without mentioning those unique to human infants. Babies need certain "preprogrammed" responses to ensure survival early in life. Examples include those useful in eating such as the "suck" and "rooting" reflexes: an object placed in a baby's mouth immediately initiates sucking, an object lightly touching an infant's cheek causes the baby to turn toward that side. Interestingly, these reflexes and many more begin to fade before the baby's first birthday. An important explanation arises from the changes that occur in the central nervous system during this time period. A baby continues to myelinate neurons—speeding conduction—and making more mature neuronal connections as learning takes place. These two factors lead to a slow dampening and eventual cessation of these reflexes.

Ultimately, the example of human infant reflexes drives home a final point: the conscious human brain is able to regulate reflexes. The antagonizing neurochemical from the cortex can, for example, minimize or eliminate a knee-jerk reflex. Occasionally, patients will be so focused on the knee that no reflex takes place. They might then be asked to interlock their hands and focus on pulling them apart while the rubber hammer lightly hits their knee. The shift in focus from the knee to the hands will allow the spinal cord reflex to occur in the absence of the cortex's inhibition.

A change in the corneal blink reflex with prolonged contact usage is another example of the cortex's effect on reflexes. The corneal reflex can be experienced when a hand or object comes close to or actually touches the eye. Almost without control, both eyelids blink forcefully and rapidly (approximately within 10 milliseconds). This reflex involves the sensory trigeminal nerve with a quick relay to both facial nerve nuclei in the brainstem. Interestingly, the reflex slowly diminishes with the constant touching of an eye during contact usage. A person will eventually be able to place and remove contacts without a blink. It is thought the conscious attention on this process reduces the reflex.

Reflexes in Disease and Injury

Knowledge of normal reflex patterns helps enlighten understanding of reflex patterns in disease/injury states. Spinal cord injuries are extraordinarily unfortunate, but teach a great deal about reflex concepts. Once a spinal cord is injured, any function governed below that site is affected. The vertebrae overlying the region divide the spinal cord's anatomy into four general segments: cervical, thoracic, lumbar, and sacral. Imagine a spinal cord injury around the 12th thoracic to the first lumbar section or T12–L1. At this level, the area around the waist and below would be impaired from both a sensation and motor standpoint.

Spinal shock—a term used to describe loss of motor function and sensation with eventual return of reflexes—begins instantly. The first 24 hours of injury would leave the lower limbs hyporeflexive and hypotonic. Reflexes such as the knee-jerk would return during days one to three, but then become hyperreflexive over the next few weeks. Finally, the muscles would become tighter during the weeks to years after the injury leading to a "hypertonic" state. This hypertonicity can be explained by unregulated neuron regeneration at and below the injury.

The return and progressive increase of the reflexes below the spinal cord injury reinforce concepts from normal reflexes. Polysynaptic reflexes return first due to the simple reason that more neurons contribute to these complex actions. The hyperreflexive state exists in the absence of central nervous system regulation in a manner analogous to human infant reflexes. Additionally, the attempt of spinal cord neurons to reestablish a connection leads to more connections below the injury, leading to a stronger, more powerful circuit for the mono- and polysynaptic reflexes.

Injuries within the central nervous system (CNS) are identified and localized with an understanding of cranial nerve reflexes. Cranial nerve reflexes fall into the polysynaptic category due to interneurons that take sensory signals and transmit motor signals to bilateral sides. For instance, a bright penlight in one eye causes both pupils to constrict. If the light causes only the eye with the light to constrict, there is a problem with the motor neuron on the contralateral side. If there is no pupilary constriction when a penlight is shone, the problem likely exists with that ipsilateral optic nerve. This understanding can help identify problems with the nerves or with the brain itself.

In addition to injuries to the CNS, back injuries can be localized with an understanding of reflexes. Consider a person with significant lower back pain after lifting a heavy object. Is this a medical emergency? Upon close examination, it appears there is no Achilles reflex on the right side compared to the left. This subtle finding, taken with other evidence, might compel the doctor to order a magnetic resonance imaging (MRI) of the patient's lower back. It would be feared that the heavy lifting caused an intervertebral disk to bulge outward into the spinal canal and push against the right-sided S1 nerve root. Surgery to repair the herniated disk is often warranted in these situations.

Reflexes and Prosthetics

Limb prosthetics is a field currently encountering rapid growth and improvement. The demand continues to grow for more responsive, advanced devices. Integrating reflex response into these devices is currently in the early stages of position adjustment. For example, consider picking up a can of soup. If the person's grip is not strong enough, the can will begin to slip. A typical response would be to tighten the grip or potentially rapidly lower the arm in hopes of not letting the soup can completely slip away. Current prosthetic devices are designed to give rapid muscular feedback in order to replicate the subconscious reaction to maintain the grip.

Future applications of reflex understanding to artificial devices are myriad. Could a device eventually be able to sense temperature and lead to a "flexor-extensor" reflex? Or might that same device be able to respond to signals arising from the contralateral side, leading to a completion of the polysynaptic reflex?

Nicholas Breitnauer

See also: Blink Reflex; Neurological Examination

Further Reading

Alberstone, C. D., E. C. Benzel, I. M. Najm, & M. P. Steinmetz. (2009). *Anatomic diagnosis of neurologic diagnosis.* New York, NY: Thieme.

Costanzo, Linda S. (2011). *Board review series: Physiology* (5th ed.). Philadelphia, PA: Lippincott Williams & Wilkins.

RESTLESS LEGS SYNDROME

Restless legs syndrome (RLS), also called Willis-Ekbom disease, is an increasingly common condition characterized by unpleasant sensations and an intense urge to move the legs. The symptoms associated with RLS range from mildly bothersome to unbearably painful and can change in severity from one day to another. Recognition of the disorder has become more frequent in recent years, with a current prevalence of 7–10 percent in the United States. RLS affects people of all ages, but has a higher incidence in the elderly. Additionally, the condition presents in women two times more than in men.

Etiology

RLS is categorized into two different subtypes based on how it originates. Primary RLS is idiopathic, meaning there is no identifiable cause for the disorder. However, clinical observation suggests that primary RLS may have a strong genetic component. More than 40 percent of patients with RLS report a personal family history of the condition, and twin studies have even demonstrated a high likelihood of hereditary contribution. Also, genetic research has found that a significant percentage of people with RLS possess the same defects on certain chromosomes, which appear to be passed down in an autosomal dominant pattern. Primary RLS presents more commonly in the young and slowly develops over time. The other subtype is classified as secondary RLS, which occurs when there is a known non-genetic factor contributing to the disease. Contrastingly, this form presents with a faster onset and more often in older patients.

Several different medical conditions have been implicated in the etiology of secondary RLS. One of the more common causes of worsening symptoms is iron deficiency. Pregnancy is also frequently associated with the disease, possibly due to hormonal changes. Other examples of medical conditions that may contribute to RLS are chronic kidney dysfunction, type 2 diabetes, or neurological issues. Studies have shown that people who have attention deficit disorder, Parkinson's disease, anxiety, or depression are all at a higher risk of developing symptoms. Deficiencies in many different vitamins, electrolytes, and hormones have also been linked to RLS.

Symptoms

The symptoms of RLS primarily reflect a dysfunction in both the sensory and motor regions of the brain. RLS presents with a spontaneous, uncontrollable urge to move the legs accompanied by uncomfortable sensations. Although occurring most often bilaterally between the ankles and knees, it can present in the arms, trunk, or face. The sensory component of RLS can be difficult to describe but has been expressed by many patients as tingling, itching, creeping, crawling, and burning. Some patients even compare the condition to feeling as though there is an electric current, flowing water, or moving insects under their skin. In severe cases, RLS can manifest as very painful aches and throbs.

The motor component of the disorder involves involuntary movements, described as feeling as if there is trapped energy in the legs. Patients can experience anything from subtle twitching and frequent pacing to full-extension muscle jerks. RLS is a prominent cause of insomnia, making it difficult to both initiate and maintain sleep.

Diagnosis and Management

Diagnosis is based predominantly on clinical symptoms and elimination of other causes, as there are no laboratory markers to determine if a patient has RLS. There are four cardinal criteria that must be met in order to truly diagnose a patient as having RLS: (1) a strong urge for leg movement accompanied by uncomfortable sensations; (2) symptoms that get worse with a lack of activity or while resting; (3) symptoms that get better, at least partially, with physical activity such as walking; and (4) symptoms present more often in the evening or nighttime.

While there is no definite cure for RLS, many therapies have been tried in practice and demonstrate some success with relieving symptoms. As with most medical conditions, the safest option is to begin with a nonpharmaceutical remedy. All patients with RLS report that physical movement can help reduce symptoms. Therefore, it is important to encourage patients to engage in moderate physical exercise, such as walking, for at least a few days per week. Some patients report feeling relief from leg spasms after warm showers or baths. This may be due to the influence of increased temperature, which helps in relaxing the muscles. Likewise, massage therapy and muscle-stretching exercises have been shown to help with pain. Finally, implementing lifestyle changes may help RLS patients alleviate chronic sleep disruption. Performing appropriate sleeping habits, such as going to bed at a reasonable time and avoiding caffeine in the evening, can help improve nighttime symptoms.

The next step in treating patients with RLS is to consider whether there are secondary causes that need to be addressed. Oral iron supplements should be given to people who are deficient, with close monitoring until levels are back to normal range. Other deficient substances that can be effectively normalized through oral supplementation are folate, vitamin B_{12}, and magnesium.

Vidya Pugazhenthi

See also: Attention Deficit Hyperactivity Disorder; Central Nervous System; Thermal Sense; Vibration Sensation

Further Reading

Leschziner, Guy, & Paul Gringras. (2012). Restless legs syndrome. *British Medical Journal, 344,* e3056.

Medline Plus. (2013). *Restless legs.* Retrieved from http://www.nlm.nih.gov/medlineplus /restlesslegs.html

Willis-Ekbom Disease Foundation. (2013). *About WED/RLS.* Retrieved from http://www .rls.org

RETINA

The retina is a light-sensitive tissue that is found in the inside surface of the back of the eye. The eye captures light and creates an image of the visual world on the retina. The retina's function can be compared to film in a camera. As the light hits the retina, it starts a chain reaction of chemical and electrical signals that trigger nerve impulses to be sent to various visual centers of the brain. These brain centers then interpret the signals as visual images.

Anatomy

The cells that make up the retina consist of three basic types: photoreceptor cells, neuronal cells, and glial cells. Photoreceptor cells are known as cones and rods. Cones work best in bright conditions and provide color vision. Rods function in dim light and provide black-and-white vision. There are three types of cones; each one perceives different wavelengths or colors of light and each one contains a different colored visual pigment. These pigments are called the red, blue, or green visual pigments. The center of the retina contains mostly cones while rods dominate the outer portions of the retina. The highest density of cones is at the center of the fovea—the center of the retina is the macula and the center of the macula is the fovea. There are no rods at the center of the fovea.

Neural cells include bipolar cells, ganglion cells, horizontal cells, and amacrine cells. Bipolar cells connect the photoreceptors to the ganglion cells. Ganglion cells have dendrites that connect with bipolar cells. Horizontal cells connect bipolar cells with each other. And finally, amacrine cells connect bipolar and ganglion cells with each other. Glial cells are scattered between and within the axons of the ganglion cells in the retina and optic nerve. These supporting cells of the retina include Müller cells, astrocytes, and microglial cells.

The retina comprises 10 different cell layers. The inner surface of the retina is next to the vitreous of the eye, which is the glass-like portion of the eye. The outermost layer of the retina, the retinal pigment epithelium, is attached to the choroid. Starting from the inner surface, the first layer is the inner limiting membrane. This basement membrane consists of Müller cells, which serve as support cells for the neurons of the retina. The second layer is the nerve fiber layer, which contain axons of the ganglion cell nuclei. The third layer is the ganglion cell layer. It comprises the nuclei of retina ganglion cells and axons of the optic nerve. The fourth layer is the inner plexiform layer and contains the synapse between the dendrites of the retinal ganglion cells and cells of the inner nuclear layer. The fifth layer is the inner nuclear layer. This layer is made up of three types of cells: bipolar cells, horizontal cells, and amacrine cells. The sixth layer is the outer plexiform layer that consists of the synapses between the dendrites of horizontal cells from the inner nuclear layer and the rods and cones of the outer nuclear layer. In the macular region, this is known as the fiber layer of Henle. The seventh layer is the outer nuclear layer and contains the cell bodies of rods and cones. The eighth layer is the external limiting membrane. This layer separates the inner segment of the rods and cones from their nucleus. The ninth layer is the photoreceptor layer, also known as the layer of rods and cones or Jacob's membrane. As its name implies, it comprises both rods and cones. Lastly, the tenth and outermost layer is the pigmented layer or retinal pigment epithelium. This layer is filled with densely packed pigmented hexagonal cells.

Physiology

The main function of the retina is to convert light into neural signals. This involves four basic processes: photoreception, transmission to bipolar cells, transmission to ganglion cells, and transmission along the optic nerve. Damage to any of these cells or processes can cause different visual problems including blindness.

In photoreception, light passes through the inner layers of the retina to reach the rods and cones. The photoreceptors contain a photopigment, which captures individual photons of light and turns them into neural signals. The rods and cones transfer the light and relay the signal to their cell bodies and out to their axons. These axons then contact the dendrites of both bipolar cells and horizontal cells. Horizontal cells are parallel interneurons that help with signal processing. The bipolar cells then pass the signal from photoreceptors to their axons. In the inner plexiform layer, bipolar axons contact ganglion cell dendrites and amacrine cells. The final step involves transmission along the optic nerve. The ganglion cells send their axons through the nerve fiber layer and meet at the center of the retina. This forms the optic nerve. The ganglion cell axons leave the eye, making up the optic nerve. These axons then travel along with the signal all the way to the lateral geniculate nucleus in the brainstem.

Disease

Macular degeneration is a major disorder of the retina and describes a group of diseases characterized by the loss of vision in the center of the visual field caused by macula cell death. It is mainly age related and usually comes in two forms: wet and dry. In the dry form, cellular debris builds up between the retina and the choroid, which may cause the retina to become detached. Retinal detachment involves the retina peeling away from the choroid. In the more severe wet form, blood vessels form behind the retina, which may also cause the retina to become detached. Retinal detachment may also be caused by trauma, such as a blow to the eye or head. When a retina begins to detach, the patient's visual field may have one or more signs such as "floaters," bright flashes of light, or a black curtain over a portion of the field of vision. Retinal detachment can be repaired if it is done quickly before the retina is devoid of oxygen. If the retina does lose too much oxygen, its cells will die, causing blindness. An ophthalmologist can repair retinal detachments or tears with a laser.

Retinopathy is a disorder caused by damage to the blood vessels that supply the retina. High blood pressure or hypertension can cause damage, which leads to hypertensive retinopathy. Diabetes mellitus can also cause damage that leads to diabetic retinopathy. Retinoblastoma is a cancer of the retina. It most commonly affects young children, but can occur rarely in adults.

Mario J. Perez

See also: Optic Nerve; Retinopathy; Visual Perception; Visual System

Further Reading

Kolb, Helga, Ralph Nelson, Eduardo Fernandez, & Bryan Jones (Eds.). (2011). *Webvision: The organization of the retina and visual system.* Retrieved from http://webvision.med.utah.edu/book/

Machemer, Robert, & Georg Michelson. (2012). *The atlas of ophthalmology: Online multimedia database.* Retrieved from http://www.atlasophthalmology.com/atlas/frontpage.jsf

RETINOPATHY

Retinopathy or diabetic retinopathy is an eye condition that develops in individuals that have either Type 1 or Type 2 diabetes. This condition occurs when the blood vessels from the light-sensitive tissue at the retina are damaged. The blood vessels in the eye provide the necessary nutrients to the retina so that when light hits the eye, the retina processes the light rays into electrical impulses to travel to the visual cortex. The brain then converts these impulses into images with depth and distance. Diabetes is normally associated with complications of the body's ability to properly store and utilize sugar. Increased levels of sugar affect the circulatory system of the retina or glucose that eventually causes damage to the blood vessels. According to the Centers for Disease Control and Prevention, millions of Americans ages 40 years and older have retinopathy due to either Type 1 or Type 2 diabetes. Americans who are 20 years and older are also at high risk, especially due to the correlation of increasing obesity rates in this age group within the United States. Women who have diabetes and are also pregnant have a greater rate of developing retinopathy.

Symptoms

With prolonged diabetes, retinal blood vessels start to leak fluid that distorts the curve of the lens in the eyes. This leads to blurry vision, spots, or floaters in the center or field of vision, and difficulty with night vision. Sudden loss of vision in one eye and seeing rings or flashing lights are also attributed to diabetic retinopathy. Risk factors for developing these symptoms include poorly controlled diabetes, poorly controlled blood pressure, high cholesterol levels, and sleep apnea. Macular edema is one prominent change to the eye in which there is swelling or thickening of the macula due to leaking fluid. Macular ischemia can also occur and is due to capillaries collapsing, causing blurry vision. There are several stages to diabetic retinopathy, including mild nonproliferative, moderate nonproliferative, severe nonproliferative, and proliferative retinopathy.

Stages

There are two main stages of diabetic retinopathy: nonproliferative retinopathy, in which the blood vessels start to leak fluid; and proliferative retinopathy, a later stage of the condition in which new blood vessels grow around the retina and the vitreous humor. Without treatment, the blood vessels might burst, resulting in cloudy sight or scars on the retina. In the beginning stages of this condition, swelling in blood vessels (microaneurysms) can occur. In moderate nonproliferative retinopathy, some of the blood vessels are blocked, causing the progression to severe nonproliferative retinopathy as more blood vessels are blocked. During proliferative retinopathy, new but fragile blood vessels are stimulated to grow in order to provide nourishment to the retina. When these new blood vessels pop due to their fragility, the released blood can lead to vision loss and blindness. In the later stages of the condition, leaks in the blood vessels can alter the eye's jelly-like vitreous humor (located in the vitreous body between the lens and retina) and cause blindness.

Diagnosis and Treatment

Doctors can examine the state of the condition using a test called fluorescein angiography. A dye is injected through the veins and as the blood flows, the dye appears in the retina. Photographs of the retina are then evaluated to detect the progression of the disease. Individuals with diabetes can monitor the rate at which this condition progresses by adjusting their blood glucose intake and lowering their risk by controlling levels of blood sugar, blood pressure, and blood cholesterol to decrease the progression. If untreated, the scars on the back of the retina can pull the retina away from the back of the eye, leading to retinal detachment and resulting in permanent blindness. There are several options to treat the condition as shown in the accompanying table.

Type	Treatment	Results
Anti-VEGF (vascular endothelial growth factor) therapy	An injection to the back of the eye that contains an antibody to remove the VEGF.	Prevents the growth of new vessels.
Intraocular steroid injection	Treats diabetic macular edema.	Reduces the amount of leaking fluid.

| Laser surgery | Treats the retina through a laser procedure. | Removes scar tissue or repairs tears in the retina once the vitreous gel is removed (see Vitrectomy). |
| Vitrectomy | Vitreous gel is surgically removed from the eye. Usually performed in cases of advanced proliferative diabetic retinopathy. | May be needed to repair retinal detachment or to remove blood from a vitreous hemorrhage. |

Simi Abraham

See also: Blindness; Retina; Visual System

Further Reading

Chee Wai Wong, Tien Yin Wong, Ching-Yu Cheng, & Charumathi Sabanayagam. (2014). Kidney and eye diseases: Common risk factors, etiological mechanisms, and pathways. *Kidney International, 85,* 1290–1302.

National Eye Institute. (2015). *Facts about diabetic eye disease.* Retrieved from https://nei .nih.gov/health/diabetic/retinopathy

RILEY-DAY SYNDROME: *See* Familial Dysautonomia

RODS

The human eye senses light via specialized nerve cells called photoreceptor cells. There are two types of photoreceptor cells: rods and cones. Together these photoreceptor cells have the ability to sense light, color, movement, and other visual stimuli. Rods function best at low levels of light and are responsible for night (scotopic) vision. These cells are incredibly sensitive and under optimal conditions a single unit of light, or photon, may activate rod photoreceptors. This property of having high sensitivity allows rods to have fine light and motion detection. Rods are far more numerous than cones and account for 95 percent of the photoreceptors in the retina (Lamb, 2015). Rods are located at the edge of the retina (inner surface of the eye), which allows for peripheral vision but does not allow for the ability to focus on fine details.

An important functional component of rods is the protein rhodopsin. Rhodopsin is densely packed inside of rod cells; it is estimated that a single rod cell contains 10^8, or 100 million, rhodopsin molecules (Milo & Philips, 2015). Rhodopsin is extremely photosensitive (sensitive to light), and its high concentration means that a single photon of light can hit a single rhodopsin molecule in one of the millions of rod cells in an eye to elicit a cellular response.

Rods have different reactions to different levels of light. When a small amount of light hits a rod cell, rhodopsin is activated and, through a series of events known as phototransduction, the signal is transmitted via neurons to the primary visual cortex (the area responsible for processing visual information) located in the occipital lobe of the brain. Once the cell response ends, rods enter a deactivated stage that can last several minutes. There are balanced amounts of activated and deactivated cells in standard lighting conditions, which allows visual perception to proceed normally. An extreme amount of light in the environment can lead to overactivation of rhodopsin, and it can take several minutes for enough cells to "reset" themselves to resume normal visual function. An example of this is walking into a dim room after being in bright sunlight: the strong light deactivates a majority of rod cells, and the room may appear darker than it really is because there are not enough rods available to immediately respond to the dim surroundings.

The high sensitivity of rod cells can also be illustrated in nonhumans. Nocturnal animals rely on rod photoreceptors to hunt prey or spot predators at night. Rod function is preserved across species, meaning humans and animals have similarly functioning rods. The main difference is the presence of the tapetum lucidum under the retina, which "bounces" unabsorbed photons around until they hit a rod rather than leave the eye as in humans (Milo & Philips, 2015). This small anatomical difference allows nocturnal animals to use rods more efficiently.

Disease

Rod photoreceptor function can be impaired by a class of genetic diseases called rod-cone dystrophies. Rod-cone dystrophies are usually inherited from a child's parents but may also occur randomly. Retinitis pigmentosa and Leber's congenital amaurosis are examples of diseases in which rods and cones either develop abnormally or break down over time. The severity and visual deterioration speed of rod-cone dystrophies can vary greatly between affected individuals. To date, there are no known treatments for such diseases.

Rhodopsin function can be impaired due to vitamin A deficiencies. In the simplest terms, a form of vitamin A functions with rhodopsin for the process of phototransduction. Deficiencies in vitamin A can affect both rods and cones to cause vision problems from night blindness to total vision loss. Many side effects can be reversed with vitamin A supplements as long as permanent damage has not taken place to the photoreceptors or other eye components, such as the epithelial tissue.

Kendra DeHay

See also: Cone Dystrophy; Cones; Visual Fields; Visual Motor System; Visual Perception; Visual System; Visual Threshold

Further Reading

Lamb, T. D. (2015). Why rods and cones? *Eye*, 1–7. http://dx.doi.org/10.1038/eye.2015.236

Milo, Ron, & Rob Phillips. (2015). *Cell biology by the numbers*, pp. 47–50, 183–187. New York, NY: Garland Science, Taylor & Francis Group.

S

SACCADES

A saccade is a small, rapid adjustment of the eye in order to bring an object into better focus. These movements are so rapid and small that they are hardly ever noticed. Typically, another person needs to watch in order to observe saccades.

Generally, these movements are necessary due to the small area of detailed vision in the eye named the fovea. This area contains the largest concentration of high-resolution retinal cells and allows for detailed vision. A saccade relies on complicated neurological connections between the frontal cortex, superior colliculus, and three pairs of ocular muscles. Ultimately, this quick motion helps build a rich, dynamic interpretation of the visual world.

Anatomy and Physiology

A typical scenario of saccade initiation would be a new stimulus in the visual field. Imagine a balloon became loosened on a windy day. This mobile, bright object would enter the visual field and information from the retina would be transmitted to different parts of the brain. Once this new piece of information was recognized, both the frontal eye field and superior colliculus would coordinate eye movement toward the object.

Prior to the fovea centering on an object, peripheral retinal cells become activated. These neurons are especially sensitive to movement and make up peripheral vision. In this part of the retina, a higher concentration of rod cells exists. Interestingly, the information gathered from these cells is only black and white. New information (such as the balloon) in the visual field is then sent to the frontal eye field.

It is believed that in this region of the cortex, attention is given to new information. This information—requiring further processing—is relayed to other portions of the visual pathways. One important connection from the frontal eye field is the superior colliculus, a region in the midbrain responsible for initiating saccades.

A detailed map of the visual world exists in this part of the brain. Information from the retina is linked to specific portions of the superior colliculus, with the front portion dedicated to the fovea. This part of the brain exists in the rostral and posterior parts of the midbrain. Neuron bodies in this region directly control the muscles that move the eye.

Within the detailed visual map of the superior colliculus, the direction and speed of a saccade are dictated. In the case of the balloon, imagine this image is toward the left side of the visual field. The superior colliculus neurons are able to discern where the fovea is currently pointed and where the new stimulus exists. Based on the distance, a saccade is initiated at speeds usually around 400 degrees/second, but can go as fast as 700 degrees/second. The total right-to-left visual field, for reference, is typically 160 degrees.

The signal to initiate a saccade is a highly coordinated movement of ocular muscles. A leftward saccade is managed by the paramedian pontine reticular formation (PPRF). Here, the signal to activate leftward movement of the left eye is controlled by the abducens nerve and lateral rectus muscle. Simultaneously, the right eye is moved left through the median longitudinal fasciculus. Both the oculomotor nerve and the medial rectus muscle facilitate this movement.

Once the saccade has completed, the image should now be directly placed on the fovea. This portion of the retina contains a higher proportion of cone cells than rod cells. This information is transmitted to the occipital cortex in the back part of the brain and the image is interpreted.

Interestingly, saccades also occur in the dark. This unique feature highlights the various functions of the superior colliculus. Not only does this part of the brain respond to signals from the frontal eye field, but it also receives somatic (peripheral sensory) stimulation. Touching an arm could also be enough to trigger a saccade toward the stimulus.

Diseases and Drugs

An exaggerated, biphasic (fast and slow) saccade is known as nystagmus. There are instances where this type of movement is normal, such as with the rotation of the head, following a repetitively moving object with your eyes, and so forth. Brain lesions or the presence of drugs and/or alcohol can bring on this type of saccade.

Active substance usage or abuse can be detected with the aid of observing for nystagmus. Alcohol, for instance, specifically contributes to horizontal or lateral gaze nystagmus. An intoxicated person following a finger or pen light from left to right will reveal quick lateral saccades with a slow correction opposite of the fast movement. Phencyclidine (PCP) is an illegal drug known to induce vertical nystagmus.

Lesion or tumors within the brain, brainstem, or cerebellum can also be associated with nystagmus. Downbeat nystagmus is associated with lesions of the brainstem at the level of the foramen magnum. A person afflicted with this malady will experience a fast downbeat with a slow upbeat saccade when focusing on an object in the center of the visual field.

Nicholas Breitnauer

See also: Nystagmus; Superior Colliculus; Visual Motor System; Visual System

Further Reading

American Optometric Association. (2014). *Nystagmus.* Retrieved from http://www.aoa.org/patients-and-public/eye-and-vision-problems/glossary-of-eye-and-vision-conditions/nystagmus

Purves, Dale, George J. Augustine, David Fitzpatrick, William C. Hall, Anthony-Samuel LaMantia, James O. McNamara, & S. Mark Williams (Eds.). (2001). Neural control and saccadic eye movements. In *Neuroscience* (2nd ed.). Sunderland, MA: Sinauer Associates. Retrieved from http://www.ncbi.nlm.nih.gov/books/NBK10992/

Wisconsin University. (2006). *Unit No. 2, brain stem: Superior colliculus.* Retrieved from http://www.neuroanatomy.wisc.edu/virtualbrain/BrainStem/23Colliculus.html

SACCULE

The vestibular system is found bilaterally within the inner ears and performs tasks to help maintain the orientation of the body with respect to gravity and forces exerted from the outside world. It provides the leading contribution about the sense of balance and spatial orientation to help with the coordination of movement with balance. The vestibular system consists of the semicircular canal system (to detect rotational movements of the head) and the otolithic organs (to detect linear movement and acceleration of the head).

The word "otolith" means "ear stone," and the saccule is one of the two otolithic organs within the inner ear. The other otolithic organ is the utricle. Both otolithic organs are part of the balancing apparatus located in the vestibule of the bony labyrinth, which is a small oval chamber that consists of the vestibule (a swelling next to the semicircular canals), three separate semicircular canals, and the cochlea (necessary for the sense of hearing). Within the vestibule is the utricle, which is located between the semicircular canals and the cochlea. The saccule is closer to the cochlea compared to the utricle.

Within the saccule are small stones (called otoconia that consist of calcium carbonate and a matrix protein) and a viscous fluid that are used to stimulate the sensory hair cells that line the saccule's epithelial layer. It is the bending of the stereocilia on the sensory hair cells that detect motion and orientation of the head. The saccule specifically detects linear movement in the vertical direction. It also detects the effect of gravity on the head and body.

Anatomical Structure

Comparatively, the saccule is the smaller of the two otolithic organs and is globular in shape. The saccule lies in the recessus sphaericus (the spherical recess) of the bony labyrinth, near the opening of the scala vestibule of the cochlea. Within the anterior portion of the saccule is a thickening called the macula acustica sacculi, which contains filaments of the vestibular portion of the vestibulocochlear nerve (cranial nerve VIII) and the sensory hair cells that detect changes in acceleration and gravitational force. Superior to the macula acustica sacculi is the otolithic membrane, which contains a gelatinous layer, and superior to that the statoconia layer. The statoconia layer is a bed of otoconia. Each sensory hair cell has stereocilia (mechanoreceptors that respond to changes in pressure) and a true kinocilium (the only sensory cilium that can depolarize and produce an action potential) at its apical end. The tips of the stereocilia and kinocilium are embedded within the otolithic membrane.

Function

The saccule has mechanoreceptors that can distinguish between the different degrees that the head tilts, particularly in the vertical direction. Because of gravity, the otolithic organ pulls on the embedded stereocilia and causes them to tilt. This shift in the direction of the stereocilia stimulates the kinocilium and induces an action potential that is sent to cranial nerve VIII, to the brainstem, and then to the brain. The brain interprets all head movements by comparing inputs from the direction of the tilt, detected by the kinocilium, to inputs from the eyes and stretch receptors in the neck. By doing so, the brain can determine if just the head is tilted or if the entire body is tilted.

Disorders of the Otolithic Organs

Damage to the otolithic organs can have an impact on the ocular (vision) function and body stabilization. Until recently, there has not been a way to measure how severely these organs could be damaged. Recent studies have developed the Vestibular Evoked Myogenic Potential (VEMP) test, which can determine the health of the saccule as it is inferior to the utricle and more proximal to the cochlea. To date, VEMP tests are employed to quantify otolithic organ input to the right and left vestibular systems. The purpose of VEMP is to determine if the saccule and the inferior vestibular nerve are functioning properly and are intact. The output of the saccule can be recorded using a sound generator. In addition, surface electrodes can be used to detect neck muscle activation or other muscles of interest.

Renee Johnson

See also: Otoliths; Semicircular Canals; Stereocilia; Utricle; Vestibular System; Vestibulocochlear Nerve

Further Reading

Drummond, Meghan C., et al. (2015). Live-cell imaging of actin dynamics reveals mechanisms of stereocilia length regulation in the inner ear. *Nature Communications, 6*, 6873. Retrieved from http://www.ncbi.nlm.nih.gov/pmc/articles/PMC4411292/

Hain, Timothy C. (2014). Otoliths. *Dizziness-and-balance.com*. Retrieved from http://www.dizziness-and-balance.com/anatomy/ear/otoliths.html

Purves, Dale, George J. Augustine, David Fitzpatrick, William C. Hall, Anthony-Samuel LaMantia, James O. McNamara, & Leonard E. White. (2008). *Neuroscience* (4th ed.). Sunderland, MA: Sinauer Associates.

SACKS, OLIVER WOLF

Oliver Wolf Sacks, MD, was a British American neurologist and best-selling author. He was a professor of neurology at New York University (NYU) School of Medicine, and his 12 books explored various neuroscience subjects, including *The Man Who Mistook His Wife for a Hat* (1985), about various neurological disorders; *Musicophilia: Tales of Music and the Brain* (2007), which was made into a PBS Nova series called *Musical Minds*; *The Mind's Eye* (2010), about vision; and *Hallucinations* (2012). Many of his books are largely collections of his patients' neurological case histories and are known for being accessible and interesting to the lay public and neuroscientists alike. Sacks won many awards for his books including the Lewis Thomas Prize by Rockefeller University, which recognizes the scientist as a poet.

Oliver Sacks was born in London, England, on July 9, 1933, to physician parents. He received his medical degree at Oxford University in 1958 and completed his residencies and fellowship at Mt. Zion Hospital in San Francisco and at the University of California–Los Angeles. He moved to New York City in 1965 pursuing a career in research. After a year, Sacks realized that he did not like lab work and accepted a position at Beth Abraham Hospital in 1966 as a consulting neurologist until 2007. Sacks worked as a consulting neurologist at several hospitals during this period and began teaching neurology in 1975 at Albert Einstein College of Medicine. He was a professor of neurology at NYU from 1992 to 2007, Columbia University from 2007 to 2012, and then returned to NYU. Sacks died in 2015.

Sacks is known for his groundbreaking work in 1966 at Beth Abraham Hospital in the Bronx where he "awakened" a group of patients who had not moved or talked in decades. He discovered that these frozen patients had all survived encephalitis lethargica and their frozen state was due to the resulting brain damage. He experimentally treated them with L-dopa, a drug that had recently been discovered as a treatment for Parkinson's disease. Sacks recounted this experience in his book *Awakenings* (1973), which was made into the 1990 movie *Awakenings* starring Robin Williams and Robert DeNiro.

Sacks appeared frequently on several news programs, and his essays and articles have been published in magazines, newspapers, medical journals, and in several "Best of" anthologies. He had many hobbies and interests including chemistry and the periodic table of elements, botany, stereoscopic vision, and swimming. Sacks had a visual disorder called prosopagnosia, which impaired him from recognizing people by their faces. He discussed this disorder and his experience of recently losing vision in one of his eyes in his book *The Mind's Eye*. Sacks's work was supported by the Guggenheim Foundation and the Alfred P. Sloan Foundation. He was an honorary fellow of the American Academy of Arts and Letters and the

American Academy of Arts and Sciences, and held honorary degrees from many universities, including Oxford, Georgetown, Bard, Gallaudet, Tufts, and the Catholic University of Peru.

Emma Boxer

See also: Heightened Senses; Neurologist; Visual System

Further Reading

Sacks, Oliver. (2010). *The mind's eye.* New York, NY: Alfred A. Knopf.
Sacks, Oliver. (2014). *Oliver Sacks, M.D.* Retrieved from http://www.oliversacks.com

SALTY SENSATION

Salty sensation, the detection of sodium ions (Na^+), is one of the five basic tastes. It is unique among the five basic tastes in that it can be both appetitive and aversive depending on the concentration of Na^+. At low salt concentrations (10–100 millimolar, mM) it is generally considered pleasant, but higher concentrations (100–500 mM) are unpleasant. Detection of Na^+ has likely been advantageous through human evolution by identifying dietary sources of Na^+ while simultaneously avoiding excessive intake to maintain body salt levels within a limited physiologic window. Proper Na^+ levels in the body are critical for homeostasis, as neurologic function, cardiac and skeletal muscle contraction, fluid balance, and just about every physiologic process is dependent on proper Na^+ concentrations. While salty sensation is primarily elicited by Na^+ ions, other monovalent cations, such as potassium (K^+) and lithium (Li^+) ions, can also be perceived as salty, especially at higher concentrations.

The receptor for saltiness in humans has proven to be elusive, in part because the primary ligand, Na^+, is both simple and ubiquitous. Though a definitive receptor has yet to be identified, it has long been known that the appetitive salty taste can be inhibited by amiloride (an organic compound with a guanidinium group containing pyrazine derivative), which has no effect on the aversive taste of high salt concentrations. This suggests that there are two distinct pathways for detecting Na^+, and that amiloride inhibits the receptor for the low concentration pathway. Based on the effect of amiloride, the best candidate for the Na^+ taste receptor is the epithelial sodium channel (ENaC), as it is a Na^+ channel expressed in taste receptor cells (TRCs) and is inhibited by amiloride.

The differential responses to high and low salt concentrations were an interesting paradox, though a mechanism of the switch from appetitive to aversive salt sensation has recently been identified in mouse models. While amiloride inhibits appetitive salt sensing by ENaC-expressing TRCs, high concentrations of Na^+, as well as K^+ and Li^+, cross-activate the bitter and sour receptors on their respective TRCs. Bitter and sour are both aversive, and their receptors are not inhibited by amiloride, so this mechanism explains both the change in the perception and the inability of amiloride to affect aversive salt sensation.

Though the exact identity of the receptors for the TRCs have not been identified, the salty TRCs are thought to signal through the same pathways as the TRCs corresponding to the other basic tastes.

Depolarization of the salty TRCs following a signaling cascade triggered by the taste receptor transmits a signal to afferent neurons. The signal is relayed by the facial nerve (cranial nerve VII) in the anterior two-thirds of the tongue and glossopharyngeal nerve (cranial nerve IX) in the posterior one-third of the tongue. Sensory afferents synapse in the rostral portion of the nucleus of the solitary tract in the brainstem, and are relayed to the thalamus with projections to the primary gustatory cortex.

Salt sensation, along with the other five tastes, decreases with age, which means that salt is not detected at lower concentrations, which may lead to the ingestion of saltier foods. Higher salt intake could exacerbate hypertension in older individuals.

Michael S. Harper

See also: Facial Nerve; Glossopharyngeal Nerve; Supertaster; Taste Aversion; Taste Bud; Taste System; Type 1 Taste Cells; Type III Taste Cells

Further Reading

McLaughlin, Susan K., & Robert F. Margolskee. (1994). The sense of taste. *American Scientist, 82*(6), 538–545.
Toshi Matsuda & Richard L. Doty. (1995). Age-related taste sensitivity to NaCl: Relationship to tongue locus and stimulation area. *Chemical Senses, 20*, 283–290.

SATIETY

Satiety is the state of satisfaction after consuming food. It is the inhibitory response that stops a person from consuming more food after he or she is full. It is one of the necessary controls for maintaining homeostasis in many organisms. The limbic region and the cerebral cortex are the main structures of the central nervous system responsible for the regulation of satiety (Ahima & Antwi, 2008). As more research emerges in this field, it is becoming apparent that many peripheral organs play an integral role in communicating with the brain regarding a person's satiety.

History and Function

Eating is necessary for survival. It is the most efficient way of providing the body with all the calories and nutrients required for optimal function. Food is broken down into small molecules that drive metabolism. Some food is processed and used immediately, while other food goes into storage as fat. The brain is responsible for monitoring energy expelled by daily activities as well as signaling hunger when supplies of energy are quickly being depleted. Food has rewarding qualities that consequently increase appetite beyond metabolic needs (Ahima & Antwi, 2008). Hypotheses on peripheral satiety signals have been proposed since the 1960s (Sharkey, 2009). It was thought that biomolecules such as glucose and fat could trigger a signal that would alert the brain whenever enough food had been consumed to meet metabolic needs. Since then, the discoveries of leptin and leptin receptors have been key in studying how satiety is regulated.

Anatomy and Physiology

Currently, neuronal and hormonal signals from the gastrointestinal tract are thought to control satiety (Ahima & Antwi, 2008). As food is consumed, the gastrointestinal tract will send signals to the central nervous system. The nucleus tractus solitarii (NTS) is a cluster of nerves that run through the medulla oblongata. These nerves will project these signals to the visceral sensory thalamus (part of the limbic system), which will then relay the information to the visceral sensory cortex (Ahima & Antwi, 2008). The visceral sensory cortex is part of the cerebral cortex. It is the structure that facilitates the perception of gastrointestinal satiety.

Leptin is a primary hormonal signal that controls satiety. It is a hormone secreted by adipocytes in the adipose tissue, also known as fat. Leptin levels directly correlate to fat levels in the body. This hormone is thought to be the long-term control of energy homeostasis whereas insulin has been shown to only have a short-term effect on satiety and energy homeostasis. Higher leptin levels mean that a lot of adipose tissue is present. There are two types of leptin receptors: short leptin receptors and long leptin receptors. Short leptin receptors are not extensively studied, but are thought to help the hormone cross the brain capillaries (Ahima & Antwi, 2008). Long leptin receptors are located in several regions of the brain, including the hypothalamus, the brainstem, and the regions of the brain that control feeding and energy outflow (Ahima & Antwi, 2008). High leptin levels will decrease appetite and increase energy expenditure whereas low leptin levels will decrease energy expenditure and increase appetite. In other words, high leptin levels will increase satiety.

Disease and Disorder

Lack of satiety results in many health problems including obesity, diabetes, and depression. Current studies in obesity indicate findings relating overeating with possible leptin resistance. Resistance to leptin will cause leptin levels to be high without the body realizing it. Satiety is not achieved in this case, which will keep appetite from decreasing. Leptin levels will undergo a net increase in these individuals if voluntary controls are not used to stop eating.

Overabundance of satiety can also result in health problems. Individuals with congenital leptin deficiency have low appetite due to the overactivity of brain regions associated with satiety (Ahima & Antwi, 2008).

Melissa Tjandra

See also: Ageusia; Dysgeusia; Hunger; Supertaster; Thirst

Further Reading

Ahima, Rexford S., & Daniel A. Antwi. (2008). Brain regulation of appetite and satiety. *Endocrinology and Metabolism Clinics of North America, 37*(4), 811–823. Retrieved from http://www.ncbi.nlm.nih.gov/pmc/articles/PMC2710609/

Murphy, Kevin G., & Stephen R. Bloom. (2006). Gut hormones and the regulation of energy homeostasis. *Nature, 444*, 854–859.

Sharkey, K. A. (2009). Peripheral satiety signals: View from the chair. *International Journal of Obesity, 33*, S3–S6. Retrieved from http://www.nature.com/ijo/journal/v33/n1s/full/ijo20098a.html

SCOTOMA: *See* Blind Spot

SEIZURES

A seizure is a sudden, erratic increase of abnormal electrical activity in the brain that temporarily affects actions and/or cognition and perception. Seizures can last for a few seconds as in absence seizures (formerly called "petit mal" seizures) or up to a few minutes as seen in complex-partial seizures. Symptoms can be as mild as a momentary blank facial expression caused by impaired consciousness in absence seizures, or as severe as the violent convulsions of tonic-clonic seizures (formerly called "grand mal" seizures). In some cases, seizures can be life threatening. A condition in which seizures last longer than five minutes or when one seizure immediately follows another is called status epilepticus. This can cause significant brain damage and death if not promptly treated. A seizure is not a disorder itself, but rather a symptom indicating an underlying central nervous system (CNS) disturbance. Individual symptoms and prognosis vary depending on the type of seizure and causative agent.

While most seizures occur as part of an epileptic disorder, sometimes they can be isolated events. Seemingly unrelated conditions like a high fever (febrile seizures) can lead to seizures, particularly in young children. A stroke can cause single-incident seizures in adults as well. Approximately 5 percent of the population has experienced a single-incident seizure, whereas only 1–2 percent of the population has epileptic seizures. The risk of developing recurrent epileptic seizures can increase after an individual has a single-incident seizure. There are many different types of epilepsy, and they can come from genetic, structural-metabolic, or unknown sources.

Subtypes and Symptoms

The wide variation not only in seizures, but also in etiology has led to the opinion that "epilepsy" is more accurately termed "the epilepsies." The International League against Epilepsy (ILAE) is currently responsible for the governing of terminology and classification relating to the different types of seizures and epilepsies.

Depending on the subtype of epilepsy, seizure symptoms can vary from visible muscle contractions to sensory and psychic symptoms only perceived by the person experiencing the seizure. Focal seizures were formerly called partial seizures, and though this terminology is now outdated it is useful in describing the symptoms. Motor symptoms in simple partial seizures cause visible muscle twitches. Sequential involvement of muscle groups is called a "march" and is identified as Jackson Ian seizures. Sensory symptoms are usually not noticeable to a bystander, but can cause considerable distress to the patient. These include both somatosensory and special sensory disturbances. Tingling, visual, auditory, olfactory, and gustatory hallucinations may ensue. The sensory aspect of the partial seizures preceding the generalized tonic-clonic seizure is called an "aura." People with this type of epilepsy often come to recognize an aura as an indicator before the start of a seizure. Psychic symptoms include senses of déjà vu and jamais vu (failure to recognize familiar scenes, people, or words). When the autonomic nervous system is involved, changes in blood pressure and heart rate have been observed along with diaphoresis and pupil dilation.

Absence seizures are a subtype of epilepsy and are typically only seen in children. Victims of this type of epilepsy will either outgrow the seizures or the seizures will progressively worsen. Symptoms present as almost unnoticeable blank stares or unresponsiveness, but can also include some autonomic and mild clonic symptoms. Increased disturbances in muscle tone and more gradual onset are atypical traits of this type of seizure.

Atonic seizures are characterized by momentary loss of muscle tone, whereas myoclonic seizures are brief involuntary muscle contractions. Tonic seizures are rigid contraction of muscles, particularly those of the limbs. Major muscle groups repeatedly contract and relax during clonic seizures. The notorious tonic-clonic seizures involve nearly immediate loss of consciousness followed by both tonic and clonic symptoms.

Complex-partial seizures originating in or involving the mesial temporal limbic structures are the most common type of seizures, and the most common cause is temporal lobe epilepsy (TLE). These seizures will frequently evolve into secondarily generalized seizures. Most patients with TLE have had some prior brain injury such as trauma to the head from riding a bicycle or a car accident, febrile convulsions, or status epilepticus. TLE is usually a permanent condition with variable seizure frequencies within a population of afflicted individuals.

Erin Slocum and Jennifer L. Hellier

See also: Limbic System; Somatosensory Cortex; Somatosensory System

Further Reading

Eadie, M. J. (1994). The understanding of epilepsy across three millennia. *Clinical & Experimental Neurology, 31,* 1–12.

Fisher, Robert S., & Maslah Saul. (2012). *Genetic causes of epilepsy.* Stanford School of Medicine. Retrieved from http://neurology.stanford.edu/epilepsy/patientcare/videos/e_09.html

International League against Epilepsy. (2012). Resource Center. Retrieved from http://www.ilae.org/Visitors/Centre/ctf/documents/ILAEHandoutV10_000.pdf

SELECTIVE SOUND SENSITIVITY SYNDROME: *See*

Misophonia

SEMICIRCULAR CANALS

The semicircular canals are found within the vestibular apparatus in the inner ear and are at right angles to each other. There are two sets of semicircular canals, one in the left inner ear and one in the right. The function of the semicircular canals is to sense head rotations in the X-, Y-, and Z-axes. These directions are called the yaw, pitch, and roll axes in flight. There are three semicircular canals, one for each axis, and each is a tiny fluid-filled tube attached to a larger, bony region containing the utricle and saccule. The canals are named for their orientation within the vestibular apparatus: horizontal, superior, and posterior semicircular canals. Together, these canals help animals maintain their balance by detecting acceleration in three perpendicular planes. The hair cells in the semicircular canals are similar to those in the organ of Corti (used for hearing); however, they detect movements of the fluid in the canals due to angular acceleration. The semicircular canals are connected to the vestibulocochlear nerve (the eighth of 12 paired cranial nerves) in the inner ear.

Anatomy and Physiology

The semicircular canals are part of the bony labyrinth in the skull and are different sizes. The horizontal semicircular canal (also known as the lateral or external semicircular canal) is the shortest canal (about 12 to 15 millimeters in length) and senses movement and rotation on a transverse plane or around a vertical basis—rotating the head to the left and then to the right, as if shaking your head "no." The superior semicircular canal (also known as the anterior semicircular canal) is usually 15 to 20 millimeters in length and detects rotations on a sagittal plane—as if nodding your head up and down to answer "yes." The posterior semicircular canal is the longest of the three canals (about 18 to 22 millimeters in length) and detects head rotations on the rostral-caudal (anterior-posterior) axis—bending your head to touch your ear to your shoulder.

Filled with endolymph fluid, each semicircular canal contains motion senses within the fluid. The utricle is an opening at the end of the canal that contains a dilated sac (osseous ampullae). In the sac, there are hair cells that contain many cytoplasmic projections called stereocilia, which are embedded within the cupula (a gelatinous structure). When rotating or moving your head, the duct moves; however, the endolymph lags behind, which in turn causes the stereocilia to bend. This mechanical movement of the stereocilia causes a change in their activation, resulting in a signal to the central nervous system about the new position of the head. After about 10 seconds of moving at a constant motion, the endolymph catches up and the sense of acceleration is diminished. This adjustment period is known as "the leans" and is often experienced by pilots as they enter a turn, causing the hair cells to be stimulated and alerting the brain that the aircraft and the pilot are no longer moving in a straight line.

Injury to the Semicircular Canals

Damage to the semicircular canals could be twofold. If any part of the canal does not work, then a person may seem to have lost his or her sense of balance or may feel dizzy. Damage to the vestibulocochlear nerve could also make a person lose the sense of balance and/or diminish the ability to hear. Injuries related to damage of the semicircular canals include, but are not limited to the sensation of spinning or the feeling that the room is spinning around (vertigo), the sensation of being off balance (disequilibrium), or the feeling of lightheadedness or feeling faint (presyncope).

Research

A study published by Fitzpatrick and colleagues (2006) showed that upon applying electrical currents across the heads of people while they walked, the researchers were able to better understand how the vestibular system helps maintain upright posture in bipedal animals including humans.

Renee Johnson

See also: Balance; Dizziness; Otoliths; Saccule; Utricle; Vestibular System; Vestibulocochlear Nerve

Further Reading

Fitzpatrick Richard C., Jane E. Butler, & Brian L. Day. (2006). Resolving head rotation for human bipedalism. *Current Biology, 16*(15), 1509–1514.

Kandel, Eric R., et al. (Eds.). (2012). *Principles of neural science* (5th ed.). New York, NY: McGraw-Hill.

Purves, Dale, et al. (2008). *Neuroscience* (4th ed.). Sunderland, MA: Sinauer Associates.

SENSES OF ANIMALS

Humans and animals have the same sensory systems including auditory (hearing), gustatory (taste), kinesthesia/proprioception (touch), olfactory (smell), and vision (sight). However, the acuity of these senses for animals may be increased or decreased compared to humans' senses. For example, rats and mice have a limited visual ability but their sense of smell is increased when the ability is compared to humans'. Additionally, some animal species have other sensory abilities that humans do not have such as echolocation, electroreception, infrared detection, ultraviolet detection, and whisking.

Echolocation

One of the most notable animal senses is echolocation, which is used by microchiropteran bats, dolphins, toothed whales, shrews, and a few cave-dwelling birds. These animals use echolocation for navigation purposes and communication as well as for hunting or foraging for food. Echolocation is a type of bio sonar. The animal will make its own high-pitched sound—above the hearing range for humans—and wait for the echo to return to its ears. In animals that use echolocation, their ears are slightly apart so that when the echo from the environment returns, the sounds are received at different time points for each ear. The auditory cortex uses this time difference to determine the distance of the object. Some blind humans have learned to use echolocation to navigate their movements by either using a clicking device or making sounds by mouth.

Electroreception

Electroreception is the ability to sense electrical fields in the environment. It is mostly used by aquatic or amphibious animals who live in the ocean, as saltwater is a good conductor of electricity. Recent studies, however, have shown that bees, cockroaches, and land monotremes (echidnas) have the ability to use electroreception as well. Lampreys, sharks and other cartilaginous fish, catfish, platypus (aquatic monotremes), and others use electroreception to detect their location, the location of their prey, and to communicate. In active electrolocation, some aquatic animals have a specialized organ that consists of modified muscles or nerves. This electric organ produces an electric field around the animal's body. The animal also has sensors to detect if an object distorts the electric field. The electric field in most cases is very weak, less than one volt. Other animals use a passive form of electrolocation. They are able to detect a nearby animal's bioelectric field in the environment by the changes of ion flow through the gills.

Infrared and Ultraviolet Detection

Some animals and insects use wavelengths that are outside of visual light, either infrared (very long wavelengths) or ultraviolet (very short wavelengths), to locate prey or food. In the cases of infrared, snakes have air-pocket pits that are covered with a membrane containing heat-sensing receptors or a pit organ. These structures are located within the head and are able to detect infrared heat to help in locating prey and to regulate the snake's body temperature. Bees have compound eyes that can use ultraviolet wavelengths to help find flowers. Scientists have shown that when flowers are viewed under ultraviolet light, the flowers reveal a pattern we humans do not see. This helps bees to identify flowers with different types of pollen.

Whisking

Many land mammals—mice, rats, cats, dogs, and others—have specialized whiskers that are necessary to detect spatial sensing such as the width of an opening or for object identification. These are called vibrissae, a Latin word meaning to vibrate. Mammals will move their facial whiskers (vibrissae), sweeping them back and forth quickly and repetitively to explore their external environment. Vibrissae are grown in groups and are located in different parts of the head or body, which may lead to different specialized tasks. Vibrissae on the head are found above the eyes (supraorbital), on the cheeks (genal), around the mouth (mystacial), and on the jaw (mandibular). Vibrissae are also found on the wrist (carpal) on the underside of the leg just above the paw. The mystacial vibrissae are divided into groups based on their size: macrovibrissae and microvibrissae. The macrovibrissae are stiff and protrude to the side of the face. These are used to detect spatial openings. For instance, if the macrovibrissae are stimulated when a cat puts its head into a small opening, the cat will know that the rest of its body would not be able to fit. In rodents, these whiskers are generally the same size as the width of the animal's body. The microvibrissae are below the nostrils and are used to identify objects.

Patricia A. Bloomquist and Jennifer L. Hellier

See also: Pheromones; Vibration Sensation; Vomeronasal Organ

Further Reading

Bedore, Christine N., Stephen M. Kajiura, & Sonke Johnsen. (2015). Freezing behaviour facilitates bioelectric crypsis in cuttlefish faced with predation risk. *Proceedings. Biological Sciences/The Royal Society*, 282(1820), pii: 20151886. http://dx.doi.org/10.1098/rspb.2015.1886

Thé, Lydia, Michael L. Wallace, Christopher H. Chen, Edith Chorev, & Michael Brecht. (2013). Structure, function, and cortical representation of the rat submandibular whisker trident. *Journal of Neuroscience, 33*(11), 4815–4824.

Xiong Guo, Bo Luo, Ying Liu, Ting-Lei Jiang, & Jiang Feng. (2015). Cannot see you but can hear you: Vocal identity recognition in microbats. *Dong wu xue yan jiu (Zoological Research), 36*(5), 257–262.

SENSORY DEPRIVATION

Sensory deprivation is the purposeful removal of one or more sensory stimuli. Alternative forms of medicine may prescribe sensory deprivation for decompressing from our society's need to be digitally connected, which can result in overstimulation of several senses. Sensory overload is the opposite of sensory deprivation and is associated with urbanization, crowding, mass media, technology, and noise.

Sensory deprivation has also been used in experimental psychology to study stress in humans. Examples of sensory deprivation include chamber restricted environmental stimulation therapy, an isolation pool, or a sensory deprivation tank. Less inclusive tools have been developed to isolate only one sensory stimulus at a time. For instance, to remove visual stimuli, a blindfold or hood will be placed over the eyes and/or head of an animal or person. Hooding raptors and birds of prey allows their handler to have better control of the bird, as the bird relaxes. Blindfolding a person can help improve his or her sleep. Similarly, headphones, earplugs, or earmuffs can be placed over or in a person's ears to remove external sound stimuli.

Short-term sensory deprivation (about 30 minutes up to 24 hours) has shown to be successful in producing rest in people and is often used in meditation. Furthermore, it has been reported to produce a sense of relaxation. However, if sensory deprivation is extended or forced upon an individual, it generally results in increased anxiety, hallucinations, depression, stress, and abnormal thoughts. Thus, sensory deprivation can have both positive and negative effects, depending on how it is being used, either as a way to help calm animals or humans, or as a practice of inhumane treatment.

Restricted Environmental Stimulation Therapy

The two most common forms of sensory deprivation are (1) chamber restricted environmental stimulation therapy—where a person lies on a bed in a completely dark and soundproof room for 24 hours, and (2) flotation restricted environmental stimulation therapy—where a person lies in an enclosed, water-filled tub with the water at skin temperature for 60 minutes. Both of these therapies remove light and sound stimuli as well as reduce touch sensations. In chamber restricted environmental stimulation therapy the person is allowed to use the bathroom, eat, and drink but goes back to lie on the bed. The individual is not encouraged to sleep, as this therapy is to help the person to focus on the lack of stimuli in the surroundings. For the flotation restricted environmental stimulation therapy, the tank is filled with water and enough Epsom salts to allow the person to float easily. The size of the tank is small so that it is restrictive and difficult for the floating person to turn over. This extended weightlessness in a dark, enclosed tank often results in changes of brainwave activity as well as relaxation for the person. Thus, some people use this therapy to help them with solving a problem in their work or life or to increase their mental creativity.

Sensory Deprivation and Experimental Psychology

Prior to formal studies of experimental isolation, only anecdotal observations were reported on solitary sailors, polar inhabitants, prisoners, and hermits. These reports show that isolation induces similar symptoms of mental illness, such as experiencing hallucinations or depression. However, wide variations were observed between people. Some were able to handle the isolation whereas others had extreme reactions.

In the early 1950s, experimental psychology researchers began sensory deprivation or perceptual isolation studies. Over the next few decades, Zuckerman and colleagues (1964) studied the different aspects of sensory deprivation, including sensory restriction, social isolation, and confinement. Additionally, they looked at sex differences between men and women. They found that women generally showed more effects than men, particularly in increases in anxiety and feelings of surrealism.

Jennifer L. Hellier

See also: Auditory System; Discriminative Touch; Olfactory System; Taste System; Touch; Vibration Sensation; Visual System

Further Reading

Goldberger, Leo. (1966). Experimental isolation: An overview. *American Journal of Psychiatry, 122*(7), 774–782.

Stronks, H. Christiaan, Amy C. Nau, Michael R. Ibbotson, & Nick Barnes. (2015). The role of visual deprivation and experience on the performance of sensory substitution devices. *Brain Research, 1624,* 140–152.

Zuckerman, Marvin. (1964). Perceptual isolation as a stress situation: A review. *Archives of General Psychiatry, 11,* 255–276.

SENSORY RECEPTORS

Living organisms have the ability to sense stimuli from the environment around them and respond in an appropriate manner. The sensory system deals with information being delivered to the nervous system by neurons that have receptors for various stimuli. A receptor is defined as either a specialized protein that detects chemical signals or as a specialized cell that detects environmental stimuli and generates a response. A stimulus is defined as a change in one or more conditions in the environment, both internal as well as external. A stimulus can be one of a variety of changes in the environment such as temperature, pressure, pain, or visible light, to name a few.

Sensory receptors are important because they provide the necessary information about the environment and allow the appropriate response to follow. They are

Neuron-Building with Clay

There are several different types of neurons such as unipolar (sensory neurons), bipolar (interneurons), multipolar (e.g., motor neurons, inhibitory neurons, etc.), and pyramidal cells (primary neurons of a specific brain circuit). You can make any of these types of neurons with clay; however, this sidebar focuses on the unipolar neurons that are the most common form of sensory neurons. Unipolar neurons, named for their appearance, are specialized neurons that act to bring sensory neural signals from the body to the central nervous system. The most common unipolar cells are found in the dorsal root ganglion, just outside of the dorsal spinal cord. Unipolar cells have a single input/output that come together at the soma. The dendrites (input) are branched at that location where it picks up the signal, and its axon may branch where it terminates in the spinal cord. This allows it to act on many neurons. Like most biological cells, unipolar neurons contain but are not limited to cell membrane, cytoplasm, nucleus, ribosomes, endoplasmic reticulum (ER), and mitochondria.

Materials:

Four colors of clay (red, green, yellow, and blue), waxed paper, tabletop, paper towels, and toothpick

Directions:

Roll a walnut-sized ball of red clay; this represents the cell membrane and cytoplasm together forming the cell body (soma). Flatten this into a quarter-inch-thick, two-inch-diameter pancake. Roll a pecan-sized ball into a long worm and a very short worm. Attach the middle of the long worm with the very short worm to one edge of the soma (making a T-shape). The long worm on one side represents the dendrites and the other side represents the axon. Create a few branches off both ends of the worm. Clean your hands each time you switch colors.

Flatten a pecan-sized ball of green clay to one inch in diameter and an eighth of an inch thick. This represents the ER. Place the clay on top of the soma, relatively in the center. With a toothpick, poke several small holes into the central section of the ER. These holes represent ribosomes, used to make proteins.

Slightly flatten one side of a peanut-sized ball of yellow clay. This represents the nucleus of the neuron. Nuclei house the genetic material. Place on top of the ER; the nucleus is not always in the center of the cell.

Finally, make four to five Tic-Tac-sized ovals. These are mitochondria, which generate energy for the cell. Place throughout the cytoplasm.

Jennifer L. Hellier

involved in an animal's, and particularly a human's, sense of taste, smell, sight, touch, and hearing. Sensory receptors are also involved with an animal's ability to breathe and move. Sensory receptors have different-sized receptive fields—the area or region where an external or internal stimulus will activate the neuron. In general, large receptive fields cover a large area but tend to have less perception while small receptive fields cover a small area and have strong perception. For example, in touch sensation, small receptor fields in the fingers allow for discriminative touch, giving the ability to sense detailed structures.

Types of Sensory Receptors

To date, sensory receptors have been categorized into five groups: mechanoreceptors, chemoreceptors, thermoreceptors, photoreceptors, and nociceptors. Some of these different receptor types are found throughout the body or in almost every sensory system.

Mechanoreceptors

Mechanoreceptors respond to a physical stimulus such as mechanical pressure or distortion. This mechanical change in position produces an electrical signal that is transmitted to the central nervous system. Mechanoreceptors are important for discerning between different sensations such as light touch, touch, positional change (balance), and pressure. Perhaps the most notable stimuli that mechanoreceptors respond to are sound waves (used for hearing) and proprioception.

Chemoreceptors

Chemoreceptors are receptors that respond to chemical stimuli in the environment. The two prominent classes of chemoreceptors are those involved in olfactory and gustatory systems. Olfactory receptors are found in the membranes of olfactory sensory neurons located in the olfactory epithelium, which lines the insides of the nose. Volatile odor molecules in the environment enter the nose when breathed in and bind to receptors specific for that odor molecule. In the gustatory system, taste cells located in taste buds of the tongue operate in the same way as olfactory sensory neurons, except these respond to aqueous chemical stimuli.

Thermoreceptors

Thermoreceptors are specialized sensory receptors that determine temperatures that are generally not painful (not too hot and not too cold). Thermoreceptors are considered to be free nerve endings or free nonspecialized endings. These receptors are found throughout the skin, cornea (the covering of the eye), and the bladder.

Photoreceptors

Photoreceptors are specialized sensory receptors that convert visible white light into the sense of vision. Specifically, these receptors absorb photons of light and transduce that absorption into a membrane potential, which activates the neuron. Photoreceptors are found in neurons located in the retina, which is the photosensitive lining of the back of the eye. There are two main types of photoreceptors: cones and rods.

Cone cells are short, wide, and have a tapering end. Cone cells need bright light to be activated and can absorb all short, medium, and long wavelengths of visible light, which represent different colors within the visible light spectrum. Rod cells are long and thin. Rod cells are activated with dim lighting, meaning they can absorb a single photon of light to be activated. This makes rod cells more sensitive to light compared to cone cells. Thus, rod cells are the main photoreceptor neurons used for night vision.

Nociceptors

Pain receptors or nociceptors are specialized sensory receptors that determine when a stimulus is painful. These receptor types are free nerve endings or free nonspecialized endings. Nociceptors send their signal to the brain and spinal cord so that the body can respond appropriately, such as letting go of a hot handle. Nociceptors are found in all locations of the body, both internally (such as the gut, heart, joints, and muscles) and externally (like the cornea, mucosa, and skin—also known as cutaneous nociceptors). This is because pain is an important signal that should not be ignored.

Jennifer L. Hellier and Roberto Lopez

See also: Cones; Mechanoreceptors; Nociceptors; Rods; Taste Bud; Thermoreceptors

Further Reading

Abraira, Victoria E., & David D. Ginty. (2013). The sensory neurons of touch. *Neuron, 79*(4), 618–639.

Fetsch, Christopher R., Gregory C. DeAngelis, & Dora E. Angelaki. (2013). Bridging the gap between theories of sensory cue integration and the physiology of multisensory neurons. *Nature Reviews: Neuroscience, 14*(6), 429–442.

Kinnamon, Sue. (2013). Neurosensory transmission without a synapse: New perspectives on taste signaling. *BMC Biology, 11*, 42.

SMELL: *See* Olfactory System

SOCIETY FOR NEUROSCIENCE

Neuroscience is the study of the structure and function of the brain. Thus, the Society for Neuroscience (www.sfn.org) is a professional group that supports scientists who are interested in furthering scientific research of the brain, nervous systems, and diseases of the nervous systems. Ralph W. Gerard created the Society for Neuroscience in 1969 so that neuroscientists and physicians throughout the world could share their scientific findings with one another. By integrating basic scientists and physicians from diverse cultures, members of the group are able to improve their knowledge as well as develop professional collaborations that might not have occurred otherwise. Members of the Society for Neuroscience range from undergraduate and graduate students to postdoctoral fellows and faculty from all stages of their career (such as middle school teachers to professors in college).

The Society for Neuroscience holds an annual meeting that occurs generally in the fall of each year in North America. During the annual meeting, members present their data during poster sessions, platform presentations, symposia, and special lectures. The Society for Neuroscience also reaches out to thousands of communities in more than 80 countries through their annual Brain Awareness Week. This week is typically held in the spring of every year; however, members present neuroscience education and outreach to their communities year round.

The Society for Neuroscience publishes the peer-reviewed *Journal of Neuroscience*. The goal of this journal is to include the most up-to-date and scientifically sound research in several neuroscience areas such as behavioral, systems (e.g., limbic, sensory, motor), cognitive (thinking), cellular, molecular, developmental, plasticity (changes induced by activity), and repair neuroscience as well as the neurobiology (the mechanisms) of neurological diseases. Another authoritative source, BrainFacts.org, is offered by the Society for Neuroscience in conjunction with the Kavli Foundation and the Gatsby Charitable Foundation. These three nonprofit organizations are leading the way to advance brain research globally. The BrainFacts.org publication and website is for students of all ages and for the layperson who is interested in learning more about the central nervous system. Furthermore, BrainFacts.org is the primary source used during Brain Awareness Week. Its scientifically correct information dispels several myths about the brain and nervous system, such as "you only use 10 percent of your brain." BrainFacts .org informs, provides, explores, and sparks ideas and understanding of the nervous system and its intricate structure and function. Specifically, it contains topics about (1) neuroscience—discusses new sophisticated tools and techniques for research; (2) brain basics—to learn how the 100 billion nerve cells connect and function together; (3) sensing, thinking, and behaving—to answer questions such as "How do brain connections allow a person to read and speak?"; (4) diseases and disorders—to discover the causes of disorders and new treatments; (5) changes across the lifespan—to learn how our brain changes from birth to old age and in response to the environment; and (6) neuroscience in society—considers how neuroscience applies to making decisions in our world. Although the website provides updated information about evidence-based research on the symptoms, causes, and prognoses of many brain diseases and disorders, it is not intended as specific medical advice. Readers needing medical advice should see their health care provider.

The Society for Neuroscience is continually working with educators to make learning about the brain and nervous system fun for everyone. Thus, through the BrainFacts.org website they host an annual educational video contest for Brain Awareness. In 2014, the top winners included videos titled *Vision and Illusion*—first place, by Leigha Phillips, affiliated with Rhode Island School of Design and Brown University, with Helen Tang and Lily Benedict; *Three Lesions, Three Lives*—second place, by Alison Caldwell, graduate student at University of California, San Diego, and Micah Caldwell; *Brainbows—Mixing Colors to Map the Brain*—third place, by Vania Cao, application scientist; and *Neuroscience Minds*—Best Song, by Michael Stendardi, student at the City University of New York.

Jennifer L. Hellier

See also: Axel, Richard; Bartoshuk, Linda; Buck, Linda; Hubel, David H.; Neurologist; Wiesel, Torsten N.

Further Reading

Society for Neuroscience. (2013). *Mission and strategic plan.* Retrieved from http://www.sfn .org/about/mission-and-strategic-plan

SOMATOSENSORY CORTEX

In the mammalian central nervous system, the somatosensory cortex is crucial to senses such as pain, touch, temperature, and spatial orientation—a sensation termed *proprioception*. The somatosensory cortex consists of a network of neurons that work together to sense and then to process this information.

Anatomy

The somatosensory cortex is the most anterior portion of the parietal lobe and is demarked as the gyrus that is just posterior to the central sulcus, which separates the parietal lobe from the frontal lobe. The central sulcus is a prominent landmark in the mammalian brain as it is the longest, uninterrupted, "straight" groove on the lateral aspect of the cerebral hemisphere. The postcentral gyrus is the somatosensory cortex with the function of integrating and processing all sensory information from the body's surface and the underlying viscera. This is where the neuronal cell bodies are found, making the cortex look gray, and why the cerebral cortex is also called "gray matter." It is also important for the perception of the senses, particularly of touch, pain, and temperature. The somatosensory cortex is often referred to as Brodmann areas 3, 1, and 2. The number order for the somatosensory cortex may seem strange to the reader. This is because when German anatomist Korbinian Brodmann (1868–1918) first sectioned the brain, he did so at an oblique angle. The first area he studied was named Brodmann area 1. As he continued his research, he continued to number the regions based on the order he studied them. Today, when looking at the somatosensory cortex from the midline to lateral direction, the somatosensory cortex is numbered 3, 1, and 2.

Along the surface of the postcentral gyrus, the body is mapped from the midline to the temporal lobe. This means that a specific body region is located in a specific region of the postcentral gyrus. This map is called a homunculus, meaning "little man." The purpose of the thalamus is to act as the relay center from the spinal cord or brainstem to the homunculus. This is the same as the reticular formation, but the reticular formation acts as a relay for the spinal cord or brainstem to the thalamus. The homunculus is the main processing center of the somatosensory system. It processes the sensory impulses from the body that were sent to the thalamus for modulation, which in turn are sent to the somatosensory cortex. If a reaction is necessary, such as to move away from a heat source, this sensory information in the cerebral cortex will be transferred to the motor cortex to respond.

Sensory Homunculus

For the sensory homunculus, the most medial and deep portion of the postcentral gyrus maps to the genitals. Just superior to that are the toes and foot. At the bend of the gyrus, the leg is represented. From the medial superior surface moving laterally the following are mapped: hip, trunk, neck, head, shoulder, arm, elbow, forearm, and wrist. The hand and fingers come next, but these are connected to a much larger area of the sensory cortex than any other previously described body part. This is because humans have significantly large numbers of sensory receptors in their hands and fingers, which helps produce discriminative touch. The specific mapping continues as: hand, little finger, ring finger, middle finger, index finger, and thumb. Now on the lateral surface superior to the temporal lobe, the next body regions are recorded: eye, nose, and face. As with the hands and fingers having a largely mapped region of the sensory cortex, so do the lips. This is because humans have many sensory receptors around the mouth that are mainly used for sensing taste, temperature, and proprioception. Thus, the following are represented: upper lip, lips, and lower lips. Nearing the final downward mapping are the teeth, gums, tongue, and pharynx. The very last body region that is demarcated, where the postcentral gyrus meets the temporal lobe, is the intra-abdominal. It is important to note that the viscera are not mapped to the postcentral gyrus.

Jennifer L. Hellier

See also: Discriminative Touch; Homunculus; Nociception; Sensory Receptors; Somatosensory System; Thalamus; Thermal Sense; Touch

Further Reading

Kandel, Eric R., James H. Schwartz, Thomas M. Jessell, Steven A. Siegelbaum, & A. J. Hudspeth. (Eds.). (2012). *Principles of neural science* (5th ed.). New York, NY: McGraw-Hill.

Kell, Christian A., Katharina von Kriegstein, Alexander Rösler, Andreas Kleinschmidt, & Helmut Laufs. (2005). The sensory cortical representation of the human penis: Revisiting somatotopy in the male homunculus. *Journal of Neuroscience, 25*(25), 5984–5987.

Purves, Dale, et al. (Eds.). (2004). *Neuroscience* (3rd ed.). Sunderland, MA: Sinauer Associates.

SOMATOSENSORY SYSTEM

In the mammalian central nervous system, the somatosensory system is crucial to senses such as pain, touch, temperature, and spatial orientation (a sensation termed *proprioception*). The system consists of a network of neurons that work together to sense and then to process this information. The network of neurons will be described in three different divisions called first-order neurons, second-order neurons, and third-order neurons.

Location

To begin with the sensing portion of the system, it involves a somatic (body) receptor that is within the skin, bones, muscles, joints, eyes, and ears. These specialized receptors will pick up sensory information and begin a sensory impulse. This sensory receptor is on a neuron that is considered the first-order neuron or primary afferent neuron for sensory information. This neuron comes from the periphery and travels the afferent pathway (toward the central nervous system). For most of the sensory neurons, their cell body is located in the dorsal root ganglion (a group of cell bodies outside the central nervous system) just lateral of the spinal cord. For sensation to the head, neck, and face, these nuclei (a group of cell bodies inside the central nervous system) are found in the brainstem and are named for the cranial nerve that carries the sensory and/or motor information to the central nervous system.

The secondary neuron is an interneuron that receives information from the first-order neuron's synapse, where neuronal information is transferred from one neuron to another. Some of these second-order neurons may send their axons to cross over to the other side of the spinal cord or brainstem before carrying the information to the thalamus, a deep relay structure within the brain. All second-order neurons will synapse in the thalamus, except for the sense of smell.

Lastly, the second-order neuron synapses on the third-order neuron, which is located in the thalamus. Here the sensory information is transferred and then carried to the correct sensory area of the cerebrum, such as the primary visual cortex for vision and the somatosensory cortex for pain, temperature, touch, and proprioception.

In the brain the somatosensory system involves the thalamus, reticular formation, and postcentral gyrus, which is found posterior to the central sulcus in the parietal lobe of the cerebral cortex. Along the surface of the postcentral gyrus, the body is mapped from the midline to the temporal lobe. This means that a specific body region is located in a specific region of the postcentral gyrus. This map is called a homunculus, meaning "little man." The purpose of the thalamus is to act as the relay center from the spinal cord or brainstem to the homunculus. This is the same as the reticular formation, but the reticular formation acts as a relay for the spinal cord or brainstem to the thalamus. The homunculus is the main processing center of the somatosensory system. It processes the sensory impulses received from the thalamus. If a reaction is necessary, such as moving away from a heat source, this sensory information in the cerebral cortex will be transferred to the motor cortex to respond.

Pathways

The somatosensory system has specific ascending pathways that are dependent on the information carried and how they ascend. One of the pathways is the anterolateral tract, which contains the (1) lateral spinothalamic tract, (2) anterior spinothalamic tract, and (3) spinoreticulothalamic tract. The lateral spinothalamic tract carries pain and temperature information while the anterior spinothalamic pathway carries crude touch sensory information. Lastly, the spinoreticulothalamic tract carries persistent aching or dull pain signals. In addition, it differs from all the ascending pathways because it synapses into the reticular formation in the brainstem rather than going straight to the thalamus.

Another ascending pathway is the posterior column or lemniscus pathway, which contains two main tracts in the spinal cord. The fasciculus gracilis tract carries highly localized information that involves fine touch, proprioception, vibration, and pressure from the inferior half of the body (legs and trunk), while the fasciculus cuneatus tract sends those same impulses but from the arms and upper body to the central nervous system.

Since these pathways involve multiple relay stations, they can be vulnerable to injury. If there were damage to an area anywhere along these pathways, it could lead to the loss of sensation. However, these paths act as a type of anastomosis of the nerves and provide backup routes for pain and temperature impulses, as these sensations are important for survival. For example, if the spinal cord is damaged on one side, the person would still be able to feel pain and possibly temperature. However, if the spinal cord is damaged completely through, the person might not be able to sense anything.

Aaron Jones

See also: Afferent Tracts; Discriminative Touch; Homunculus; Nociception; Sensory Receptors; Somatosensory Cortex; Thalamus; Thermal Sense; Touch

Further Reading

Dougherty, Patrick, & Chieyeko Tsuchitani. (1997). Somatosensory systems. In *Neuroscience Online, an electronic textbook for the neurosciences* (Chap. 2). Retrieved from http://neuroscience.uth.tmc.edu/s2/chapter02.html

Kandel, Eric R., James H. Schwartz, Thomas M. Jessell, Steven A. Siegelbaum, & A. J. Hudspeth (Eds.). (2012). *Principles of neural science* (5th ed.). New York, NY: McGraw-Hill.

Purves, Dale, et al. (Eds.). (2004). *Neuroscience* (3rd ed.). Sunderland, MA: Sinauer Associates.

SOUND LOCALIZATION

For animals, it is very important to determine the direction of a sound as it can help with survival. This ability is called sound localization and it is a function of the auditory system. The brain is able to localize sound by using several components of the sound wave, such as interaural intensity (the amount of energy flowing in a sound wave between the ears); spectral information (a continuous series); and time differences in sounds, to name a few. Just like how a GPS (global positioning system) works, sound localization uses three dimensions for best results including horizontal (azimuth), vertical (elevation), and distance positions. If a sound is traveling, then velocity is also used for positioning the sound wave.

Humans are able to hear different sound frequencies (or wavelengths, from peak to peak of the sound) ranging from high to low sounds. However, this is dependent on the individual's hearing ability of each ear and the quality of the sound. Specifically, for high frequencies (shorter wavelengths), the brain can detect the time of arrival by how the sound wave was reflected (or bounced) off the person's torso, shoulders, and outer ears (pinnae). When the wave is reflected, some of the higher frequencies are lost and the brain can detect the minute differences between the original wave and the reflected wave. This information can help position and localize the sound source. For low frequencies (longer wavelengths), the brain uses the change in phase (peak to peak or valley to valley) of a sound to identify its position. This means that the brain determines if one ear received the sound's peak and the other ear received the sound's valley. This difference would be a shift of the phase that is used for localizing the source.

Patricia A. Bloomquist

See also: Auditory System; Cochlea; Cochlear Implants; Deafness; Vestibulocochlear Nerve

Further Reading

Blauert, Jens. (1996). *Spatial hearing: The psychophysics of human sound localization* (2nd ed.). Cambridge, MA: MIT Press.

SOUR SENSATION

Sour sensation, the detection of acidity, is one of the five basic tastes. Sourness is an aversive taste in that it is generally regarded as unpleasant, though there is some evidence that sour is less aversive in children compared to adults. It has likely been advantageous through human evolution by facilitating the detection of spoiled foods, as bacterial growth and fermentation produce acidic compounds. The standard substance used for the definition of sour taste is diluted hydrochloric acid (HCl), which produces hydrogen ions (H^+) in solution. Many foods contain organic compounds that are weak acids, including citric acid in fruits and acetic acid in vinegar. Sour sensation is specifically the detection of H^+, as opposed to the molecules from which the H^+ has dissociated.

The cells responsible for the detection of sour have been identified as taste receptor cells (TRCs) that express the PKD2L1 receptor, which is part of the transient receptor potential (TRP) family. While PKD2L1 is a marker of sour-responsive TRCs, it is not conclusively the sour receptor. The mechanism of sour detection has yet to be fully elucidated, and it is still unclear whether the taste is the sensation of extracellular or intracellular H^+ levels. The ambiguity stems from the fact that HCl and acetic acid sensation are discordant with their acidity. It has been proposed that since acetic acid can diffuse into cells, it is detected more sensitively despite being a weaker acid.

The detection of carbonation is also mediated through sour TRCs, but is dependent on the presence of carbonic anhydrase 4 (Car4), an extracellular carbonic anhydrase that reversibly converts carbon dioxide (CO_2) gas and water (H_2O) into bicarbonate (HCO_3^-) and H^+. This receptor is expressed on sour TRCs, suggesting that its activity and the local production of H^+ allows carbon dioxide and acidic compounds to be sensed as the same taste.

Only TRCs that express the PKD2L1 sense sourness, and TRCs that detect sourness do not detect other tastes. Different TRCs are responsible for all five of the primary tastes. TRCs are organized into taste buds, which contain 50–150 TRCs each. Taste buds throughout the tongue contain TRCs for all five basic tastes; therefore, there is no topographic taste map. The specificity of the TRC to one taste alone is essential for the way that the different taste sensations are encoded.

Depolarization of the sour TRCs following stimulation of the unidentified receptor transmits a signal to afferent neurons. The signal is relayed by the facial nerve (cranial nerve VII) in the anterior two-thirds of the tongue and glossopharyngeal nerve (cranial nerve IX) in the posterior third of the tongue. Sensory afferents synapse in the rostral portion of the nucleus of the solitary tract in the brainstem and are relayed to the thalamus with projections to the primary gustatory cortex.

Despite this delineation of taste reception, sour receptors may mediate the aversive taste of high-salt solutions. At high concentrations, salt switches from appetitive to aversive, and it has been shown that high salt concentrations may stimulate sour receptors as well as bitter receptors.

Michael S. Harper

Lemon Test

Foods and beverages provide calories and nutrients that are essential for humans to survive. Sour foods generally have an aversive taste that is determined by the amount of acidity (pH) they contain. This sidebar focuses on the perception of sour foods and how this perception changes when a natural agonist—miraculin—binds to sweet taste receptors when the pH of the mouth changes.

Miraculin is a glycoprotein dimer that can be isolated from the red berries of the West African plant *Richadella dulcifica*. These berries are often called Miracle Berry or Magic Fruit. Miraculin on its own has no taste at a neutral pH. However, it can elicit an intense and persistent sensation of sweet when the tongue is exposed to an acidic pH, such as that of a lemon. Thus, miraculin converts sour-tasting foods (e.g., lemons, vinegar) to be perceived as sweet.

Materials:

1 Miracle Berry/Magic Fruit tablet (this can be purchased online from Amazon.com)
1 small paper cup
2 to 4 tablespoons of soda (such as a cola type)
2 pieces of lemon (cut the lemon into 6 to 8 wedges)

Directions:

Pour the soda into the paper cup and set it aside. As a control for this experiment, bite into or eat one of the lemon wedges. This should taste sour. Next, drink some of the soda. This should taste sweet. Next, for about 1 minute, chew/dissolve, swish, and coat your mouth with the Miracle Berry/Magic Fruit tablet. You want to ensure that the miraculin binds to your sweet receptors, which are located on the tongue, cheeks, and the roof of the mouth. Gargling the chewed tablet with your saliva will also work. For best results, ensure you take your time with this step. Swallow the chewed Miracle Berry/Magic Fruit tablet with your saliva. You may take a small drink of water (about 1 to 2 tablespoons) to wash down any remaining liquid in your mouth.

Next, bite into or eat the last piece of lemon. This should now taste sweet and not sour! In fact, it should taste like lemonade. It is because the miraculin has bound to sweet taste receptors because of the acidity of the lemon, and everything will now taste sweet. Next, drink some of the soda. For most persons, this should taste even sweeter than before. If the experiment was done right, food will have a sweet(er) perception for about an hour.

Jennifer L. Hellier

See also: Facial Nerve; Glossopharyngeal Nerve; Supertaster; Taste Aversion; Taste Bud; Taste System; Type III Taste Cells

Further Reading

Kataoka, Shinji, Ruibiao Yang, Yoshiro Ishimaru, Hiroaki Matsunami, John C. Kinnamon, & Thomas E. Finger. (2008). The candidate sour taste receptor, PKD2L1, is expressed by type III taste cells in the mouse. *Chemical Senses, 33*(3), 243–254. http://dx.doi.org/10.1093/chemse/bjm083

McLaughlin, Susan K., & Robert F. Margolskee. (1994). The sense of taste. *American Scientist, 82*(6), 538–545.

SPATIAL SEQUENCE SYNESTHESIA

Synesthesia is the cross-integration of two or more sensory systems at the same time. There are two main categories used to classify synesthesia: perceptual, which is triggered by sensory stimuli such as sights and sounds, and conceptual, which involves abstract concepts such as time and calendars. The most prevalent conceptual form of synesthesia is spatial sequence synesthesia, which involves the synesthetes seeing units of time or mathematical concepts as shapes in their extrapersonal space or their mind's eye. These shapes can include being surrounded by the months of the year as a flat ribbon, each unit of time having a distinct shape and arranged like a Ferris wheel, or seeing the days of the week like a spiral staircase directly in front of you. It is estimated that approximately 20 percent of synesthetes experience spatial sequence synesthesia.

Synesthetic Experience

As with other forms of synesthesia, spatial sequence synesthesia is individual, consistent over time, idiosyncratic, and can evolve. There is a rich variety of detailed visual content that can be experienced by an individual with spatial sequence synesthesia such as associated visual images, color, texture, and written text. This variation reflects a distinction between spatial imagery and visual imagery. Spatial imagery can take the form of a spatial map with flexible viewpoints and is detailed and complex. Visual imagery represents visual surface properties and depicts visual appearance. The majority of synesthetes with spatial sequence synesthesia experience both spatial and visual images as opposed to experiencing only one of the two. Spatial sequence synesthetes typically experience numerical sequences as floating in the space around them. This can include visualizing the months of the year in some pattern in space. One suggested idea is that this is part of the reasoning behind visualizing the calendar from left to right. This is based on a directional bias for reading in Western nations. Some synesthetes describe what they experience as having a mental map of sequences within their head.

Spatial Sequence Synesthesia and Memory

Spatial sequence synesthetes have also been shown to have superior memories over their nonsynesthete counterparts. This is in stark contrast to the historical viewpoint that all forms of synesthesia are a product of overactive imaginations or a sign of mental illness. Spatial sequence synesthetes have an automatic, built-in mnemonic reference that helps them to remember a sequence and as such they do not have to create one for themselves. Recently spatial sequence synesthesia has been linked to a superior ability to form memories. This type of synesthesia has also been linked to hyperthymestic syndrome where individuals can recall events with perfect clarity from any point in their lives. Scientists are now looking at the possible benefits of synesthesia. Does it improve memory or help in learning a musical instrument or in composing music? Research has indicated that synesthetes show a marked tendency to spend more time engaging in creative disciplines. It is believed that certain aspects of synesthesia could be taught. This is an exciting possibility that has far-reaching benefits for augmenting memory and working with some mental health disorders such as autism, dyslexia, and attention deficit hyperactivity disorder (ADHD).

Carolyn Johnson Atwater

See also: Auditory-Tactile Synesthesia; Grapheme-Color Synesthesia; Lexical-Gustatory Synesthesia; Mirror-Touch Synesthesia; Proprioception; Synesthesia

Further Reading

Jonas, Clare N., & Mark C. Price. (2014). Not all synesthetes are alike: Spatial vs. visual dimensions of sequence-space synesthesia. *Frontiers in Psychology, 5,* 1171. http://dx.doi.org/10.3389/fpsyg.2014.01171. Retrieved from http://journal.frontiersin.org/article/10.3389/fpsyg.2014.01171/full

Rothen, Nicolas, Kristin Jünemann, Andy D. Mealor, Vera Burckhardt, & Jamie Ward. (2015). The sensitivity and specificity of a diagnostic test of sequence-space synesthesia. *Behavioral Research.* http://dx.doi.org/10.3758/s13428-015-0656-2

Simner, Julia, Neil Mayo, & Mary-Jane Spiller. (2009). A foundation for savantism? Visuo-spatial synaesthetes present with cognitive benefits. *Cortex, 45*(10), 1246–1260.

STEREOCILIA

A cilium is a hair-like cellular protrusion found in eukaryotic cells. Long segments of microtubules pair to form a framework that gives structure to the cilium. Cilia can be motile or primary (nonmotile) depending on the arrangement of microtubules and accompanying proteins; cells with primary cilia can be found in many places in the human body and serve as sensory cells, such as the highly specialized stereocilia found in the inner ear's hair cells. Stereocilia are the apical end of hair cells. Hair cells are mechanosensory cells, meaning they respond to mechanical stimuli, which are physical forces such as sound waves. Stereocilia in the inner ear are responsible for two different detecting senses: hearing and balance.

Auditory Pathway

The inner ear contains an organ called the cochlea. The cochlea is a small bone with a cone-shaped body and a spiral tip, resembling a snail shell; the entire structure is hollow. The inner surface of the cochlea is lined with a delicate layer of epithelial (skin) tissue and the entire structure is filled with fluid. This fluid, or perilymph, aids in the transmission of sound, which travels into the ear in waves. Sound waves make their way into the cochlea where the waves' vibrations disturb stereocilia on hair cells. The hair cells turn the mechanical stimulus into a neural impulse that is sent to the auditory cortex in the temporal lobe of the brain. It has been found that healthy hair cells are capable of amplifying faint sounds by disturbing the perilymph and mechanically activating surrounding stereocilia.

Vestibular Pathway

Connected to the cochlea are three fluid-filled tubes called the semicircular canals. The fluid contained in these tubes is referred to as endolymph. The semicircular canals are oriented in such a way that they can detect head movement in any direction. One of the canals detects side-to-side motion, another detects front-to-back motion, and the third detects angular acceleration (tilt or spin). Stereocilia in the semicircular canals detect mechanical forces like those in the cochlea but, rather than sound wave detection, these stereocilia sense changes in endolymph flow. Mechanical stimulus results in transmission of a neural impulse from the hair cell to the cerebellum, an area at the base of the brain responsible for balance, movement, and coordination. Neural input from a change in head orientation lasts approximately 10 seconds into the movement. After this, if no additional change in position occurs, the input is terminated. This is why you do not feel dizzy when turning your head or feel as if you are falling when you lie on a flat surface. In contrast, vertigo is a feeling of constant dizziness that occurs due to problems that impair the function of the stereocilia, endolymph, neural impulse, or a combination of these.

Stereocilia Damage

Stereocilia are incredibly fragile portion of the hair cells and can be easily damaged by exceptionally loud noise, illness, toxins, aging, or head trauma. Damaged or destroyed stereocilia are incapable of regeneration, so any hearing loss associated with stereocilia injury is permanent. This sensorineural hearing loss begins with the inability to hear faint noises and progresses as the level of damage increases. It is estimated that the number of Americans with any type of hearing loss has doubled since 1970. In fact, hearing loss due to environmental noise is such a prevalent occurrence that the U.S. Environmental Protection Agency passed the Noise Control Act of 1972 as a means of protecting U.S. citizens from hazardous levels of urban noise.

Kendra DeHay

See also: Age-Related Hearing Loss; Auditory System; Cochlea; Semicircular Canals; Vestibular System; Vestibulocochlear Nerve

Further Reading

American Speech-Language-Hearing Society. (2016). How we hear. Retrieved from http://www.asha.org/public/hearing/How-We-Hear/

Ciliopathy Alliance. (2014). Structure and function of cilia: What are cilia? Retrieved from http://www.ciliopathyalliance.org/cilia/structure-and-function-of-cilia.html

Martin, Laura J. (2014). Hearing and the cochlea. *Medline Plus*. Retrieved from https://www.nlm.nih.gov/medlineplus/ency/anatomyvideos/000063.htm

Noise Control Act of 1972, 42 U.S.C. 4901 to 4918. (1972). Retrieved from http://www.gsa.gov/graphics/pbs/Noise_Control_Act_of_1972.pdf

STEREOPSIS

Stereopsis refers to binocular vision, which results from the brain integrating images from both eyes to form one image. As a result of stereopsis humans have depth perception. If one eye is not functioning normally or lacks normal vision, the brain may not interpret images from that eye. The resulting visual input lacks depth. Approximately 10 percent of the population lacks stereopsis. Treatment to restore stereopsis includes addressing the underlying cause and training the eyes to work together through vision therapy. Younger patients may be able to gain stereopsis, whereas older patients have lower rates of success.

History

Knowledge of the concept of stereopsis dates back to artists such as Leonardo da Vinci (1452–1519) who struggled to render the three-dimensional (3D) world on a two-dimensional canvas. Yet stereopsis was not defined until the mid-1800s when Charles Wheatstone published a paper on binocular vision and later created a stereoscope for observing two-dimensional pictures in 3D.

Understanding the concept of stereopsis has opened the door to many types of entertainment in the past century. By the late 1800s many homes had a stereo viewer and sets of photos called stereographs were widely available. In the 1920s, 3D movies were created. View-Master, familiar to many children, allows the viewer to experience 3D scenes including national monuments, landmarks, and animals. In the 1990s, Magic Eye pictures (stereograms that do not require a stereoscope) became popular and allowed viewers to see 3D images without a stereoscope.

Tests for Stereopsis

A variety of tests are used to measure stereoacuity; most of these tests rely on stereograms that can be viewed with polarized glasses. With polarized glasses, a person with stereoacuity will see a 3D image floating above a field of random dots. For children, a picture of a fly is viewed wearing polarized lenses. If the child has stereovision, the fly's wings will appear to be above the image. For the test, the child will be asked to pinch the fly's wings. A child with stereopsis will attempt to grab the wings above the image, whereas a child lacking stereopsis will touch the image itself. More detailed tests have been designed for adults that can measure the degree of stereoacuity a person has.

Significance of Stereopsis

Many people who lack stereopsis have amblyopia (lazy eye), strabismus (crossed eye), lack vision in one eye, or have another reason why their eyes are unable to work together. Lack of stereopsis causes a lack of 3D vision and may make sports, some manual tasks, and driving more difficult. Vision training can help a person learn to succeed at any of these tasks. Wiley Post (1898–1935) was the first pilot to fly around the world solo, and since he had only one eye, he lacked stereopsis. Despite a lack of stereopsis he was able to undergo vision training and successfully take off, fly, and land a plane (Elshatory & Siatkowski, 2014).

There may, however, be an advantage for the estimated 10 percent or more of the population lacking stereopsis. Blakeslee (2011) tested art students and compared them to other students and discovered artists have poorer stereopsis. Furthermore, the same study discovered that based on photographs of established artists, a higher percentage of artists have misaligned eyes than persons with "normal" vision (Blakeslee, 2011).

Regaining Stereopsis

Treatment is focused on restoring stereopsis. In order to have stereopsis a patient must have two eyes with similar visual acuity that are in alignment, transmitting images to the brain in a way that the images can be interpreted. Treatment, therefore, may involve wearing eyeglasses to balance the visual input being sent to the brain, having surgery to align the eyes, or patching the stronger eye to allow the brain to interpret input from the weaker eye. Additional types of vision therapy including eye exercises may restore stereopsis.

If a lack of stereopsis is discovered early and the underlying cause is treated, stereopsis can be restored. There may be a critical age range during which stereopsis can be recovered, but this concept has been challenged by the reports of a neuroscientist dubbed "Stereo Sue" who was able to regain stereopsis in her 50s (Sacks, 2006). Stereo Sue's story has caused speculation that the adult brain is more plastic than once thought.

Future

Future studies will help us understand the complex mechanism of stereopsis. Further understanding of the adult brain may reveal techniques that allow people who lack stereopsis to regain stereopsis later in life.

Lisa A. Rabe

See also: Amblyopia; Blindness; Optic Nerve Hypoplasia; Strabismus

Further Reading

Blakeslee, Sandra. (2011, June 14). A defect that may lead to a masterpiece. *New York Times*, p. D6. Retrieved from http://www.nytimes.com/2011/06/14/health/views/14vision.html?_r=2&

Elshatory, Yasser M., & R. Michael Siatkowski. (2014). Wiley Post, around the world with no stereopsis. *Survey of Ophthalmology*, *59*(3), 365–372. Retrieved from http://dx.doi.org/10.1016/j.survophthal.2013.08.001

Sacks, Oliver. (2006, June 19). Stereo Sue. Why two eyes are better than one. *The New Yorker*. Retrieved from http://www.newyorker.com/magazine/2006/06/19/stereo-sue

STRABISMUS

Strabismus is the medical term for crossed eyes. This is when a person's eyes will not look at the same place at the same time, which can cause the person to have double vision. One eye may be turned inward (esotropia), outward (exotropia), upward (hypertropia), or downward (hypotropia) compared to the other eye.

Signs and Symptoms

Strabismus occurs when the six extraocular muscles are weak and have poor motor control or when a person has severe farsightedness. The extraocular muscles are controlled by three cranial nerves: oculomotor (cranial nerve III), trochlear (cranial nerve IV), and abducens (cranial nerve VI). These nerves work together to keep a person's eyes focused on the same location. Strabismus can cause double vision or diplopia in both eyes (binocular diplopia) as well as uncoordinated eye movements, a loss of vision, and/or a loss of depth perception. This occurs because the extraocular muscles do not align the eyes properly so that convergence cannot occur. For instance, one eye will focus on an object but the other eye is turned inward or outward and will focus on a completely different object. Thus, two different images are sent to the brain, which can be confusing for visual perception. In young children, their brains may learn to ignore the image from the weaker eye—usually the turned eye. If the turned eye is only slightly askew, then both eyes may focus on the same object but the images are focused on different regions of the two retinas.

Causes

In general, strabismus is the result of an underlying systemic disease, damage to the cranial nerves serving the eye muscles, or inherited. Some diseases resulting in strabismus include but are not limited to cerebral palsy, Down syndrome, stroke, and trauma to the head. Persons with strabismus may have the same eye always turned in the same direction. This can be present all the time or only occurs when the person is tired or ill. In other cases, some patients' eyes alternate in turning.

In some cases, a person may have "lazy eye," or amblyopia, where the eye does not focus well. If amblyopia is untreated, it may cause strabismus. As previously stated, the brain may ignore images from the turned eye, which can cause that eye to never see well. Thus, it is imperative to provide treatment as soon as possible.

Diagnoses and Treatments

A health care provider will determine the severity of the strabismus. The provider will perform a general eye exam that tests a person's visual acuity and corneal light reflex, and perform a retinal exam. The health care provider may also perform a general physical exam to determine if there is an underlying cause for the strabismus.

Treatments for strabismus depend on the cause of the crossed eyes. The underlying cause must be treated first for best results. Many persons with strabismus are prescribed eyeglasses or contact lenses to correct the farsightedness. Treatment for amblyopia will include a patch to be worn over the strong eye. This will force the weaker eye to work hard and should improve its vision. An optometrist may also prescribe eye exercises (vision therapy), prism lenses (to reduce the amount of light into the eye so that it does not turn as much), and/or eye surgery (for severe cases).

In the majority of cases, strabismus can be corrected if treatment is provided as soon as possible. However, if treatment is delayed, then permanent vision loss in the weak eye can occur. In cases of strabismus caused by amblyopia, patching of the good eye should be done prior to age 11. Otherwise the amblyopia may become a permanent condition.

Jennifer L. Hellier

See also: Amblyopia; Cranial Nerves; Diplopia; Visual Perception

Further Reading
American Association for Pediatric Ophthalmology and Strabismus. (2014). Strabismus. Retrieved from http://www.aapos.org/terms/conditions/100
Blumenfeld, Hal. (2010). *Neuroanatomy through clinical cases.* Sunderland, MA: Sinauer.
Olitsky, S. E., D. Hug, L. S. Plummer, & M. Stass-Isern. (2011). Disorders of eye movement and alignment. In R. M. Kliegman, R. E. Behrman, H. B. Jenson, & B. F. Stanton (Eds.). *Nelson Textbook of Pediatrics*, 19th ed. (Chapter 615). Philadelphia, PA: Elsevier Saunders.

SULLIVAN, ANNE

Anne Sullivan was a gifted teacher, best known for being an instructor and lifelong companion of Helen Keller (1880–1968), a deaf, blind, and mute child. As a young child Sullivan contracted trachoma, an eye disease caused by bacteria, which left her blind and without reading or writing skills. Overcoming many personal challenges, she received her education as a student of the Perkins School for the Blind. Soon after graduation she became a teacher to Keller and together they dramatically changed the world's perception of individuals with disabilities.

Born April 14, 1866, in Feeding Hills, Agawam, Massachusetts, Johanna Mansfield Sullivan was the oldest child of illiterate, unskilled, and impoverished immigrants who came to the United States in 1860 from Ireland. Her mother died when she was eight and her father abandoned Sullivan and her siblings shortly thereafter. Sullivan was sent to live at the Tewksbury Almshouse, a home for the poor. In 1880, Sullivan approached a visiting inspector at the home and told him that she wanted to go to school. Later that year, she entered the Perkins School for the Blind. While there, Sullivan developed a friendship with and learned from Laura Bridgman (1829–1889), a graduate of Perkins and the first blind and deaf person to be educated there. Additionally, Sullivan underwent several eye operations that significantly improved her vision. In 1886 she graduated from Perkins as valedictorian of her class. A short time later, Sullivan was recommended to go to Tuscumbia, Alabama, to tutor young Keller.

Over 49 years, Sullivan and Keller's relationship grew from one of teacher and student to companion and friend. Sullivan began to teach Keller vocabulary, spelling each word out into her palm. Over the course of several months, Keller learned 575 words, some multiplication tables, and the braille system. A well-known accounting details how Sullivan finger-spelled the word "water" on one of Keller's hands as she ran water over her other hand. This moment was a breakthrough, allowing Keller to connect the concept of sign language with the world and people around her.

In 1888, Sullivan traveled with Keller to Perkins to continue Keller's education, spelling class lectures into Keller's hand and spelling out information from textbooks to her. As a result, Keller became the first deaf-blind person to graduate from college.

Sullivan met John A. Macy (1877–1932), a Harvard University instructor, who helped edit Keller's autobiography. The two married in 1905 and in 1914 they broke up, never officially divorcing.

Despite Anne's declining health, the women traveled widely, giving lectures, performances, and appearing in the film *Deliverance*. At the age of 70, Sullivan died on October 20, 1936, at her home in Forest Hills, New York. Her ashes were placed in the National Cathedral in Washington, D.C.—a distinct honor, as it is also the final resting place of President Woodrow Wilson and other distinguished individuals.

Sullivan's story continues to inspire through film and theatrical productions. Her work with Keller was showcased in the play *The Miracle Worker*, which was later turned into the 1962 film starring Patty Duke (1946–2016) as Keller and Anne Bancroft (1931–2005) as Sullivan.

Lin Browning

See also: Blindness; Braille; Keller, Helen

Further Reading

Braddy, Nella. (1933). *Anne Sullivan Macy: The story behind Helen Keller*. New York: Doubleday.

Keller, Helen. (1955). *Teacher, Anne Sullivan Macy: A tribute by the foster child of her mind*. New York: Doubleday.

Perkins School for the Blind. (n.d.). Anne Sullivan. Retrieved from http://www.perkins.org /history/people/anne-sullivan

SUPERIOR COLLICULUS

Processing a visual stimulation involves multiple areas of the brain. One important component is the superior colliculus. This structure—located deep within the brainstem—helps process both visual and somatic tactile sensations. It is involved in specific eye movements called "saccades," head movements, and in interpreting body position relative to somatic sensation.

Studying this structure across different species reveals varying functions of this structure. Certain snakes possess the ability to sense infrared signals. This sense is aided by neurons from the trigeminal nerve (cranial nerve V) in contrast to the optic nerve (cranial nerve II) in primates or humans. The trigeminal nerve senses stimulations such as touch, temperature, and pain for the face and helps to explain how these reptiles are able to detect heat signals.

Anatomy

The superior colliculus is located on the uppermost part of the brainstem in the posterior aspect. Surrounding structures include the pineal gland, thalamus, and cerebellum. Piercing through this structure is the cerebral aqueduct responsible for connecting the flow of cerebrospinal fluid from the ventricles to the exterior of the cortex and spinal cord. Within the structure of the superior colliculus, there exist multiple individual structures. Surrounding the cerebral aqueduct is the periaqueductal gray. This area plays a role in the sensation and modulation of pain signals from the periphery. Additionally, the oculomotor nucleus and the Edinger-Westphal nucleus are present. The oculomotor nucleus is responsible for multiple eye movements facilitated by the medial, superior, and inferior rectus muscles. Also, this area controls the opening and closing of the eyelid. The Edinger-Westphal nucleus is responsible for constricting the eye and aiding in accommodation of the lens (seeing close) and convergence of the eye (ensuring both eyes are pointed in similar directions).

Directly inferior to this structure is the inferior colliculus. It is similar in structure but different in function. The major function is processing of auditory information. The location of a sound source can be triangulated utilizing the shorter relay time from the side a sound originates compared to the longer relay time on the opposite side. Taken together, these two structures are known as the tectum or roof of the midbrain.

Physiology

The visual input from the retina is rapidly conducted via the optic nerve to the occipital cortex, the frontal eye field, and subsequently the superior colliculus. This frontal eye field is specifically responsive to new visual stimulus. For example, consider what happens when another person walks into a room at the periphery of your right visual field. Your brain will give more attention to this new stimulus with the signal being transmitted to neurons within the superior colliculus.

Before the signal arrives, it first had to cross to the contralateral side via the optic chiasm. Similar to the left occipital cortex processing information from the right visual field, the left superior colliculus reflects a map of the right visual field.

The signal from the person walking into the right visual field is processed in the left superior colliculus. At this point, the position of the new stimulus is compared to the location of the fovea in the retina. A calculation of direction and distance is made in order to align the fovea and the new visual stimulus. The next step is to initiate rapid movement of both eyes known as a saccade and head positioning to facilitate this alignment.

In order for the rightward saccade to occur in a horizontal manner, the paramedian pontine reticular formation (PPRF) is engaged. This structure relays a signal to the right eye lateral rectus muscle to contract, allowing for a deviation to the right. Simultaneously, the left eye quickly moves left via a signal relayed by the median longitudinal fasciculus. This structure signals the left oculomotor nerve to facilitate a contraction of the left medial rectus muscle. Ultimately, this coordinated effort brings the new visual stimulus into the focus of both foveas.

Interestingly, the superior colliculus also directs rapid movement of the head and neck. This process takes place via the tectospinal tract. Nerve cell bodies responding to the visual or somatosensory signal on the right will again initiate in the left within the superior colliculus. These tectospinal neurons will decussate (or cross over) at an area called the medulla pyramid in the brainstem. The motor signal will exit at the level of the cervical spinal cord toward musculature in the right periphery. At this point, neck muscles quickly contract to help adjust the visual field to the new stimulus.

Taken together, the superior colliculus is a region within the brainstem responsible for reflexive adjustments to new visual or tactile stimulation, arising from an evolutionarily old portion of the brain (the brainstem itself). It is clear that an animal's survival can be dependent on quickly processing and adjusting to new information.

Nicholas Breitnauer

See also: Accommodation; Inferior Colliculus; Occipital Lobe; Optic Nerve; Retina; Saccades; Senses of Animals; Thalamus; Visual Fields; Visual System

Further Reading

Dragoi, Valentin, & Chieyeko Tsuchitani. (1997). Visual processing: Cortical processing. In *Neuroscience Online, an electronic textbook for the neurosciences* (Chap. 15). Retrieved from http://neuroscience.uth.tmc.edu/s2/chapter15.html

Wisconsin University. (2006). *Unit No. 2, brain stem: Superior colliculus.* Retrieved from http://www.neuroanatomy.wisc.edu/virtualbrain/BrainStem/23Colliculus.html

SUPERIOR SALIVATORY NUCLEUS

The superior salivatory nucleus is a structure associated with cranial nerve VII or the facial nerve that innervates the submandibular and sublingual salivary glands and is important in the secretion of saliva for digestion. It works together with the inferior salivatory nucleus to allow for full function of the parotid gland. The superior salivatory nucleus has portions that are also part of the lacrimal nucleus, which innervate the lacrimal and mucosal glands.

Basic Salivary Gland Anatomy

The major salivary glands in humans are responsible for the synthesis and secretion of saliva, a product that helps with the initial steps of digestion of food. There are three major paired salivary glands that make up this system: (1) the sublingual glands, which are the smallest of the major salivary glands and are located under the tongue, and which secrete saliva into the floor of the mouth through the duct of Rivinus; (2) the submandibular glands, which are somewhat larger than the sublingual glands and are located under the mandible (or jaw bone) and also

SUPERIOR SALIVATORY NUCLEUS 381

secrete saliva into the floor of the mouth; and (3) the parotid glands, which are the largest of the salivary glands and are located just below and behind the ear. The parotid glands are the glands that become inflamed when a person has the mumps. Saliva is secreted into the mouth from the parotid gland through the Stensen duct (or parotid duct). Sensory and autonomic nerves including cranial nerve IX or the glossopharyngeal nerve, which is composed in part by the inferior and superior salivatory nuclei, regulate the parotid gland.

Autonomic Innervation of the Submandibular and Sublingual Glands

The peripheral nervous system in humans is composed of the somatic nervous system, which sends nerves to many of the muscles that we control voluntarily and exits the central nervous system from the spinal cord, and the autonomic nervous system, which regulates the organs and structures of the body that we do not voluntarily control. In the autonomic nervous system there are two neurons that are important to the function of this system: (1) the preganglionic neuron, which passes from the spinal cord or brain to a peripheral autonomic "ganglion," where a synapse is formed with the second neuron known as the (2) postganglionic neuron, which passes from the autonomic ganglion after forming a synapse with the preganglionic neuron to the organ or other structure innervated by the nerve.

Cranial nerve VII is responsible for the innervation of the submandibular and sublingual glands. It is composed of two neurons, both a preganglionic and a postganglionic neuron. The first neurons, or the preganglionic neurons, are distributed partly via the chorda tympani and lingual nerves to the submandibular ganglion. The postganglionic fibers then travel to the submandibular gland and sublingual gland to innervate the secretory cells. When these secretory cells are activated they release saliva, which is required for early digestion in the mouth.

Autonomic Innervation of the Lacrimal and Mucosal Glands

Some of the preganglionic fibers of the superior salivatory nucleus travel with the greater petrosal nerve through the pterygoid canal. These fibers stimulate the pterygopalatine ganglion, which has postganglionic fibers that travel to the lacrimal and mucosal glands. Activation of these postganglionic fibers produces tears from the lacrimal gland in the eye as well as mucus from the mucosal glands in the nose, palate, and pharynx.

Pathology of the Superior Salivatory Nucleus

The superior salivatory and its adjoining lacrimal nuclei are dispersed and lie just medial of the motor portion of the facial nucleus. Thus, damage to the facial nucleus generally results in damage to the superior salivatory nucleus. This would result in the lack of ability to produce saliva from the submandibular and sublingual glands, tears from the eye, and mucus on the same side of the lesion. This is often seen in Bell's palsy, which may be caused by edema (swelling) and inflammation of the facial nerve. It is characterized by unilateral (one side) and temporary weakness or total paralysis of the facial nerve

Jennifer L. Hellier and Charles A. Ferguson

See also: Autonomic Nervous System; Bell's Palsy; Chorda Tympani Nerve; Facial Nerve; Inferior Salivatory Nucleus; Taste Bud; Taste System

Further Reading

Holsinger, F. Christopher, & Dana T. Bui. (2007). Anatomy, function, and evaluation of the salivary glands. In Eugene N. Myers and Robert L. Ferris (Eds.), *Salivary gland disorders* (pp. 1–16). Berlin and Heidelberg: Springer-Verlag.

Kiernan, John A. (2005). *Barr's The human nervous system: An anatomical viewpoint* (p. 150). Baltimore, MD: Lippincott Williams & Wilkins.

SUPERTASTER

A supertaster is an individual who experiences the sensation of taste to a far greater intensity than that of the average person. Taste can be defined in terms of the lowest detectable concentration, known as the threshold, and at the highest detectable concentration, known as the suprathreshold response. Supertasters are members of a phenotype whose tasting abilities stretch past that of the average suprathreshold response. In the past, this phenomenon has been tested through individuals using the bitter chemical propylthiouracil (PROP) in order to determine the bitterness suprathreshold response in individuals of the supertaster phenotype. Recent studies have shown, however, that supertasting stretches beyond the scope of just bitterness and may involve somatosensation, as well as retronasal olfaction.

History

The term *supertaster* was coined in 1991 by American psychologist Linda Bartoshuk (1938–) in an article she published in the journal *Food Technology*, after she and her research team noticed that people with the ability to taste would report perceived perception to a highly variable degree. The initial test used to test for supertasters was the PROP suprathreshold response, however, recent studies have suggested that bitterness is not the only taste sensation involved in supertasting, suggesting that general supertasters may have different sensory responses than those of the PROP supertasters.

Beyond Bitterness

New evidence has emerged to suggest that supertasting is not only limited to orosensory functions, but may also be linked to chemosensory function as well. Most notably, supertasters are able to differentiate between smaller changes in ingredient levels than a "normal" taster. A challenge arises in determining whether supertasting is linked with liking and disliking food in the sense that many people tend to report a distaste for a certain flavor when that taste increases in intensity, whereas others report proportionality between the two. There is currently a hypothesis reported by Calò and colleagues (2011) that a polymorphism in the TAS2R38 bitterness receptor in addition to polymorphisms in the *gustin* gene known as the gustin polymorphism may act as a genotypic marker for the PROP supertaster phenotype, which, if true, would provide for great advancement in studying the chemosensory influences in supertasting and on eating behavior.

Taste Mechanism

The majority of the oral cavity is lined with papillae, which contain taste receptors. These taste receptors synapse with afferent fibers and are activated whenever a chemical enters the oral cavity. After stimulation of the taste receptors, the afferent fibers project information to the cortex of the brain, encoding an impulse for taste perception. It is believed that it is somewhere in this pathway that the increased perception in supertasters lies. It was long believed that the increase in taste sensation was simply due to the fact that supertasters may have had a higher density of taste receptor genes. However, new evidence shows that polymorphisms in RAS2R38 and gustin genes, both involved in bitterness taste perception, lead to a much higher degree of taste perception to low concentrations of PROP in individuals identified as supertasters.

Associated Issues

Rutgers University food scientist Beverly Tepper found a correlation between supertasters and excessive weight loss, especially in women. She found that women in their 40s who were known to be supertasters were 20 percent thinner than nontasters (people without the ability to taste). This is likely due to the fact that many people who are known supertasters report that foods and beverages that the general public tends to enjoy are too sweet or too bitter. Because of this sensation that normally perceived tastes are too strong for their liking, many supertasters are more likely to limit their eating. This has led many researchers to further develop their knowledge of the correlation between taste sensation disabilities and body mass.

Gage Williamson

See also: Bartoshuk, Linda; Hyperguesia; Hypoguesia; Taste Aversion; Taste Bud; Taste System

Further Reading

Calò, Maria Carla, Alessandra Padiglia, Andrea Zonza, Laura Corrias, Paolo Contu, Beverly J. Tepper, & Iole Tomassini Barbarossa. (2011). Polymorphisms in TAS2R38 and the taste bud trophic factor, gustin gene co-operate in modulating PROP taste phenotype. *Physiology & Behavior, 104*(5), 1065–1071.

Hayes, John E., & Russell S. J. Keast. (2011). Two decades of supertasting: Where do we stand? *Physiology & Behavior, 104*(5), 1072–1074.

Webb, Jordannah, Dieuwerke P. Bolhuis, Sara Cicerale, John E. Hayes, & Russell S. J. Keast. (2015). The relationships between common measurements of taste function. *Chemosensory Perception, 8*(1), 11–18.

SWEET SENSATION

Sweet sensation, the detection of sugars, is one of the five basic tastes. Sweet tastes are appetitive, in that they are generally regarded as pleasant. The ability to detect sugars has likely been advantageous through human evolution by facilitating the identification of substances with high caloric value. The standard substance that is used to measure sweetness is sucrose (table sugar), which is designated as having a sweetness index of 1. Common sugars range in sweetness from 0.15 (lactose) to 1.7 (fructose), and common artificial sugars range from 180 (aspartame; brand name Equal®) up to 8,000 (neotame; brand name NutraSweet®).

The relative sweetness of a molecule is determined by its affinity for the receptor for sweet sensation, the heterodimer of the Taste Receptor 1 Member 2 (T1R2) and Taste Receptor 1 Member 3 (T1R3) G-protein coupled receptors. The T1R2+R3 receptor is expressed on the surface of taste receptor cells (TRCs). TRCs that express the T1R2+R3 receptor sense sweetness, and TRCs that detect sweetness do not detect other tastes.

Different TRCs are responsible for all five of the primary tastes. TRCs are organized into taste buds, which contain 50–150 TRCs each. Taste buds throughout the tongue contain TRCs for all five primary tastes; therefore, there is no topographic taste map. The specificity of the TRC to one taste alone is essential for the way that the different taste sensations are encoded.

Depolarization of the sweet TRCs following a signaling cascade triggered by the taste receptor transmits a signal to afferent neurons. The signal is relayed by fibers of the facial nerve (cranial nerve VII) in the anterior two-thirds of the tongue and the glossopharyngeal nerve (cranial nerve IX) in the posterior third of the tongue. Sensory afferents synapse in the rostral portion of the nucleus of the solitary tract in the brainstem and are relayed to the thalamus with projections to the primary gustatory cortex.

The T1R2+R3 receptor broadly detects different sugars and artificial sweeteners. In general the sensation of one sugar is indistinguishable from another, though

Chocolate Test

Foods and beverages provide calories and nutrients that are essential for humans to survive. Sweet foods generally are more calorie-rich than others and are considered appetitive or pleasant in taste. This sidebar focuses on the perception of sweet foods and how this perception changes when a natural antagonist—gymnemic acid—blocks sweet taste receptors.

Gymnemic acid is a glycoside that can be isolated from the leaves of the *Gymnema sylvestre* plant, which grows in central and southern India. Gymnemic acid reduces the taste of sugar when placed in the mouth by blocking sweet receptors found in taste buds. *Gymnema sylvestre* leaves are often chewed in India to fight sweet cravings.

Materials:

1 *Gymnema sylvestre* capsule (it should contain at least 450 milligrams of *Gymnema sylvestre* leaf extract, 25% gymnemic acid in each capsule. This can be purchased from an organic food store and found in the vitamin aisle.)
2 small paper cups
1 to 2 tablespoons of water
2 to 4 tablespoons of soda (such as a cola type)
2 pieces of chocolate (dark chocolate will have a more pronounced effect than milk chocolate)

Directions:

Pour the water into one of the paper cups. Open the *Gymnema sylvestre* capsule and dump the powder into the water. Stir until mostly dissolved and set aside. This will look like an herbal tea mix and may have a bitter taste. Pour the soda into the other paper cup and set aside. As a control for this experiment, eat one of the pieces of chocolate. This should taste sweet. Next, drink some of the soda. Again, this should taste sweet. Next, for about 1 minute, swish and coat your mouth with the *Gymnema sylvestre* liquid. You want to ensure that the gymnemic acid binds to your sweet receptors, which are located on the tongue, cheeks, and the roof of the mouth. Gargling will also work. If the taste of the liquid is too pungent, plug your nose to reduce the bitterness. For best results, ensure you take your time with this step. Swallow the *Gymnema sylvestre* liquid. You may take a small drink of water (about 1 to 2 tablespoons) to wash down the remaining *Gymnema sylvestre* liquid in your mouth.

Next, eat the last piece of chocolate. This should now taste bitter and not sweet! It is because the gymnemic acid has blocked the sweet taste receptors, and the sugar in the chocolate can no longer bind. Next, drink some of the soda. Again, this should taste bitter or very acidic. If the experiment was done right, sweet perception will be blocked for about an hour.

Jennifer L. Hellier

artificial sweeteners may produce a slightly different taste than natural sugars. It is possible that the homodimer of T1R3 can detect natural sugars but not artificial sweeteners, or bitter receptors may be cross-activated by artificial sweeteners at high concentrations.

The T1R2+R3 receptor detects sugars with relatively low affinity when compared to the affinities of the bitter receptors and bitter tastants. This means that substances need relatively high concentrations of sugar to be identified as sweet, consistent with the need to identify foods that are sufficiently nutritive.

The ability to detect sweet, along with the other tastes, declines with age. This may result in the ingestion of more sweet foods, which could exacerbate obesity and diabetes in older individuals. More recently, it has been identified that sugars can be detected by taste receptors in the gut, but not consciously sensed. Gut sensing of sugar may have important implications for regulation of appetite and metabolism.

Michael S. Harper

See also: Facial Nerve; Glossopharyngeal Nerve; Supertaster; Taste Aversion; Taste Bud; Taste System; Type II Taste Cells

Further Reading

Joesten, Melvin D., John L. Hogg, & Mary E. Castellion. (2007). Sweetness relative to sucrose (table). *The World of Chemistry: Essentials* (4th ed., p. 359). Belmont, CA: Thomson Brooks/Cole.

Mayo Clinic. (2015). Artificial sweeteners and other sugar substitutes. Retrieved from http://www.mayoclinic.org/healthy-lifestyle/nutrition-and-healthy-eating/in-depth/artificial-sweeteners/art-20046936

McLaughlin, Susan K., & Robert F. Margolskee. (1994). The sense of taste. *American Scientist, 82*(6), 538–545.

SYNCOPE: *See* Fainting

SYNESTHESIA

Erica Goode wrote in the *New York Times*, "Most people experience the sensory world as a place of orderly segregation. Sight, sound, smell, taste, and touch are distinct and separate. With synesthesia, in which the customary boundaries between the senses appear to break down, sight mingles with sound, or taste with touch" (1999). The word *synesthesia* derives from the Greek words *syn* meaning together and *aesthesis* meaning perception. Synesthesia is a perceptual condition whereby sensations from one sense are simultaneously perceived together by one or more additional senses in unusual ways. A person who has this condition is referred to as a synesthete. Some synesthetes hear, smell, or taste in color; some taste shapes; some see people surrounded by color; and others perceive written digits, letters, and words in color. Examples of this "joined perception" are seeing the number 7 as being purple or the sound of your mother's voice as being green; seeing a yellow border around your best friend; seeing units of time as shapes; and feeling music as a tickling sensation on the back of your neck.

History and Indicators

Synesthesia has been known to exist for the past 300 years and was thought to be quite rare, mainly because people with the condition maintained silence about their experiences when they realized theirs were not typical. There are probably many people who have the condition but do not know it; estimates range from 1 in 200–300 to 1 in 100,000 people having some variation of the condition. Besides synesthesia, synesthetes have some other similarities: they tend to be female with three times as many women as men in the United States having synesthesia, while the number jumps to eight times as many women as men in the United Kingdom; they tend to be left-handed; they are of normal to above average intelligence and have normal standard neurological exams. Synesthesia runs in families and seems to be a dominant trait, possibly residing on the X-chromosome. The writer Vladimir Nabokov (1899–1977) and the physicist Richard Feynman (1918–1988) reputedly were synesthetes, as is the singer Mary J. Blige (1971–).

More Common Types of Synesthesia

It is estimated that there are more than 70 different types of synesthesia. These depend on the way that the synesthete's brain processes sensory information. Rarely, synesthetes experience more than one type of synesthesia. Following are a few of the most common types:

1. Grapheme-color synesthesia—Individuals with this type of synesthesia experience letters or numbers as a color.
2. Chromesthesia—These synesthetes associate sounds with colors.
3. Lexical-gustatory synesthesia—These synesthetes experience words as taste.
4. Auditory-tactile synesthesia—Synesthetes with this synesthesia experience sensations on their bodies when hearing certain sounds.
5. Spatial sequence synesthesia—Individuals with spatial sequence synesthesia experience sequences at various different points in space.

Further Research

Synesthesia presents an intriguing problem because logically it should not be a product of the human brain, where the evolutionary trend has been for increasing anatomical separation of function. Studies have confirmed that synesthesia is biological, automatic, and apparently unlearned, distinct from both hallucination and metaphor. Researchers ascribe synesthesia as "crossed wires" in the brain. Neurologist Richard E. Cytowic (1952–) hypothesized in the 1980s that the condition's cause rested in the limbic system, the more emotional and primitive part of the brain. His case studies and book written in 1993, *The Man Who Tasted Shapes*, brought attention to the condition and prompted psychologists and neuroscientists to research various hypotheses. Research teams found that synesthetes' experiences are consistent across time. They also established that synesthesia is concretely measurable in the brain, using positron emission tomography (PET) and functional magnetic resonance imaging (fMRI). Other studies demonstrate that synesthetic perception occurs involuntarily and interferes with ordinary perception. Studies have also shown an interesting effect in the cortex. When colored-hearing synesthetes hear certain words, they display activity in the areas of the visual cortex associated with processing color. Nonsynesthetes do not show activity in these areas, even when asked to imagine colors or to associate certain colors with certain words (Nunn et al., 2002).

It is unclear which parts of the brain are involved in synesthesia. It is proposed that synesthetes' brains are genetically equipped with more connections between neurons, which causes the usual limited sensory communication to break down. Other speculations are that we all may be born with abundant connections but most of us lose those connections as we mature. Modern behavioral, molecular, genetic, and brain-imaging tools hold exciting promise for uncovering how synesthesia operates and for better understanding how the brain normally organizes perception and cognition.

Synesthesia may reveal something about human consciousness. No one knows how we bind all of our perceptions together into one complete whole, one complete concept. The additional perceptions that synesthetes have add to the concept. Studying synesthesia might help us understand the nature of human cognition and perception and how the concept of similarity is embedded within the nervous system. Equally important is the idea that synesthesia can bring unique abilities to a creative person, which might help bring significant contributions to the world.

Carolyn Johnson Atwater

See also: Auditory-Tactile Synesthesia; Grapheme-Color Synesthesia; Lexical-Gustatory Synesthesia; Mirror-Touch Synesthesia; Spatial Sequence Synesthesia

Further Reading

Cytowic, Richard E. (2003). *The man who tasted shapes*. Cambridge, MA: MIT Press.

Goode, Erica. (1999). When people see a sound and hear a color. *New York Times.* Retrieved from http://www.nytimes.com/1999/02/23/science/when-people-see-a-sound-and-hear-a-color.html?pagewanted=all

Nunn, J. A., L. J. Gregory, M. Brammer, S. C. Williams, D. M. Parslow, M. J. Morgan, . . . J. A. Gray. (2002). Functional magnetic resonance imaging of synesthesia: Activation of V4/V8 by spoken words. *Nature Neuroscience, 5*(4), 371–375.

TACTILE CORPUSCLES: *See* Meissner's Corpuscles

TASTE AVERSION

Taste aversion is a strong dislike for a certain food or flavor. A taste aversion or a conditioned taste aversion develops when an animal or a human associates a certain food with symptoms of sickness (vomiting and nausea) that were caused by toxic, poisonous, or spoiled food. Taste aversions can be so strong that it only takes one episode of associating a food with sickness for the taste aversion to develop.

Taste aversions are common in persons receiving chemotherapy, which can be dangerous as each time the patient eats a new food, he or she develops a new taste aversion. This is because the medicine caused the nausea or vomiting, but the patient associated the sickness with ingesting the food. Eventually, chemotherapy patients do not want to eat, which can slow down their recovery as well as be dangerous to their overall health.

Taste Aversion Experiments

American psychologist John Garcia (1917–2012) was most noted for his conditioned taste aversion experiments performed in the 1950s. Garcia was observing a rat's behavior following a session of radiation. He found that the rat would develop a taste aversion to the food it ate just prior to the radiation treatment. At the time, scientists believed that taste aversions would develop after a single trial with a long delay between the ingestion of the food and the sickness. Thus, to better understand the occurrence of taste aversion, Garcia gave three groups of rats sweetened water and then followed it with Group 1 receiving no radiation, Group 2 receiving mild radiation, and Group 3 receiving strong radiation. He then measured the amount of sweetened water they would drink after the radiation or no radiation session. The rats with both mild and strong radiation drank significantly less sweetened water compared to nonirradiated rats. This finding showed that a long delay was not required to develop a taste aversion and that an event causing nausea could produce the association with the food. Thus, the study of conditioned taste aversion began.

Behavior and Physiology

Survival of a species is a paramount trait that is innate in all animals. Behavioral scientists and psychologists posit that taste aversions are a type of survival mechanism or an adaptive trait that teaches the animal to avoid toxic or poisonous foods, such as poisonous plants (e.g., oleander, foxglove, and rhubarb leaves) and berries (e.g., nightshade, holly, and pokeweed berries). By causing the animal to vomit or be nauseated, the animal will stop eating the plant or berry before it causes severe harm or death. This strong association of a food with sickness will protect the animal so that it will avoid other similar plants or berries and ultimately avoid future toxicities or poisonings.

The development of a taste aversion, however, can be unintentional. Specifically, a taste aversion can occur because of other events or other substances and not because of the food itself. Consider the following example of an event causing the taste aversion. A person at an amusement park eats a hot dog. Right after he eats, the person rides a fast spinning ride like the Tea Cups at Disneyland, which makes him vomit. The spinning ride actually caused the nausea or sickness, but the person associates the hot dog as the cause of the vomiting. For an example of another substance causing a taste aversion, consider a young child with a very loose tooth eating corn on the cob. The child bites into the corn, which results in the tooth falling out and the gum bleeding. The mixture of blood with the corn can cause a sickening taste or feeling. Thus, the child will develop a taste aversion to the corn, when it was the blood that caused the nausea. Both of these types of instant taste aversion can last for years and may never become extinct.

Disease and Treatments

Patients with cancers often receive chemotherapy and/or radiation to treat their disease. As shown by Garcia, this can lead to taste aversions. It is important to note that a person does not need cognitive awareness for a taste aversion to develop. This means that the person does not have to recognize the connection of the cause and the effect or the food and the sickness. Chemotherapy patients are hungry and hope to enjoy their food, but the drugs make them sick and cause their body to reject the food. Thus, research has focused on developing strong antiemetic (antinausea and antivomiting) drugs to counteract and prevent the development of taste aversions for cancer patients as well as for motion sickness.

Jennifer L. Hellier

See also: Dizziness; Emesis; Hypergeusia; Hypogeusia; Nausea; Taste System

Further Reading

Bernstein, Ilene L. (1999). Taste aversion learning: A contemporary perspective. *Nutrition, 15*(3), 229–234.

Carelli, Regina M., & Elizabeth A. West. (2014). When a good taste turns bad: Neural mechanisms underlying the emergence of negative affect and associated natural reward devaluation by cocaine. *Neuropharmacology, 76*(B), 360–369.

Garcia, J., D. J. Kimeldorf, & R. A. Koelling. (1955). Conditioned aversion to saccharin resulting from exposure to gamma radiation. *Science, 122*(3160), 157–158.

TASTE BUD

Taste buds are the peripheral sensory organs of the gustatory system. They are garlic-shaped clusters of cells that sense five basic tastes: sweet, bitter, umami, salty, and sour.

Anatomy

Taste buds contain 50–100 elongate cells that sense chemical tastants and communicate this information to taste nerve fibers. Each taste bud has an apical pore, where a small opening in the epithelial tissue allows the apical ends of taste receptor cells to access chemicals in the oral cavity. At its base, a taste bud is innervated by taste nerves that contact the taste receptor cells inside.

Taste buds are found in specialized regions both on the tongue and in separate tissues in the oral cavity. On the tongue, taste buds are housed in the fungiform, circumvallate, and foliate papillae. Fungiform papillae are small, rounded protrusions scattered across the top of the anterior tongue. These bumps are more concentrated at the very tip of the tongue, and each contains one to five taste buds. The circumvallate papillae are located at the back of the tongue—these large bumps mark semicircular troughs in the tongue epithelium, which are lined with taste buds. Taste buds in the circumvallate papillae are much more concentrated than in the fungiform papillae. The foliate papillae house taste buds in several pits lining each side of the posterior tongue—taste buds here are highly concentrated, as in the circumvallate papillae. Taste buds even exist outside the tongue—humans have a few taste buds on the soft palate, the tissue posterior to the hard palate on the roof of the mouth, as well as in the larynx.

Development

Taste bud tissue patterning and development occurs during gestation, such that we are born with our first functioning taste buds. Unlike sensory cells in the auditory and visual systems (hair cells and retinal neurons, respectively), which are quite limited in their ability to regenerate, taste buds are constantly turning over and renewing throughout the life of an organism. Taste buds are repopulated by a population of basal progenitor cells that are capable of differentiating into either taste cells or epithelial cells. Some of these cells then migrate into the base of the taste bud, becoming taste-specific progenitor cells, which eventually differentiate into one of the three types of mature taste cells: Type I, Type II, or Type III.

While taste bud turnover tends to remain stable throughout a lifetime, the ability of taste buds to regenerate can be perturbed—chemotherapeutic drugs, for example, can disrupt taste in head and neck cancer patients. It is thought that these drugs disrupt or eliminate the sense of taste by disabling proper taste cell renewal (Barlow, 2015).

Function

Taste buds throughout the oral cavity are responsible for sensing at least five basic tastes: sweet, bitter, umami, salty, and sour. Each of these tastes indicates important information about ingested foods. Sweet foods are high in sugars, suggesting nutritional content. Umami, a Japanese term for "savory," generally indicates the protein content of food, which is also of nutritional importance. Salt is important for many processes in the body—with taste buds that sense salt content, the body can regulate salt intake. Bitter and sour are generally thought to be aversive qualities—taste buds help us to avoid ingesting poisonous and perhaps rotten foods by recognizing bitter and sour compounds. Many plants produce toxic chemicals. To avoid these, organisms evolved a sense of bitter taste, which recognizes a wide array of toxic molecules we might find in our diets. Foods that are too high in acid may be rotten or rancid and will taste sour, allowing us to avoid ingesting potentially damaging foods. All of these taste qualities are sensed by specialized taste receptor cells in taste buds. Bitter, sweet, and umami qualities are sensed by Type II cells, sour and some salty substances are sensed by Type III cells, and some salt sensation may occur through Type I cells, though these cells are primarily support cells. Taste buds may also sense fatty acids and calcium, but whether these are primary taste qualities have not yet been confirmed.

Contrary to the popularized "taste map" of the tongue, the five tastes are *not* strictly segregated to specific regions of the tongue. Some taste buds have more of one particular cell type than another—for example, there are more Type III cells per bud in the circumvallate papillae than in fungiform papillae. But most, if not all, taste buds contain cells to detect all five taste qualities.

Courtney E. Wilson

See also: Taste System; Type I Taste Cells; Type II Taste Cells; Type III Taste Cells

Further Reading

Barlow, Linda A. (2015). Progress and renewal in gustation: New insights into taste bud development. *Development, 142*(21), 3620–3629. http://dx.doi.org/10.1242/dev.120394.

Kandel, Eric R., James H. Schwartz, Thomas M. Jessell, Steven A. Siegelbaum, & A. J. Hudspeth (Eds.). (2012). *Principles of neural science* (5th ed., Chap. 32). New York, NY: McGraw-Hill.

TASTE SYSTEM

Taste, or gustation, is the sensation that occurs when a substance in the mouth, a tastant, reacts chemically with receptors to send a signal to the brain. Taste is distinguished from flavor, a term that generally describes a broader experience, which includes gustation, olfaction, trigeminal nerve stimulation (texture, pain, temperature), and even sight and sound. There are five basic categories of taste: bitter, sweet, sour, salty, and umami (a Japanese word that loosely translates as "savory" in English). Other possible basic tastes, such as fatty acids, calcium, carbon dioxide, and even water, are being investigated.

Taste has evolved to help humans distinguish between nutritious and toxic foods. Foods with sugar have evolved to taste good because sugar is essential for survival. Umami tastes delicious because proteins are essential. Salt is an essential nutrient that must be consumed in a specific amount to maintain proper levels in the body; this is why a little bit of salt tastes good, but too much salt tastes bad. Sour appears to have both aversive and pleasant qualities that function to alert us when foods have spoiled or when plants are not yet ripe, but also to encourage the consumption of sour fruits that contain important vitamins and nutrients. Bitterness has evolved to be a generally aversive taste because most foods that taste bitter tend to be poisonous. However, the bitter molecules in many edible plants are toxic only in high concentrations and these edible plants contain anticarcinogenic nutrients. Thus, it makes sense that these edible plants taste pleasant to many people.

Anatomy

Taste stimulants are detected via taste organs, called taste buds, which are located in the mucosa of the tongue, soft palate, inner cheeks, pharynx, and epiglottis. It is important to note that taste buds are not the bumps on a person's tongue; these are called papillae. Each person has about 3,000–10,000 taste buds, most of which are on the surface of the tongue (Bartoshuk & Snyder, 2013). Each taste bud is a cluster of 50–100 elongated epithelial cells arranged like the segments of an orange. The cells are renewed about every 12 days. They are divided into three main groups: Type I are support cells; Type II are the receptor cells, which contain the G protein–coupled receptors that bind sweet, bitter, and umami tastants; and Type III react to sour stimuli, which involve ion channels. Type III are also known as presynaptic cells because, unlike Type II, they have identifiable synapses with the nerve fiber and release neurotransmitters, such as serotonin and GABA (gamma-aminobutyric acid), onto the afferent nerve fiber. The mechanism that Type II cells use to excite the nerve fiber is unknown; however, it is speculated that ATP (adenosine triphosphate) acts as a transmitter. The cells that contain receptors for salty taste have not been clearly delineated.

The receptor proteins are located in the plasma membrane of long microvilli called gustatory hairs that extend from the taste cells through a taste pore to the

Doritos® Experiment

The flavors of foods and beverages are perceived through both the taste and olfactory systems. In fact, the sense of smell is the most important chemical sense for flavor to be distinguished. This is why food does not taste as flavorful when a person has a stuffy or runny nose from a head cold, flu, or sinusitis. This sidebar focuses on isolating one of the five basic tastes, umami.

Umami is a Japanese word that is best translated into English as "savory." It detects amino acids that are appetizing, such as meat, mushrooms, tomatoes, and cheese. Humans have taste receptors that are specific for L-glutamate, an amino acid that is found in high-protein foods and that binds to the umami taste receptors. The most common salt form of L-glutamate is monosodium glutamate (MSG). It is a common misconception that MSG is bad for humans and that it causes headaches, allergies, and childhood obesity. In fact, most taste researchers agree the notion that MSG causes sickness in humans is unfounded.

Materials:

1 Lay's® Potato Chip—Classic
1 Doritos® Tortilla Chip—Nacho Cheese flavor

Directions:

You will need to eat the potato chip first so that you will saturate the salt receptors and be able to isolate the umami receptors that the Doritos® Tortilla Chip will stimulate. These brand-named chips are necessary for the experiment to work the best, as each chip has the same amount of salt. For best results, make sure your nasal passage is clear and that you can take a deep breath. Place the Lay's® Potato Chip in your mouth and eat it very slowly. You should take about a minute to dissolve the salt and potato chip in your mouth before you swallow the chip. Swish the dissolved salt and melted potato chip throughout your mouth—as you have taste buds on your cheeks, inside of lips, and roof of the mouth—and then swallow. With one hand plug your nose. Note: you can breathe through your mouth during this experiment. Place the Doritos® Tortilla Chip in your mouth and chew about 5–10 times with your nose still plugged. If you have completely saturated the salt receptors in your mouth, then the Dorito® chip should not have any taste. Unplug your nose, as this will allow retronasal olfaction to take place. Instantly, the cheesiness of the Dorito® should be detected as the MSG should have bound to your isolated umami receptors.

Jennifer L. Hellier

surface of the papillae. The taste pores are filled with saliva, which transports the dissolved tastants to the receptors. The epithelial taste cell then generates impulses in the sensory nerve fibers that innervate them.

Most taste buds are contained in papillae. There are three types of papillae: the relatively large circumvallate, found at the back of the tongue in an arc; foliate, found on the edges of the medial tongue; and fungiform, found at the tip of the tongue. The taste pores containing the protrusions of the microvilli are located on the surface of the fungiform papillae and buried in the sides of the circumvallate and foliate papillae. In order for food molecules to be tasted, they must be dissolved in saliva because only then can they flow into the taste pores.

The popular tongue map that shows each of the five tastes being perceived on a certain region of the tongue, specifically bitter on the back, sweet on the tip, is a successfully propagated myth that was started in 1942 by a textbook author who misunderstood a research paper on the subject. Contrary to this popular belief, all five tastes can be perceived anywhere there are taste buds.

To the Brain

Taste information travels to the brain via three cranial nerves. The chorda tympani branch of the facial nerve (cranial nerve VII) carries impulses from taste receptors in the anterior two-thirds of the tongue; the glossopharyngeal nerve (cranial nerve IX) from the tongue's posterior third and pharynx; and the vagus nerve (cranial nerve X) from the few taste buds on the epiglottis and lower pharynx. These three cranial nerves synapse in the solitary nucleus located in the medulla. From there, impulses are transmitted to the ventral posterior medial nucleus of the thalamus and then to the gustatory area of the cerebral cortex in the insula lobe. The orbitofrontal cortex receives projections from the insular cortex, as well as information about touch, temperature, and smell, suggesting it is an integration area for flavor. The three nerves partially inhibit one another. This provides a means to retain taste perception if one nerve is damaged, for the other two nerves will have amplified signals. When a nerve is damaged, this delicate inhibition process is tampered with and this can sometimes result in "phantom taste."

The lingual branch of the trigeminal nerve (cranial nerve V) has nerve endings surrounding taste buds. It sends sensory information about touch, temperature, and pain. These nerves can be irritated by certain chemicals, such as capsaicin, and send a signal of pain and heat to the brain, giving us the sensation of spiciness, or pungency. Menthol works the same and elicits a feeling of coolness. These are both chemesthetic sensations.

Theories of Transduction

There are two theories that explain how taste sensations are encoded from receptor to brain: the labeled line hypothesis and pattern coding theory. Labeled line theorizes that each individual nerve fiber encodes only one of the five basic tastes. Pattern coding, also known as across fiber coding or population coding, theorizes that nerve fibers receive information from more than one of the five tastes, and the overall pattern of many nerve fibers firing is interpreted by the brain to be a particular taste or tastes.

In fungiform papillae, the nerve fibers that innervate taste cells branch so they innervate multiple cells, and each cell can also be innervated by multiple different fibers. Recordings show that the taste cells innervated by branches of the same taste fiber have similar specificities to tastants. This supports the labeled line theory. However, recordings also show that nerve fibers can respond to more than one taste class, evidence supporting the pattern coding theory. A general consensus is beginning to arise that both theories are partially correct: nerve fibers are "best" at transducing one taste. So while they may weakly respond to another taste, "sucrose" best fibers, for example, are best at sending the "sweet" message to the brain.

Bitter

Bitterness is a "bad" taste that is believed to have developed to preserve life. Thus, when a person or animal eats something that is bitter, they do not like the taste and spit it out. Substances that are bitter include coffee, beer, aspirin, quinine, peels of citrus fruits, and many vegetables. There are about 25 different known receptor proteins that bind with bitter tastants. They are called the T2R receptors and are encoded from a family of genes called Tas2r.

Sweet

Sweetness is the taste of simple carbohydrates, which are the body's source of energy. It is important for survival and eating sweet foods signals reward pathways in human brains so that everyone is encouraged to eat these energy-rich foods. There are about 25 variants of the T2R bitter receptors but only 3 variants of the T1R G protein–coupled receptors for sweet and umami. This makes sense, for while there are many different molecules that are poisonous, there are only a few different carbohydrates that are biologically important to humans.

Umami

Umami is a savory taste that is elicited by the amino acid glutamate that is found naturally in meat, aged cheeses, and tomatoes. In its salt form, glutamate is the flavor enhancer monosodium glutamate, or MSG. There was controversy about the safety of MSG, but the consensus today is that aside from a few sensitive people, MSG is safe.

Salty

Saltiness is the taste elicited by salts, which are molecules made up of oppositely charged particles. Table salt, or sodium chloride (NaCl), dissolves into positive and negative ions, Na^+ and Cl^-. Sodium ions enter taste cells through sodium ion channels and depolarize the taste cells, causing them to transduce a signal to the afferent nerve fiber.

Sour

Sour is the taste of acid, such as hydrogen chloride (HCl) or organic acids, like lactic and citric acids. Sour foods include many citrus fruits, vinegar, yogurt, and spoiled dairy (cheese and sour cream). Acids release hydrogen ions (H^+) that interact with ion channels on taste cells and depolarize them. The exact mechanisms of H^+ detection, however, are not completely understood.

Emma Boxer

See also: Bitter Sensation; Chorda Tympani Nerve; Cranial Nerves; Facial Nerve; G Proteins; Glossopharyngeal Nerve; Interrelatedness of Taste and Smell; Salty Sensation; Sensory Receptors; Sour Sensation; Sweet Sensation; Taste Bud; Trigeminal Nerve; Umami; Vagus Nerve

Further Reading

Bartoshuk, Linda M., & Derek J. Snyder. (2013). Taste. In D. W. Pfaff (Ed.), *Neuroscience in the 21st century, from basic to clinical* (pp. 781–813). New York, NY: Springer Science+Business Media.

Mueller, Ken L., Mark A. Hoon, Isolde Erlenbach, Jayaram Chandrashekar, Charles S. Zuker, & Nicholas J. Ryba. (2005). The receptors and coding logic for bitter taste. *Nature, 434*, 225–229.

Yarmolinsky, David A., Charles S. Zuker, & Nicholas J. Ryba. (2009). Common sense about taste: From mammals to insects. *Cell, 139*(2), 234–244.

TEMPERATURE SENSE: *See* Thermal Sense

THALAMUS

Within the brain, there are a few deep structures that are essential for normal brain functioning. One of these structures is the thalamus, which is located on the midline of the brain and consists of two symmetrical halves. The word *thalamus* is derived from Greek, meaning "chamber" or "inner room," as it receives almost all sensory and motor information. Thus, the thalamus is generally believed to act as a relay station between a variety of subcortical areas and the cerebral cortex.

Anatomy and Physiology

There are three main parts of the diencephalon: the hypothalamus, the sub-thalamus, and the thalamus. All three of these structures work closely together as a nuclear complex in many different bodily functions. The hypothalamus controls temperature, hunger, thirst, fear, anger, and the pituitary gland. The hypothalamus acts with the portion of the reticular system in the midbrain to keep the brain alert and awake. The subthalamus acts like a train depot; it carries impulses from the basal nuclei to the thalamus, and then to the hypothalamus. It is important for transporting and modulating neural impulses used for coordinating movements. Finally, the thalamus is a center that delivers or relays sensory impulses to the surface of the cerebrum, such as impulses from the cerebellum to the cerebral cortex. The thalamus provides input about ongoing movement to the motor areas of the cerebral cortex. It also contains a special part of the reticular system that helps coordinate sensory messages and helps regulate the activity of the brain.

Overall, the thalamus is the main part of the diencephalon and is the regulation of consciousness, sleep, and alertness. It is found at the most superior portion of the brainstem, near the center of the brain. It is highly connected by fiber tracts that bind it to the overlying cerebral cortex. The thalamus is about the size and shape of a walnut and is located obliquely and symmetrical on each side of the third ventricle. There are two thalami, one in each brain hemisphere, and the superior medial surface of each thalamus makes up the lateral walls of the third ventricle. The thalami are also connected to each other on the midline by the inter-thalamic adhesion.

Thalamic Nuclei

The thalamus consists of six functionally distinct nuclei, which are the lateral (ventral and dorsal tiers), medial, anterior, intralaminar, midline, and reticular nuclei. The lateral, medial, and anterior groups are named by their location relative to a large collection of axons called the internal medullary lamina. The system of lamellae is made up of myelinated fibers that separate the different subparts of the thalamus. The intralaminar, midline, and reticular groups are considered nonspecific thalamic nuclei.

The lateral nuclei are further divided into two tiers: the ventral and dorsal. The ventral tier of the lateral nucleus is further divided into six nuclei, which are named for their location within the ventral tier. These consist of relay neurons that receive limited sensory and motor input and project this information to specific sensory and motor cortical regions. The dorsal tier of the lateral thalamus and the medial group project to association cortices and thus are both considered association nuclei. The anterior group receives specific neuronal impulses and relays this information to the hypothalamus and the cingulate gyrus of the cerebral cortex. The intralaminar group is made up of a cluster of nuclei that are intermixed within the internal medullary lamina. The reticular group is found on the lateral aspect of the thalamus, and the midline group is located on the dorsal wall of the third ventricle.

Connections and Functions

Because of how integrated the thalamus is in almost all neurological functions, there are several connections and functions that are involved with these structures. An easy way to understand this is first by grouping the thalamic functions and then identifying the responsible connections. The functions are grouped by limbic, motor, somatic sensation, hearing, and vision. For limbic functions, which include emotional expression, the main inputs are from the mammillary body of the hypothalamus, the cingulate gyrus, the amygdala, the hypothalamus, and the reticular formation of the brainstem. The output fibers for limbic function terminate in the cingulate gyrus, the prefrontal cortex, and the basal forebrain.

Motor information is brought to the thalamus by the globus pallidus of the basal nuclei and the dentate nucleus of the cerebellum. The major output for motor function ends in the premotor and the motor cortices. This helps modulate ongoing movement and sends this appropriate information to the motor areas of the cortex. Sensory information of the body is received from the dorsal column and medial lemniscal pathways from the spinal cord as well as the sensory nuclei of cranial nerve V. This sensory information is then relayed to the somatosensory cortex. Research studies have shown that the somatosensory cortex and its association cortices also project back to the thalamus to further integrate sensory information. This information is then projected to the temporal, parietal, and occipital lobes.

Neurons involved with hearing project to the thalamus via the inferior colliculus. The thalamus then modulates these signals and sends them to the primary auditory cortex within the temporal lobe. Vision is transferred to the thalamus via the retinal ganglion axons that make up the optic nerve and the optic tract. The thalamus then modulates these signals and sends them to the primary visual cortex within the occipital lobe. Finally, studies have also shown that the thalamus modulates its own activity. This is done through the reticular nucleus. It receives information from the cerebral cortex and the other thalamic nuclei and projects this information after modulation of the signal back out to the remaining thalamic nuclei.

Patricia A. Bloomquist

See also: Auditory System; Brain Anatomy; Discriminative Touch; Nociception; Olfactory System; Sensory Receptors; Somatosensory Cortex; Somatosensory System; Touch; Visual System

Further Reading

Hebb, Adam O., & George A. Ojemann. (2013). The thalamus and language revisited. *Brain and Language, 126*(1), 99–108.

Jones, Edward G. (2003). History of neuroscience: The thalamus. In *IBRO history of neuro-science*. Retrieved from http://ibro.info/wp-content/uploads/2012/12/The-Thalamus.pdf

THERMAL SENSE (TEMPERATURE SENSATION)

Temperature for living organisms is essential to maintain health and homeostasis (physiological balance within the body). Animals, and particularly humans, have the ability to sense heat and cold from the environment around them, which allows them to respond in an appropriate manner. Furthermore, the brain helps maintain the animal's core temperature so that the body can protect itself during extreme temperature situations. In animals, temperature and pain sensations travel together in the nervous system. Specifically, these sensations are mediated by the same fiber types within the peripheral nervous system, travel in the spinal cord within the same pathway, and are perceived within the somatosensory cortex (postcentral gyrus of the brain). Regulation of body temperature is mediated by the hypothalamus, a deep brain structure located below the thalamus.

Anatomy and Physiology

The body's sensory systems deal with temperature information being delivered to the nervous system by neurons that have special receptors for temperature stimuli that are generally not too painful, not too hot, and not too cold. These receptors are called thermoreceptors, which are free nerve endings found throughout the skin, the cornea (the covering of the eye), and the bladder. There are two fiber types used to sense temperature: C-fibers and A delta fibers. C-fibers are usually unmyelinated, meaning they lack a covering of insulation (myelin, produced by Schwann cells) around their axons. Thus, nerve impulses (action potentials) do not travel as fast in these types of fibers. A delta fibers are lightly myelinated, meaning they have a covering of insulation around their axons, allowing action potentials to travel quicker. For warm temperatures between 32° and 48°C (or 90° and 118°F), C-fibers will increase their firing rate of action potentials in response to being warmed. For cool or cold temperatures between 10° and 30°C (or 50° and 86°F), both C-fibers and A delta fibers are activated. Specifically, the C-fibers reduce their firing of action potentials when cooled, while A delta fibers increase their firing rate of action potentials. Nociceptors (pain receptors) can act as thermoreceptors to determine pain from temperature, such as when a person burns his hand. Additionally, nociceptors are activated as thermoreceptors when temperatures are too cold and cause pain.

Temperature signals travel within the C-fibers and A delta fibers to the spinal cord where they synapse on to neurons located in the dorsal horn. These neurons then project some of their axons to the same side (ipsilateral) and the majority of their axons to the opposite side (contralateral) of the spinal cord where they join the anterolateral system, the second major ascending (afferent) pathway that ends in the somatosensory cortex. Because temperature and pain information travel on both sides of the spinal cord, it acts as a backup system so if part of the spinal cord is damaged, not all temperature and pain sensation is lost. For the head and face, temperature information travels through cranial nerve V (trigeminal nerve), synapses in the trigeminal nucleus in the brainstem, and then terminates in the somatosensory cortex.

A body's core temperature is regulated by the hypothalamus in response to peripheral and central input. The set point for human body temperature ranges from 36.4° to 37.2°C (or 97.5° to 99°F) and is called *normothermia*. Temperature regulation works by a feedback system that detects changes between peripheral thermoreceptors in the skin, spinal cord, and viscera, and central thermoreceptors in the anterior section of the hypothalamus. The central thermoreceptors in the hypothalamus change their firing rate based on the temperature of the blood or their local temperature. The hypothalamus then integrates temperature information from the autonomic nervous system, endocrine system, and skeletal muscles to determine if the core temperature is too hot (hyperthermia) and sweating needs to begin to cool down the body, or if the core temperature is too cold (hypothermia) and shivering needs to begin to burn energy and make body heat.

Jennifer L. Hellier

See also: Free Nerve Endings; Nociception; Sensory Receptors; Somatosensory Cortex; Somatosensory System; Thermoreceptors

Further Reading

Kambiz, S., L. S. Duraku, J. C. Holstege, S. E. Hovius, T. J. Ruigrok, & E. T. Walbeehm. (2014). Thermo-sensitive TRP channels in peripheral nerve injury: A review of their role in cold intolerance. *Journal of Plastic, Reconstructive, and Aesthetic Surgery, 67*(5), 591–599.

Kandel, Eric R., James H. Schwartz, Thomas M. Jessell, Steven A. Siegelbaum, & A. J. Hudspeth (Eds.). (2012). *Principles of neural science* (5th ed.). New York, NY: McGraw-Hill.

Purves, Dale, et al. (2008). *Neuroscience* (4th ed.). Sunderland, MA: Sinauer Associates.

THERMORECEPTORS

Thermoreceptors are a class of receptors responsible for thermal sensation, which stems from the relationship between the amount of heat produced by the organism's metabolism and the amount of heat expelled to the environment by that organism. These specialized cells are activated by temperature changes. A signal is then sent to the nervous system via an action potential. Different temperature thresholds trigger different classes of thermoreceptors to fire action potentials (Schepers & Ringkamp, 2009). An action potential is a signal relayed from the

Temperature Test

Temperature for living organisms is essential to maintain health and homeostasis (physiological balance within the body). Animals, and particularly humans, have the ability to sense heat and cold from the environment around them, which allows them to respond in an appropriate manner. Furthermore, the brain helps maintain the animal's core temperature so that the body can protect itself during extreme temperature situations. In animals, temperature and pain sensations travel together in the nervous system. Specifically, these sensations are mediated by the same fiber types within the peripheral nervous system, travel in the spinal cord within the same pathway, and are perceived within the somatosensory cortex (postcentral gyrus of the brain). Regulation of body temperature is mediated by the hypothalamus, a deep brain structure located below the thalamus.

Materials:

Volunteer
Tuning fork (can be purchased on Amazon.com) or other metallic instrument
Thermometer
Cold water or ice
Cup

Directions:

Skin temperature test: Use a tuning fork or other metallic instrument to test a person's ability to feel a cold sensation on the skin. *Never use heat to test temperature as it can be too hot and burn the person.* Place the tuning fork in a cup of cold or ice water for a few minutes. The metal is a good conductor of temperature and will cool down quickly. Ask the person to close their eyes and tell you when they feel a change in temperature on the skin. Place the cooled tuning fork gently on their right forearm and ask them if they feel a cold sensation. Move the cooled instrument to the person's upper right arm and ask them if they feel a cold sensation. Repeat this same test with the remaining extremities (left arm and both legs).

    Core temperature test: This test is what most people think of when talking about testing temperature and is generally taken at each health care visit. To take a person's temperature, use the thermometer as recommended by the manufacturer. Today, the most common thermometers are the instant-read type and can be used in the ear canal (tympanic) or along the forehead (temporal) to measure temperature. Normal readings are around 98.6°F (37°C), while temperatures above 100°F (37.8°C) are considered to be a fever. If you do not have a thermometer, you can use the back of your hand or your lips to test for a fever on the person's forehead or the back of his or her neck. Note that the back of the hand and lips are more sensitive to temperature than the palm of the hand. Determine if the person's forehead or neck is warmer than normal. Do not feel the person's hands or feet as often the extremities will feel cool when there is a fever.

Jennifer L. Hellier

thermoreceptor down the axons and to the central nervous system, which will then respond with an action accordingly. These receptors are important for an organism's survival because they are crucial for maintaining homeostatic temperature.

Function of Thermoreceptors

Thermoreceptors essentially function as the thermostat of a living organism. Most organisms lose their enzymatic function if they are exposed to temperatures outside their homeostatic temperature range, which can have lethal effects for the organism. Early research suggests that some organisms such as humans and primates have the ability to perform thermal adaptation after prolonged exposure to nonhomeostatic temperatures (McCleskey, 1997). Thermal adaptation suggests that thermoreceptors are still firing action potentials, but they do so in a decreased intensity because they are desensitized to their stimuli—the threshold temperature. The organism at this point will experience diminishing thermosensation and feel that it is less hot or less cold. Although the autonomous nervous system can adjust internal temperatures to a certain extent, thermal adaptation essentially silences the temperature alarms of the body. It does not necessarily mean the organism is out of danger in extreme conditions.

Anatomy and Physiology

Thermoreceptors are divided into two categories: peripheral thermoreceptors and central thermoreceptors. Peripheral thermoreceptors are located on the skin and mucous membranes. These are the first detectors of temperature changes outside (external environment) of the organism. Peripheral receptors are divided into two classes: cold receptors and hot receptors. Different temperature thresholds trigger them. In humans, the homeostatic temperature is 37°C. Cold receptors will fire action potentials when the skin is exposed to a temperature of 25°C (Schepers & Ringkamp, 2009). As temperatures continue dropping and/or as exposure to cold is prolonged, cold receptors will eventually stop firing. Hot receptors will fire an action potential when the skin is exposed to 30°C or warmer. This is technically still below homeostatic internal temperature, but hot receptors are thought to fire action potentials not only to sense hot, but also warm temperatures (McCleskey, 1997).

A different set of receptors called thermal nociceptors are activated when temperatures are so extreme that they begin to cause pain. These receptors alert the body to immediate danger. These receptors are technical pain receptors. Current research indicates that the thresholds for thermal nociceptors are far beyond those of hot or cold thermoreceptors. In these extreme cases, hot and cold thermoreceptors will no longer actively fire action potentials.

All information captured by thermoreceptors is then quickly relayed to the central thermoreceptors. Central thermoreceptors are mainly located in the anterior hypothalamus. The central thermoreceptors are responsible for responding by activating the autonomic nervous system (sympathetic nervous system) as well as communicating with the cerebral cortex. The cerebral cortex will activate a voluntary response that involves the organism consciously making a choice to react to the situation, such as to put on a jacket if the person is cold. The autonomic nervous system's response to a dropping core temperature can include vasoconstriction of the cutaneous blood vessels, neurotransmitter production such as epinephrine, and also production of hormones such as thyroid-stimulating hormone. The response to rising core temperature includes vasodilation of the cutaneous blood vessels and acetylcholine production, which activates sweat glands.

Disease and Disorders

Since thermoreceptors are the primary messengers of thermosensation, defects in these structures will inhibit the signaling pathway. This will prevent the organism from being able to feel changing temperatures. A genetic mutation in the coding region of these receptors may cause a genetic defect in which the organism can no longer sense hot or cold. Trauma and burns can also cause nerve damage and impair thermoreceptor function.

Melissa Tjandra

See also: Free Nerve Endings; Nociception; Nociceptors; Sensory Receptors; Thermal Sense

Further Reading

McCleskey, Edwin W. (1997). Thermoreceptors: Recent heat in thermosensation. *Current Biology, 7*(11), R679–R681.

Schepers, Raf J., & Matthias Ringkamp. (2009).Thermoreceptors and thermosensitive afferents. *Neuroscience and Biobehavioral Reviews, 33*(3), 205–211. Retrieved from http://www.sciencedirect.com/science/article/pii/S0149763408001206?np=y

THIRST

Thirst is the craving for fluids, which results in the basic instinct of animals to drink. Drinking is an essential mechanism that is involved in fluid balance. Thirst comes from the lack of fluids or an increase in the concentration of certain osmolytes, like salt (sodium, potassium, and chloride). Dehydration can cause many problems and is associated with disorders including but not limited to renal (kidney) problems and neurological problems, such as blurry vision and seizures. Excessive thirst, or polydipsia, could be an indication of diabetes. Receptors in the body are able to detect a decreased volume of osmolytes or an increased concentration of osmolytes. The central nervous system is then signaled to identify this change in the body, resulting in producing the desire to drink to remedy the problem.

Detection Methods

There are multiple detection methods of thirst including but not limited to (1) decreased blood volume, (2) the renin-angiotensin system, and (3) arterial baroreceptors. Hypovolemia (decreased blood volume) results from excessive blood loss, vomiting, and/or diarrhea. If the blood volume falls too low, then the heart will not be able to pump and circulate blood effectively. This will eventually result in heart failure. Loss of blood volume is detected by the kidneys and triggers the renin-angiotensin system. This system secretes an enzyme called renin into the blood stream when the kidneys detect low blood volume. Renin enters the blood and catalyzes angiotensinogen to angiotensin I, which is almost immediately converted to angiotensin II. Traveling through the blood until it reaches the posterior pituitary gland and the adrenal cortex, angiotensin II causes a cascade of hormones, causing the kidneys to retain more water and sodium to increase blood pressure and therefore blood volume.

Causes

The major cause of thirst is dehydration. When your body does not have enough water to carry out normal tasks, and thirst is the main symptom, you are already dehydrated. Dehydration can be caused by a number of factors including but not limited to exercise, diarrhea, vomiting, and too much sweating. Signs of dehydration include dry mouth, thirst, dry skin, and headaches.

Another cause of thirst is diabetes. Diabetes is a disease in which your body does not make enough insulin or is not able to use insulin properly. This results in increased sugar in the bloodstream. The kidneys excrete some of the excess sugar into the bladder for release with urination. However, due to the increased concentration of sugar in the bladder, more water is drawn in to dilute the sugar. Thus, persons with diabetes urinate more often, resulting in losing more water.

Thirst will cause dry mouth, a condition called xerostomia. With dry mouth, the salivatory glands are not able to produce as much saliva and therefore a person will feel thirsty all the time. Severe decreases in salivation can result in tooth decay and gum disease. Anemia is another condition in which your body does not have enough healthy red blood cells. Severe anemia can result in thirst.

Treatments

The first and foremost treatment for thirst is to drink more water. In the past, it was suggested that each person drink eight cups or 64 ounces of water daily. However, new research shows that to maintain hydration, a person should drink half of his or her weight in ounces of water. For example, a 150-pound person should drink at least 75 ounces of water each day. If that person is also exercising, then he or she should drink even more water each day. If drinking more water does not satisfy the craving of thirst, then the next step is to seek medical care. There could be an underlying condition or a side effect of medication causing thirst.

Renee Johnson

See also: Baroreceptors; Hunger; Visceral Sensation

Further Reading

Institute of Medicine. (2005). *Dietary reference intakes for water, potassium, sodium, chloride, and sulfate*. Washington, DC: National Academies Press. http://dx.doi.org/10.17226/10925.

Mayo Clinic. (2015). Disease and conditions: Dry mouth. Retrieved from http://www.mayoclinic.org/diseases-conditions/dry-mouth/basics/complications/con-20035499

Stanhewicz, Anna E., & W. Larry Kenney. (2015). Determinants of water and sodium intake and output. *Nutrition reviews*, 73(2), 73–82. http://dx.doi.org/10.1093/nutrit/nuv033

3D MOVIES AND TECHNOLOGY

A three-dimensional (3D) stereoscopic film enhances the illusion of depth perception, thereby adding a 3D effect. Stereoscopic photography is the most common approach in the production of 3D films. With stereoscopic photography, a regular motion picture camera is used and images are recorded in two different perspectives. Special projection hardware/eyewear must be used to view the depth illusion while watching the film. The 3D illusion is not limited to just theatrical films; it has also been used in television broadcasts, especially since the increase in 3D televisions and Blu-ray 3D movies.

History

The stereoscopic era of motion began in the 1890s, patented by William Friese-Greene (1855–1921), a British film pioneer. Two films were viewed side by side and the viewer had to look through a stereoscope to combine the two images to get the 3D look. Theatrical use was not practical with this mechanism. In 1900, Frederic Eugene Ives (1856–1937) patented a stereo camera rig, which had two lenses coupled together and were 1¾ inches apart. In 1915, Edwin S. Porter (1870–1941) and William E. Waddell tested the 3D idea with an audience in New York City. After the tests, nothing was produced in a 3D version.

3D movies have existed since 1915 but were largely relegated to a place in the motion picture industry. This was due to the costly hardware and processes required to make the depth illusion stand out. It was also due to the lack of standardized formats for all of the segments of entertainment businesses. The earliest 3D film to be shown was *The Power of Love* in 1922 due to the camera rig produced by film producer Harry Fairall. This was also the earliest film in which red/green anaglyph glasses were used. A large increase in 3D films began in the 1950s in American cinemas, and later in the 1980s and 1990s in IMAX high-end theaters and Disney-themed venues. 3D films became more and more successful throughout the 2000s with movies including but not limited to *Ghosts of the Abyss* (2003), *The Adventures of Sharkboy and Lavagirl* (2005), *Open Season* (2006), *Scar 3D* (2007), *Bolt* (2008), and *The Final Destination* (2009), and with the unprecedented success in December 2009 and January 2010 of *Avatar*. The film *Scar 3D* was the first 3D video-on-demand released through major cable broadcasters in 2010.

In 2011, there was an audience decline in 3D film interest as *Harry Potter and the Deathly Hallows—Part 2* and *Captain America: The First Avenger* were the major releases on their opening weekend and ran opposite to *Kung Fu Panda 2* in 3D and *Cars 2* in 3D. Forty-seven 3D movies were released in 2011; however, box office profits were down 18 percent from 2010.

Anaglyph Method

The anaglyph method was the first method used in presenting theatrical 3D films. Two images are superimposed in an additive light setting with two filters: red and cyan. The glasses with two different color filters for each eye separate the images by cancelling the filter color out and rendering the complementary color black. Anaglyph images are much easier to see than viewing parallel or crossed eye stereograms.

Polarization Method

The viewer wears polarized lenses, which are oriented differently, usually at 45 and 135 degrees with linear polarization or clockwise/counterclockwise with circular polarization. Each filter passes only light that is similarly polarized and blocks all other light. Circular polarization is slightly more advantageous than linear polarization as viewers do not need to hold their heads upright and aligned with the screen to allow the polarization to work properly. Polarized stereoscopic pictures have been around since 1936 and from 1952 to 1955, 3D movies were offered almost entirely with linear polarizing lenses. The polarization method was also used in the revival of 3D movies in the 1980s.

Health Effects

Some viewers complain of headaches and eyestrain after watching 3D movies. Motion sickness is also more easily introduced during the viewing of 3D films. A published study has shown that of those who watch 3D films, about 55 percent experience various levels of headaches, nausea, and disorientation. Two primary effects caused by 3D films that are unnatural to the human eye are crosstalk between the eyes (imperfect image separation) and the mismatch between convergence and accommodation (inability to see an object's position—making the person question, is it behind or in front of the scene?).

Renee Johnson

See also: Accommodation; Color Perception; Visual Perception

Further Reading

The Eyecare Trust. (n.d.). 3D Vision. Retrieved from http://www.eyecaretrust.org.uk/view.php?item_id=566

Gray, Brandon. (2011). June sees box office dip. *Box Office Mojo.* Retrieved from http://www.boxofficemojo.com/news/?id=3201&p=.htm

Variety. (2015). Filmmakers like S3D's emotional wallop. Retrieved from http://variety.com/2009/digital/features/filmmakers-like-s3d-s-emotional-wallop-1118008671/

TINNITUS

Tinnitus is defined by *Webster's Dictionary* as "a sensation of noise (as a ringing or roaring) that is caused by a bodily condition (as a disturbance of the auditory nerve or wax in the ear) and typically is of the subjective form which can only be heard by the one affected" (http://www.merriam-webster.com/dictionary/tinnitus). It has been reported that more than 50 million Americans have experienced tinnitus at some point in their lives, and today 1 in 5 people have symptoms of tinnitus that impact their lives in a negative way. Tinnitus can be either intermittent or constant and in one ear or both.

Symptoms, Causes, and Etiology

Patients experiencing tinnitus often present with varying types and severity of symptoms. Tinnitus is most commonly described as a "ringing" in the ears but can also be described variably as a buzzing sound, a whining sound, a tickling sensation, or a beeping sound among many others. The symptoms of tinnitus can be constant or intermittent with hours, days, or even weeks between events. It can affect one ear or both. In addition to the typical symptoms of tinnitus, many individuals suffer from varying degrees of hearing loss as well. Particularly frustrating to many patients is the fact that tinnitus is almost always something that only the patient can hear, which makes it a very subjective disease and one that is difficult to treat.

In many cases, the cause or etiology of tinnitus is not well known or understood. Studies have been done looking at various aspects of the auditory system as well as more systemic causes in the brain or causes that may be behavioral or psychological. Some cases of tinnitus are thought to be caused by the buildup of cerumen (earwax) within the outer ear or the external auditory canal. Often if this cerumen is in direct contact with the eardrum or tympanic membrane, it can cause the symptoms of tinnitus. Infections of the middle ear as well as a more rare condition known as otosclerosis (hardening of the middle ear bones or ossicles) have also been known to cause the symptoms of tinnitus. While middle ear infections are relatively easy to treat, otosclerosis is a condition with no known treatment. Finally, tinnitus is also thought to be caused by damage or loss of the hair cells within the inner ear that are connected directly to the auditory nerve. This damage has been shown to be caused by high volume/frequency noise, some medications, and most commonly aging.

There are a wide variety of other diseases that have tinnitus as a presenting symptom. Some of the more common include Meniere's disease, Arnod-Chiari malformation, trauma/head injuries resulting in skull fractures or concussions, metabolic diseases such as thyroid dysfunction or hyperlipidemia, vitamin B_{12} deficiency, Lyme disease, and migraine headaches. Psychedelic drugs and benzodiazepine withdrawal have also been known to cause temporary symptoms of tinnitus.

Diagnosis and Treatment

Diagnosis of tinnitus is very difficult given the subjective nature of this disease. Often, physicians will begin treating the symptoms to determine if they are transient or not. If symptoms persist, diagnostic tests such as audiograms (hearing tests), CAT (computerized axial tomography) scans, or MRI (magnetic resonance imaging) scans can be done to determine if there are any physical abnormalities within the auditory system or the brain. CAT scans and MRIs are often done when a patient complains of pulsatile tinnitus or asymmetric hearing loss as both of these symptoms can be related to significant vascular issues or acoustic neuromas.

While treatment for tinnitus varies widely depending on the duration and severity of the symptoms, there are a number of common treatments used by medical professionals to try to decrease the frequency and intensity of symptoms. Some of these include the use of (1) hearing aids, which can help individuals who are also suffering from hearing loss, (2) wearable sound generators, which are small electronic devices that emit "white noise" to mask the louder tinnitus, or (3) antidepressant/antianxiety medications, which can sometimes help patients who are suffering from loss of sleep or anxiety brought on by the constant symptoms of tinnitus; and in extreme cases (4) the use of cochlear implants or acoustic neural stimulation, which can be used either to bypass the inner ear or to provide a broadband acoustic signal that offsets the tone of the tinnitus. While many of these treatments often help patients with tinnitus, to date, there is no known effective treatment to stop the symptoms of this disease completely.

Charles A. Ferguson

See also: Auditory Hallucinations; Auditory System; Auditory Threshold; Brainstem Auditory Evoked Potentials; Vestibulocochlear Nerve

Further Reading

Langguth, Berthold, Peter M. Kreuzer, Tobias Kleinjung, & Dirk De Ridder. (2013). Tinnitus: Causes and clinical management. *Lancet Neurology, 12*(9), 920–930.

Levine, Robert A., & Yahav Oron. (2015). Tinnitus. *Handbook of clinical neurology, 129*, 409–431.

National Institute on Deafness and Other Communication Disorders (NIDCD). (2014). Tinnitus. Retrieved from http://www.nidcd.nih.gov/health/hearing/pages/tinnitus.aspx

Nicolas-Puel, Cecile, Ruth Lloyd Faulconbridge, Matthieu Guitton, Jean-Luc Puel, Michel Mondain, & Alain Uziel. (2002). Characteristics of tinnitus and etiology of associated hearing loss: A study of 123 patients. *International Tinnitus Journal, 8*(1), 37–44.

TONGUE: *See* Taste System

TONOTOPIC MAP

The auditory system is a sensory system that is responsible for the sense of hearing. The ability to hear allows animals to be able to detect sounds in their surroundings without direct contact or without seeing the source of the sound. It has been suggested that different frequencies—low-pitched and high-pitched sounds—are mapped to different regions of the auditory cortex, making a tonotopic map. The tonotopic map of the human brain is a method to provide a means of creating a function map of the auditory cortex through the use of acoustic frequencies perceived by the human ear. By interpreting different frequencies, different regions of the auditory cortex increase their activity levels. This change in activity allows researchers to create a function map of the auditory cortex by mapping the specific regions that respond to numerous different frequencies. Scientific research shows that tonotopic maps in the auditory cortex are similar to the retinotopic fields that are mapped in the visual cortex.

Mechanism

Upon receiving a sound wave, an organ within the inner ear known as the organ of Corti transduces the signal of waves into an electrical signal that the brain interprets as sound. Within the organ of Corti are several specialized sensory neurons called hair cells that use mechanotransduction to detect sound waves (movement) near the ear. These hair cells line the organ of Corti across its basilar membrane, which winds throughout the spiral-shaped cochlea. The hair cells form a functional synapse with nerve fibers that make up the vestibulocochlear nerve (cranial nerve VIII). This nerve traverses the brainstem, making a pathway that synapses in the auditory cortex, which is located in the superior portion of the temporal lobe of the brain. The functionality of each of these hair cells lies in their physical layout in the organ of Corti. Specifically, the hair cells are "tuned" to progressively higher frequencies the deeper the hair cells lie. This is due to the fact that the basilar membrane varies greatly in mechanical and physical properties along its length. This difference in the tuning frequencies of the hair cells along the basilar membrane allows the inner ear to act as a sound frequency analyzer, and therefore allows researchers to use neuroimaging to create a map of functional organization within the auditory system.

Uses

Tonotopic mapping is useful in creating a functional layout of the auditory cortex of numerous model organisms and humans through the organization of frequency-dependent responses, which are suggestive of specific tonotopically organized regions of the auditory cortex. Studies have shown that the position of the functional response in the auditory cortex varies systematically with differences in frequencies encountered, as shown by functional magnetic resonance imaging (fMRI) of the auditory cortex, located in the superior surface of the temporal lobe of the brain. Through these studies, researchers have identified seven regions in the brain specific to different frequencies encountered, three regions sensitive to high frequencies, and four regions sensitive to lower frequencies. High-pitched sounds have been mapped to the anterolateral aspect of the transverse temporal gyrus (also called Heschl's gyrus), while low-pitched sounds are mapped to the lateral fissure. The lateral fissure contains the transverse temporal gyrus. Thus, there are multiple tonotopically organized brain regions in humans. Based on these imaging studies, in which they compare differences in anatomical areas and frequency progressions, researchers are able to hypothesize as to the different functional regions within the human auditory cortex.

Gage Williamson

See also: Age-Related Hearing Loss; Auditory Processing Disorder; Auditory System; Brainstem Auditory Evoked Potentials; Deafness; Sensory Receptors; Vestibulocochlear Nerve

Further Reading

Gray, Lincoln. (2015). Auditory system: Structure and function. In John H. Byrne (Ed.), *Neuroscience Online, an electronic textbook for the neurosciences* (Chap. 12). Retrieved from http://neuroscience.uth.tmc.edu/s2/chapter12.html

Langers, Dave R. M., & Pim Van Dijk. (2012). Mapping the tonotopic organization in human auditory cortex with minimally salient acoustic stimulation. *Cerebral Cortex, 22*(9), 2024–2038.

Saenz, Melissa, & Dave R. M. Langers. (2014). Tonotopic mapping of human auditory cortex. *Hearing Research, 307,* 42–52. http://dx.doi.org/10.1016/j.heares.2013.07.016

Talavage, Thomas M., Martin I. Sereno, Jennifer R. Melcher, Patrick J. Ledden, Bruce R. Rosen, & Anders M. Dale. (2004). Tonotopic organization in human auditory cortex revealed by progressions of frequency sensitivity. *Journal of Neurophysiology, 91*(3), 1282–1296.

TOUCH

In mammals and particularly in humans, touch is the oldest, most primitive, and pervasive sense. In the uterus as early as eight weeks of gestation, touch is the first of the five sensory systems to develop and respond to stimulation. Additionally, it is the first sense humans experience as infants. Touch helps babies to grow and bond with mothers, fathers, and other caregivers, while helping animals and humans to learn about the world around them. Touch also plays an integral role in biological, cognitive, and social development. It is the physical contact of the somatosensory system to the outside world. It allows people to learn shapes and hardness of objects.

There are several million points on the human body that register cold, heat, pain, or touch. These points that register the four basic cutaneous senses are mapped within the central nervous system to the somatosensory cortex, or the postcentral gyrus. Thus, touching an object can give the feeling of warmth, cold, pain, and pressure, and that information is sent to the brain for processing. There are many kinds of touch organs, called tactile corpuscles, in the skin and mucous membranes. These touch organs are found everywhere on and within the skin: near hair, in hairless areas (like the palm and fingertips), and in deeper tissues.

Anatomy and Physiology

The somatosensory system mediates many sensations received by the skin and body. Specifically for touch, it includes crude touch—with itch and tickle—and discriminative touch. Together these modalities make up haptic perception. The term *haptic* is derived from Greek, meaning "to touch." Thus haptic perception integrates somatosensory information in recognizing objects. Texture, hardness, and temperature are material properties that are mediated through touch. It is also important to note that touch and proprioception are integrated sensations as they transmit their signals to the brain via the same pathway within the spinal cord and brainstem.

Touch is a peripheral nervous system function that transmits its information to the central nervous system. This means that the cell bodies of the neurons live in the dorsal root ganglion and the axon divides into a peripheral axon and a central axon. The peripheral axon ends in the joint, muscle, skin, or tendon while the central axon ends in the spinal cord of the central nervous system. The skin is the main touch receptor organ while joint, muscle, and tendon tissues are used in proprioception. The sensations of touch are represented by neurons that exhibit modality specificity. Modality specificity occurs when a somatosensory neuron is stimulated, which results in a perceived sensation that is specific to the information processed by the neuron.

Crude versus Discriminative Touch

The skin identifies two types of touch: crude (least sensitive) and discriminative (most sensitive) touch. The form of touch where localization is not possible is called crude touch. Crude touch or nondiscriminative touch is a sensory modality that allows the body to sense that something has touched it, without being able to localize exactly where the body was touched. For example, if a person were touched five inches below the left shoulder, the person would say he or she was touched on the back on the left side, but would not be able to give the exact location. Fine touch, then, is able to localize where the body was touched. Fine and crude touch do work in parallel, meaning a person will be able to localize touch until fibers carrying fine touch have been disrupted. When that happens, the body will feel the sensation, but will be unable to identify the exact location where it was touched.

The sensation of touch begins when an object comes in contact with the sense organ and presses it out of shape, or touches a nearby hair. The sense of touch is more sensitive in some parts of the body compared to other parts. The lips, tongue, fingers, feet, and genitals are the most sensitive. The least sensitive is the back. The reason for the difference is due to the fact that the end organs for touch are not scattered evenly over the body, but instead are arranged in clusters. This keenness of touch can easily be measured by an esthesiometer. This instrument looks like a drawing compass with two needlepoints. The tip of the tongue can feel both points when they are 1 millimeter apart. Less sensitive areas feel only one point at this distance. The back of the shoulders feels two points when the points are more than 60 millimeters apart. These differences show that certain body regions respond only to crude or fine touch. The nervous tissues from the sense organs then carry the sensation or nerve impulses to the brain.

Patricia A. Bloomquist

See also: Discriminative Touch; Homunculus; Mechanoreceptors; Sensory Receptors; Somatosensory Cortex; Somatosensory System

Further Reading
Dougherty, Patrick, & Chieyeko Tsuchitani. (1997). Somatosensory systems. In *Neuroscience Online, an electronic textbook for the neurosciences* (Chap. 2). Retrieved from http://neuroscience.uth.tmc.edu/s2/chapter02.html
Gibson, James J. (1962). Observations on active touch. *Psychological Review, 69*(6), 477–491.
Klatzky, Roberta L., & Susan J. Lederman. (2002). Touch. In A. F. Healy & R. W. Proctor (Eds.), *Experimental psychology* (pp. 147–176). Volume 4 in I. B. Weiner (Editor-in-Chief), *Handbook of Psychology.* New York, NY: Wiley.

TRIGEMINAL NERVE
The trigeminal nerve (CN V) is the fifth of 12 pairs of cranial nerves. It carries primarily somatosensory (temperature, pressure, and pain) information of the head and face, but also some motor information to the front third of the head. The nerve

is named three (*tri-*) twins (*-geminus*) in Latin after its three major branches. Because of these distinct branches, each division is named after the region it innervates. Specifically, the branches are named ophthalmic (V_1), maxillary (V_2), and mandibular (V_3). The trigeminal nerve is one of the three largest and thickest cranial nerves in mammals, the others being the optic (for vision) and vagus (for autonomic function for the gut, heart, and lungs).

The ophthalmic branch is mostly composed of sensory fibers and innervates the top half of the face, the cornea, tear duct, and part of the nasal cavity. The maxillary branch is also primarily composed of sensory fibers and innervates the nasal cavity and the upper jaw, including the roof of the mouth. The mandibular branch contains both sensory and motor fibers. The sensory fibers of the mandibular branch innervate the lower jaw, lips, tongue, and cheeks. The motor fibers of the mandibular branch innervate the muscles of the jaw responsible for chewing. Sensory trigeminal fibers originate in the trigeminal (or Gasserian) ganglia that are found in a depression in the bottom of the cranial cavity.

Chemesthesis

Chemesthesis is the stimulation of the somatosensory system by chemicals rather than by tactile stimulus. Most somatosensory nerves are protected from chemicals by a layer of keratinized skin. However, the trigeminal nerve innervates mucus membranes, which are not so protected, allowing for the stimulation of trigeminal nerve fibers. Chemesthetic chemicals are commonly used in cooking as spices. For example, capsaicin, a chemical found in chili peppers, stimulates temperature-sensitive pain fibers, creating the sensation of heat. Other spices that contain chemicals that stimulate the somatosensory system are garlic, basil, and mint. In the nasal cavity, chemesthetic stimulation is generally considered painful and results in reflexive changes in respiration rate to protect the airway. It is common for the sensations of chemesthesis and taste or smell to be confused with each other, but they are all distinct sensory modalities, mediated by entirely different cranial nerves.

Trigeminal Neuralgia

Trigeminal neuralgia is a pathological condition typified by reoccurring facial pain. The pain can occur unilaterally or bilaterally and is typically described as burning or stabbing. The sensation usually reoccurs in the same region of the face but has been reported to spread from the original location as time with the condition passes. In some cases, trigeminal neuralgia is caused by compression of the nerve by a tumor, cyst, or aneurysm. In these cases, treatment of the underlying condition can provide relief. However, in many cases, the exact cause of trigeminal neuralgia can be idiopathic, meaning the exact cause of the condition cannot be determined.

Speculative causes of this disease have included tension placed on the trigeminal nerve at points where it exits the skull, compression of trigeminal ganglia due to anomalies in local circulation, and demyelination of the nerve root. The demyelination hypothesis is supported by the occurrence of trigeminal neuralgia in many individuals with multiple sclerosis. Initial treatments for trigeminal neuralgia usually focus on alleviating the pain with a combination of narcotics, anti-inflammatories, and steroids. Anticonvulsants have been successfully used to prevent bouts of pain, but these treatments generally become less effective over time. Surgically relieving the vasculature pressure on the trigeminal ganglia can relieve the pain in some situations. In extreme cases, cutting the trigeminal ganglion or nerve can bring relief, but it carries the risk of significant side effects, including permanent facial numbness or paralyzation (complete loss of muscle function) of the muscles of mastication. This means that patients with such complications may not be able to chew on the side of mouth where the cut was made.

C. J. Saunders

See also: Central Nervous System; Cranial Nerves; Nerves; Somatosensory Cortex; Somatosensory System

Further Reading

Bryant, Bruce P., & Wayne L. Silver. (2000). Chemesthesis: The common chemical sense. In T. E. Finger, W. Silver, and D. Restrepo (Eds.), *Neurobiology of taste and smell* (pp. 73–100). New York: Wiley-Liss.

Prasad, Sashank, & Steven Galetta. (2009). Trigeminal neuralgia: Historical notes and current concepts. *Neurologist, 15*(2), 87–94.

Silver, Wayne L., Phillip Roe, & Cecil J. Saunders. (2010). Functional neuroanatomy of the upper airway in experimental animals. In J. B. Morris and D. Shusterman (Eds.), *Toxicology of the nose and upper airways* (pp. 45–64). New York, NY: Informa Healthcare.

Tizzano, Marco, Brian D. Gulbransen, Aurelie Vandenbeuch, Tod R. Clapp, Jake P. Herman, Hiruy M. Sibhatu, . . . Thomas E. Finger. (2010). Nasal chemosensory cells use bitter taste signaling to detect irritants and bacterial signals. *Proceedings of the National Academy of Sciences USA, 107,* 3210–3215.

TUNNEL VISION

Vision occurs when light from all angles of the visual fields hit the retina, the photosensitive lining of the back of the eye. However, in some cases the light from the periphery (the sides) is not seen, resulting in tunnel vision. Specifically, tunnel vision is a visual field defect where peripheral (side) vision is lost while keeping visual acuity in the central regions. If the peripheral vision is slowly lost over a period of time, a person may not realize that he or she has tunnel vision. That is why it is important to have vision checked every year by an optometrist or ophthalmologist. Glaucoma is one of the many causes of tunnel vision, which becomes more prevalent in persons over the age of 40. Glaucoma is a severe condition that can lead to blindness if left untreated.

Causes, Signs, and Symptoms

Tunnel vision can be a result of damage to the optic nerve (cranial nerve II, which is the primary nerve used for sight and connects the eyes to the brain), the retina, or the occipital lobe (part of the brain that processes visual input). When the damage is to the optic nerve it is called optic neuropathy. A specific type of optic neuropathy is optic neuritis, which is the inflammation of the optic nerve. It can occur at any length of the optic nerve and its cause is unknown. Scientists have suggested that optic neuritis may be a type of autoimmune disorder, where the body's immune system abnormally attacks itself.

Other noninflammatory causes of optic neuropathy may include glaucoma, which is associated with increased pressure within the eye; reduced blood flow to the eye; neurological diseases such as diabetes; tumors along the optic nerve; deficiencies in nutrition; and excessive tobacco or alcohol use, just to list a few. Since there are several causes of tunnel vision, this entry will only discuss the most common causes: cataracts, glaucoma, and retinitis pigmentosa (a degenerative eye disease that damages the retina).

Cataracts are a clouding of the lens within the eye. This clouding decreases normal vision as if a film were over the eye. Cataracts increase in probability as a person ages, but some infants can be born with cataracts (congenital cataracts). Cataracts are the most common cause of blindness and can be surgically corrected.

The term *glaucoma* refers to several conditions that cause damage to the optic nerve. It is a slow but steady loss of peripheral vision and can lead to blindness if not treated. The most common type of glaucoma is an abnormal increase in eye pressure, called intraocular pressure. This may happen when too much fluid is produced within the eye or if the natural drainage (outflow channels called trabecular meshwork) of this fluid is blocked. Glaucoma may also occur with normal eye pressure but there is reduced blood flow to the optic nerve. Glaucoma must be treated as soon as possible to reduce the chances of permanent blindness.

Finally, retinitis pigmentosa is a rare degenerative disease that is first identified when a person complains of night blindness. This tends to be followed by several years or even decades later of slow peripheral tunnel vision loss. This vision loss is caused by the death of photoreceptors (rods and cones) in the retina. Since these neurons are unable to regenerate, retinitis pigmentosa, an inherited disease, affects both eyes and often leads to blindness.

Treatment

It is very important to see a doctor as soon as possible if a person is experiencing tunnel vision. As in most cases, treatment for tunnel vision depends on the underlying cause. If glaucoma is detected in the early stages, medical intervention can stop the loss of peripheral vision altogether. Glaucoma is usually treated with eye drops, lasers, and/or surgery to prevent further loss of vision. Additionally, vitamin A derivatives may be beneficial in improving retinal degenerative diseases such as retinitis pigmentosa.

Patricia A. Bloomquist

See also: Optic Nerve; Retina; Visual Fields; Visual Perception; Visual System

Further Reading

Davis, Jennifer C., Heather McNeill, Michael Wasdell, Susan Chunick, & Stirling Bryan. (2012). Focusing both eyes on health outcomes: Revisiting cataract surgery. *BMC Geriatrics, 12,* 50.

National Eye Institute. (2014). Facts about retinitis pigmentosa. Retrieved from http://www.nei.nih.gov/health/pigmentosa/pigmentosa_facts.asp

Perusek, Lindsay, & Tadao Maeda. (2013). Vitamin A derivatives as treatment options for retinal degenerative diseases. *Nutrients, 5*(7), 2646–2666.

TYPE I TASTE CELLS

Taste buds are the sensory end organs of the gustatory system. They contain three basic types of cells—Type I, Type II, and Type III cells. These networks of cells allow for the detection of five distinct taste qualities: sweet, bitter, umami, salty, and sour. Type I cells are thought to play a glial-like support role in the taste bud and may participate in salt detection.

Anatomy

Type I cells are the most abundant of the three cell types—they make up approximately 50 percent of the cells in each taste bud. Unlike Types II and III cells, which are spindle-shaped, Type I cells have extensive membrane protrusions that allow them to wrap around neighboring cells in the taste bud. They extend from the base of the taste bud to the apical pore, where an opening in the tongue epithelium allows taste cells to access chemical stimuli in the oral cavity. Near the apical pore, Type I cells form "bushy" membrane structures targeted toward the pore. Type I cells are often adjacent to nerve fibers innervating the taste bud, but do not form synapse-like structures that would suggest direct chemical communication between the two cell types.

Development

Taste bud cells are continually turning over during the life of an organism. As taste cells are damaged and die, a population of renewing basal cells repopulates the taste bud with new taste cells. Type I cells renew more quickly than either Type II or Type III cells in the taste bud—they have been reported to turn over every seven days or so.

Function

In comparison with other cell types in the taste bud, relatively little is known about Type I cell function. Since Type I cells wrap around other taste cells in the taste bud, this suggests a glial-like role. Glial cells in the brain generally function as support cells for neurons, but in some cases also participate actively in signaling from one neuron to the next. They can perform many roles in the brain: some insulate axons (the wire-like parts of neurons along which electrical signals travel), others regulate blood flow in certain brain areas, still others regulate activity at synapses (the communication points between two neurons) and may provide metabolic support for adjacent neurons.

Type I cells perform another glial-like role in the taste bud. Glial cells in the brain often remove or process excess neurotransmitters released by signaling cells. Type II cells in taste buds release a small molecule, adenosine triphosphate (ATP), as a neurotransmitter, allowing them to communicate taste information to innervating nerve fibers and, ultimately, the taste centers of the brain. Type I cells express a protein on their membranes called NTPDase (ecto-nucleoside triphosphate diphosphohydrolase), which "chews up" extra ATP in the taste bud so nerve fibers receive the appropriate amount of neurotransmitter. They also express proteins that can transport neurotransmitter molecules from the extracellular space into Type I cells. Regulating neurotransmitter concentration in taste buds ensures the efficient and precise communication of taste information from the taste bud to the central nervous system.

There is also some evidence to suggest that Type I cells might play a role in taste reception itself, rather than just supporting other taste cells. They express a membrane ion channel (a protein that forms a pore in the cell membrane and lets certain charged particles pass through) that can detect salt (Vandenbeuch et al., 2008). How Type I cells might communicate this taste information to nerve fibers is still unknown.

Courtney E. Wilson

See also: Salty Sensation; Taste Bud; Taste System; Type II Taste Cells; Type III Taste Cells

Further Reading

Chaudhari, Nirupa, & Stephen D. Roper. (2010). The cell biology of taste. *Journal of Cell Biology, 190*(3), 285–296.

Kandel, Eric R., James H. Schwartz, Thomas M. Jessell, Steven A. Siegelbaum, & A. J. Hudspeth (Eds.). (2012). *Principles of neural science* (5th ed., Ch. 32). New York, NY: McGraw-Hill.

Vandenbeuch, Aurelie, Tod R. Clapp, & Sue C. Kinnamon. (2008). Amiloride-sensitive channels in type I fungiform taste cells in mouse. *BMC Neuroscience, 9*, 1. http://dx.doi .org/10.1186/1471-2202-9-1.

TYPE II TASTE CELLS

Taste buds are the sensory end organs of the gustatory system. They contain three basic types of cells—Type I, Type II, and Type III cells. These networks of cells allow for the detection of five distinct taste qualities: sweet, bitter, umami, salty, and sour. Type II cells are sensitive to sweet, bitter, and umami taste qualities.

Anatomy

Type II cells are wide and spindle shaped, extending from the base of the taste bud to the apical pore. Here, an opening in the tongue epithelium allows the finger-like tips of taste cells to access chemicals present in the oral cavity. Type II cells are more abundant in taste buds than Type III cells, but less abundant than Type I cells.

Though they communicate to nerve fibers innervating the taste bud, Type II cells do not form traditional synapse structures with adjacent nerve fibers. Instead, the nerve fibers wrap around Type II cells. At points of contact with these surrounding nerve fibers, Type II cells have atypical mitochondria. Mitochondria are the energy factories of cells—they produce ATP (adenosine triphosphate), which is used to fuel many cellular processes. Electron microscopy images show mitochondria to be generally ovoid, with layers of membrane stacked inside. The atypical mitochondria in Type II cells, in contrast, are much larger and oddly shaped, with inner membranes that appear more twisted and less orderly than typical mitochondria. Type II cells use ATP as a neurotransmitter, as well as an energy source. It is thought that these atypical mitochondria are located at contact points with nerve fibers to ensure that there is a large, available source of ATP for signaling to afferent nerves.

Development

Taste bud cells are continually turning over during the life of an organism. As taste cells are damaged and die, a population of renewing basal cells repopulates the taste bud with new taste receptor cells. Type II cells survive for approximately two weeks before being replaced by new, maturing taste cells.

Function

Each Type II cell is sensitive to bitter, sweet, or umami stimuli. While not neurons, Type II cells behave similarly to neurons. They too fire action potentials—the electrical signal that travels from one end of a neuron to the other—and release

ATP as a neurotransmitter when stimulated with bitter, sweet, and umami substances.

Any one Type II cell expresses apically located receptors for one of three stimuli: bitter, sweet, or umami. Bitter receptors belong to the Taste 2 Receptor (T2R) family and are more varied than either sweet or umami receptors. Bitter taste reception is thought to warn organisms of possible poisonous substances before ingestion. This helps explain why they are the most varied receptors—poisonous substances can come in a wide variety of molecular structures, and the receptors evolved to match them. Sweet receptors are made up of two subunits, called Taste 1 Receptor 2 (T1R2) and Taste 1 Receptor 3 (T1R3). Both of the subunits are necessary to make the sweet receptor. Some animals (cats, for example) lack functional T1R2 genes, and thus are unable to taste sweet substances. Umami can be thought of as the "savory" quality—indicating the protein content of the food. Mushrooms and meats are high on the "umami" scale. Umami receptors also involve two subunits: Taste 1 Receptor 1 (T1R1) and T1R3. T1R3 is a subunit of both the umami and sweet receptors. Like the sweet receptor, both T1R1 and T1R3 are necessary to form the umami receptor.

Regardless of whether a Type II cell expresses bitter, sweet, or umami receptors, it processes this signal via the same signaling pathway. T2Rs and T1Rs are all G protein–coupled receptors, meaning they activate G proteins when they detect the proper substrate. These activated G proteins then start a set of processes called a signaling cascade inside the cell. For taste receptor–associated G proteins in Type II cells, this cascade causes an increase in the calcium concentration inside the cell. The increase of calcium, in turn, causes calcium-activated ion channels to open. Ion channels are pores in the cell membrane that open when activated, allowing ions to pass through. There are many kinds of ion channels that pass different kinds of ions and are activated by different conditions. These particular ion channels allow sodium ions into the cell. Since sodium ions are charged, they disrupt the delicate electrical balance of the cell, ultimately causing an action potential. By an unknown mechanism, this action potential causes Type II cells to release ATP through wide pores in the membrane called hemichannels. This ATP then stimulates the afferent nerve fiber, which carries the signal to the central nervous system. Eventually, this signal reaches the insular cortex, which processes taste information.

Courtney E. Wilson

See also: Bitter Sensation; G Proteins; Sweet Sensation; Taste Bud; Taste System; Type I Taste Cells; Type III Taste Cells; Umami

Further Reading

Chaudhari, Nirupa, & Stephen D. Roper. (2010). The cell biology of taste. *Journal of Cell Biology, 190*(3), 285–296.

TYPE III TASTE CELLS

Taste buds are the sensory end organs of the gustatory system. They contain three basic types of cells—Type I, Type II, and Type III cells. These networks of cells allow for the detection of five distinct taste qualities: sweet, bitter, umami, salty, and sour. Type III cells are sensitive to sour and some salty tastes.

Anatomy

In comparison to other cells in the taste bud, Type III cells are less abundant and smaller in size. These cells are spindle shaped and extend from the base of the taste bud to the apical pore, where an opening in the tongue epithelium allows taste cells to access chemicals present in the oral cavity. Interestingly, Type III cells are the only taste cells to make traditional synapses with afferent nerve fibers. At these sites, the taste cell membrane appears thicker in electron microscope images, indicating an aggregation of proteins important in synaptic transmission. Vesicles (small membranous sacs containing signaling molecules known as neurotransmitters) are also present. Here, vesicles fuse to the outer cell membrane, allowing for the release of neurotransmitters that chemically signal the receiving nerve fiber.

Development

Taste bud cells are continually turning over during the life of an organism. As taste cells are damaged and die, a population of renewing basal cells repopulates the taste bud with new taste receptor cells. Type III cells are the slowest to undergo this process—they may even take months to die off and renew.

Function

Type III cells are sensitive to both sour and salty stimuli. While not neurons, Type III cells behave similarly to neurons. They too fire action potentials—the electrical signal that travels from one end of a neuron to the other—and release neurotransmitters when stimulated with sour and salty substances.

Acid (sour) stimuli cause action potentials and neurotransmitter release in Type III cells via two cooperative mechanisms: (1) acid sensing ion channels located in Type III cells at the apical pore, and (2) a lowering of pH inside the cell (Chang et al., 2010; Ye et al., 2015). Simply put, sour substances contain acids, which have a low pH and freely dissociating hydrogen ions (H^+, protons). Type III cells express an ion channel (a protein in the cell membrane that forms a pore and lets certain ions through when open) that allows for the passage of free protons from the oral cavity into the cell. Electrically active cells are negatively charged inside the cell— the entrance of positively charged protons into Type III cells, then, disturbs the electrical balance between inside and out, causing a depolarizing electrical signal (action potential) that travels to the base of the cell. Some acids further promote

Type III cell depolarization via intracellular acidification. Many relatively weak acids, like citric and acetic acid, can pass through cell membranes where their associated protons can dissociate and block potassium-passing ion channels. Since these potassium ion channels steady the electrical balance of the cell membrane, blocking them with protons also disturbs the electrical balance of the cell, ultimately encouraging depolarizing action potentials. For this reason, psychophysical experiments report that weak acids often taste more sour than stronger acids (like hydrochloric acid, which does not cross the cell membrane) of the same pH.

When electrical action potentials reach the base of the cell, they cause vesicle fusion to the membrane and neurotransmitter release. Type III cells release serotonin, GABA (gamma-aminobutyric acid), and norepinephrine when stimulated. These neurotransmitters may signal to the afferent nerve as well as neighboring Type II cells, but the details of neurotransmitter signaling are not well understood. Regardless, Type III cells communicate to nerve fibers, causing neurons in taste nerves to fire. These nerves carry the signal to the brainstem and, ultimately, the insular cortex of the brain, which processes taste information.

Courtney E. Wilson

See also: Salty Sensation; Sour Sensation; Taste Aversion; Taste Bud; Taste System; Type I Taste Cells; Type II Taste Cells

Further Reading

Chang, Rui B., Hang Waters, & Emily R. Liman. (2010). A proton current drives action potentials in genetically identified sour taste cells. *Proceedings of the National Academy of Sciences of the United States of America, 107*(51), 22320–22325. http://dx.doi.org/10.1073/pnas.1013664107

Chaudhari, Nirupa, & Stephen D. Roper. (2010). The cell biology of taste. *Journal of Cell Biology, 190*(3), 285–296.

Wenlei Ye, Rui B. Chang, Jeremy D. Bushman, Yu-Hsiang Tu, Eric M. Mulhall, Courtney E. Wilson, . . . Emily R. Liman. (2016). The K+ channel KIR2.1 functions in tandem with proton influx to mediate sour taste transduction. *Proceedings of the National Academy of Sciences of the United States of America, 113*(2), E229–238.

U

UMAMI

Umami, the detection of amino acids, is one of the five basic tastes. The word *umami* is Japanese for "delicious taste"; perhaps the best English equivalent is "savory." It is an appetitive taste, in that it is generally regarded as pleasant. It has likely been advantageous in human evolution by facilitating the detection of foods rich in amino acids, some of which cannot be synthesized by humans and are thus essential components of nutrition. The standard substance used to define umami is L-glutamate. L-glutamate is an amino acid, and as such is abundant in high-protein foods, but it is only sensed in its free form. Therefore, substances that are high in protein that are partially metabolized have the strongest umami taste, including fish sauce, soy sauce, and tomatoes. Monosodium glutamate (MSG) is a salt of L-glutamate and was developed as a food additive to enhance the umami flavor of foods. Another amino acid, L-aspartate, can be sensed as umami as well, but most other amino acids are not detected to an appreciable degree in humans. The narrow specificity of the receptor for glutamate is intriguing, considering that glutamate itself is not an essential amino acid, but suggests that glutamate is sufficiently indicative of the amino acid content of food.

While umami was the most recently recognized primary taste, the umami receptors were identified more readily. The receptor responsible for umami sensation is the heterodimer of Taste Receptor 1 Member 1 (T1R1) and Taste Receptor Member 3 (T1R3; Nelson et al., 2002). Additionally, the metabotropic glutamate receptors mgluR4 and mgluR1 may be involved in umami sensation. The receptors are expressed on the surface of taste receptor cells (TRCs). Only TRCs that express the T1R1+R3 receptor sense umami, and TRCs that detect umami do not detect other tastes. Different TRCs are responsible for all five of the primary tastes and are organized into taste buds, which contain 50–150 TRCs each. Taste buds throughout the tongue contain TRCs for all five primary tastes; therefore, there is no topographic taste map. The specificity of the TRC to one taste alone is essential for the way that the different taste sensations are encoded.

Depolarization of the umami TRCs following a signaling cascade triggered by the receptor transmits a signal to afferent neurons. The signal is relayed by the facial nerve (cranial nerve VII) in the anterior two-thirds of the tongue and the glossopharyngeal nerve (cranial nerve IX) in the posterior third of the tongue. Sensory afferents synapse in the rostral portion of the nucleus of the solitary tract in the brainstem and are relayed to the thalamus with projections to the primary gustatory cortex.

The T1R1+R3 receptor detects glutamate with relatively low affinity when compared to the affinities of the bitter receptors and bitter tastants. This means that substances need relatively high concentrations of glutamate to be sensed as umami, consistent with the need to identify foods with sufficient amino acid content. Though the primary taste of umami is defined as sensing of glutamate, it has been suggested that the full taste classically described as umami is not elicited by glutamate alone, but rather is a complex taste elicited by potentiation from the ribonucleotides inositol monophosphate or guanine monophosphate.

Michael S. Harper

See also: Facial Nerve; Glossopharyngeal Nerve; Supertaster; Taste Aversion; Taste Bud; Taste System; Type II Taste Cells

Further Reading

McLaughlin, Susan K., & Robert F. Margolskee. (1994). The sense of taste. *American Scientist, 82*(6), 538–545.

Nelson, Greg, Jayaram Chandrashekar, Mark A. Hoon, Luxin Feng, Grace Zhao, Nicholas J. P. Ryba, & Charles S. Zuker. (2002). An amino-acid taste receptor. *Nature, 416*(6877), 199–202. http://dx.doi.org/10.1038/nature726

UTRICLE

The utricle is one of the two otolithic organs within the inner ear. The other otolithic organ is the saccule. Both of the otolithic organs are part of the balancing apparatus located in the vestibule of the bony labyrinth, which is a small oval chamber that consists of the vestibule (a swelling next to the semicircular canals), three separate semicircular canals, and the cochlea (necessary for the sense of hearing). Within the vestibule is the utricle, which is located between the semicircular canals and the cochlea. The saccule is closer to the cochlea compared to the utricle. Within the utricle are small stones (called otoconia, consisting of calcium carbonate and a matrix protein) and a viscous fluid that are used to stimulate the sensory hair cells that line the utricle's epithelial layer. It is the bending of the stereocilia on the sensory hair cells that detects motion and orientation of the head. The utricle specifically detects linear accelerations such as coming to an abrupt stop in a car, or tilting the head on the horizontal plane.

Anatomical Structure

Comparatively, the utricle is larger than the saccule and is an oblong shape. It is compressed and occupies the upper and posterior part of the vestibule. The utricle makes a true contact with the recessus ellipticus labyrinthi ossei (also known as the elliptical recess of the bony labyrinth), which helps maintain its structure. Within the utricle is the macula utricle, which is a thickening on the wall and the epithelium that lines the utricle. The epithelium contains the sensory hair cells that detect changes in acceleration. Superior to the epithelium is the otolithic membrane, which contains a gelatinous layer, and superior to that the statoconia layer. The statoconia layer is a bed of otoconia. Each sensory hair cell has stereocilia (mechanoreceptors that respond to changes in pressure) and a true kinocilium (the only sensory cilium that can depolarize and produce an action potential) at its apical end. The tips of the stereocilia and kinocilium are embedded within the otolithic membrane.

Function

The utricle has mechanoreceptors that can distinguish between the different degrees that the head tilts. Because of gravity, the otolithic organ pulls on the embedded stereocilia and causes them to tilt. This shift in the direction of the stereocilia stimulates the kinocilium and induces an action potential that is sent from the vestibular portion of the vestibulocochlear nerve (cranial nerve VIII) to the brainstem and then to the brain. The brain interprets all head movements by comparing inputs from the direction of the tilt, detected by the kinocilium, to inputs from the eyes and stretch receptors in the neck. By doing so, the brain can determine if just the head is tilted or if the entire body is tilted.

Disorders of the Otolithic Organs

Damage to the otolithic organs can have an impact on ocular (vision) and body stabilization. Until recently, there has not been a way to measure how severely these organs could be damaged. Recent studies have developed the Vestibular Evoked Myogenic Potential (VEMP) test, which can determine the health of the saccule as it is inferior to the utricle and more proximal to the cochlea. To date, VEMP tests are employed to quantify otolithic organ input to the right and left vestibular systems. The purpose of VEMP is to determine if the saccule and the inferior vestibular nerve are functioning properly and are intact. The output of the saccule can be recorded using a sound generator. In addition, surface electrodes can be used to detect neck muscle activation or other muscles of interest. More research is needed to improve this technique as well as to determine how to test the integrity of the utricle.

Renee Johnson

See also: Saccule; Semicircular Canals; Stereocilia; Vestibular System; Vestibulocochlear Nerve

Further Reading

Drummond, Meghan C., et al. (2015). Live-cell imaging of actin dynamics reveals mechanisms of stereocilia length regulation in the inner ear. *Nature Communications, 6,* 6873. Retrieved from http://www.ncbi.nlm.nih.gov/pmc/articles/PMC4411292/

Hain, Timothy C. (2014). Otoliths. *Dizziness-and-balance.com.* Retrieved from http://www.dizziness-and-balance.com/anatomy/ear/otoliths.html

Purves, Dale, et al. (2008). *Neuroscience* (4th ed.). Sunderland, MA: Sinauer Associates.

V

VAGUS NERVE

The vagus nerve (cranial nerve X) is a mixed nerve, meaning that it contains both sensory and motor components. Specifically, it has an extensive motor and sensory distribution to thoracic and abdominal viscera, as well as to structures in the pharynx and larynx. It emerges from the brainstem as a bundle of small rootlets. From there, it wanders inferiorly below the head and neck to enter the chest and abdomen. This is how it received its Latin term, *vagus*, which means "wandering." There are two major roles of the vagus nerve. First, it functions as the parasympathetic motor output of the autonomic nervous system; and second, it functions to relay information about the viscera to the brain via sensory neurons. These sensory neurons are called primary visceral sensory neurons. In fact, most of the nerve fibers in the vagus nerve are sensory in nature.

Anatomy and Physiology

The vagus nerve originates in the medulla oblongata from four main nuclei: the nucleus solitarius, nucleus ambiguus, dorsal nucleus of the vagus nerve, and spinal trigeminal nucleus. The fibers from the nucleus solitarius receive sensory taste information along with sensory input from organs. The nucleus ambiguus fibers send parasympathetic output to the heart, which is used to lower heart rate. Fibers from the dorsal nucleus of the vagus nerve send parasympathetic output to abdominal organs, which results in increased secretory activity of glands and increased rates of peristalsis. Finally, the spinal trigeminal nucleus receives sensory information from the outer ear and the mucus layer of the larynx. It travels a long distance from its point of origin in the brainstem to the various organs of the neck, thorax, and abdomen that it innervates.

In its journey, cranial nerve X exits the skull through the jugular foramen along with cranial nerves IX and XI. The vagus nerve then descends in a covering (called the carotid sheath) with the internal jugular vein and internal carotid artery, inferiorly through the neck and eventually into the chest and abdomen. Along the way, the vagus nerve gives off several branches on both sides of the body to innervate various organs and/or skeletal muscles. It has two enlargements: the superior ganglion—which is near the opening of the foramen that receives general sensory information and connects with neurons from cranial nerves IX and XI—and the inferior ganglion—which receives sensory input from various organs. Because the vagus nerve carries so many different afferent fibers from so many different visceral organs, it is a very large and thick nerve that is easily identified within the neck, thorax, and abdominal cavity.

In the thorax, the right and left vagus nerves take different paths on their way to the abdomen. The left vagus nerve is closely aligned with the arch of the aorta and gives off a branch, the left recurrent laryngeal nerve. This branch then hooks around a ligament under the arch before ascending up into the neck to supply motor function and sensory sensation to the larynx. On the right side, the right recurrent laryngeal nerve comes off the right vagus nerve much higher up, hooking around the right subclavian artery before ascending up the neck.

The recurrent laryngeal nerves innervate the intrinsic muscles of the larynx, such as the thyroarytenoid, posterior and lateral cricoarytenoid, and arytenoid muscles. Because the left recurrent laryngeal nerve passes under the aortic arch, it is longer than the right recurrent laryngeal nerve. Along the way, both recurrent branches give off smaller branches to the heart, esophagus, trachea, and pharyngeal constrictor muscles before reaching their destination, the larynx.

The vagus nerves enter the abdomen through a natural hole in the diaphragm called the esophageal hiatus, which allows the esophagus, vagus nerve, and a few vessels to pass through the diaphragm. This section of cranial nerve X supplies motor parasympathetic fibers to all organs (except the adrenal glands) from the neck down to the latter third of the transverse colon. It also innervates some muscles in the larynx that are involved in speech, the throat, and the palate. Based on the location of the vagus nerves braches, cranial nerve X is responsible for a variety of tasks that include the control of heart rate and blood pressure, gut peristalsis, speech, and breathing.

Clinical Symptoms and Disease

Isolated lesions of the vagus nerve are uncommon, but damage to the recurrent nerves can occur. Cancers of the larynx or thyroid glands or thyroid surgery can injury these nerves. The result is decreased movement of the vocal fold on the damaged side, causing hoarseness. Bilateral damage to the recurrent branch can result in difficulty in swallowing, reduced gag reflexes, and dysarthria (problems with speaking due to the lack of muscle control). To test which vagus nerve is damaged, an easy clinical diagnostic assessment is to see if the patient's uvula deviates to one side. If it does, the uvula will move away from the side of the lesion. In addition, patients will not be able to elevate their palate.

Robin Michaels and Jennifer L. Hellier

See also: Autonomic Nervous System; Cranial Nerves; Nerves; Peripheral Nervous System; Seizures

Further Reading

Liang, Barbara. (2012). *The 12 cranial nerves.* Retrieved from http://www.wisc-online.com
    /objects/ViewObject.aspx?ID=AP11504

Moore, Keith L., Anne M. R. Agur, & Arthur F. Dalley (Eds.). (2010). *Essential clinical
    anatomy* (4th ed.). Baltimore, MD: Williams and Wilkins.

Yale University School of Medicine. (1998). *Cranial nerves.* Retrieved from http://www.yale
    .edu/cnerves/

VERTIGO: *See* Dizziness

VESTIBULAR SYSTEM

The vestibular system is a sensory system that detects the position and movement of the head. By monitoring the position and movement of the head, the vestibular system contributes to the sense of balance and equilibrium. The main organs of the vestibular system are located within the inner ear on both sides of the head, just posterior to the cochlea of the auditory system. There are two components in the vestibular system: the semicircular canal system and the otoliths. Each component is responsible for detecting different types of movement. The semicircular canals detect rotational movement, and the otoliths detect gravity and linear acceleration. The vestibular system is closely tied to the visual centers of the brain that control eye muscle movement as well as areas of the autonomic nervous system within the cerebellum that maintain subconscious muscle tension. When the vestibular system is malfunctioning and the subconscious muscle tension is abnormal, it may cause symptoms like motion sickness, vertigo, or uncontrolled eye movements.

Anatomy and Physiology

The vestibular system has two portions: the otolith organs and the semicircular canals. The otolith organs are two fluid-filled, round structures that detect the force of gravity, tilts of the head, and linear acceleration. The semicircular canals are made up of three half-circle, fluid-filled tubes that detect rotational and head tilt movements. Both of these organs are found in the inner ear just posterior to the cochlea. The otolith organs are found centrally between the cochlea and the semicircular canals, and the semicircular canals loop out posteriorly from the otolith. There is a set of vestibular organs located on each side of the head within the temporal bone.

The three semicircular canals detect head rotations such as nodding vertically, shaking horizontally, or movement from shoulder to shoulder. The semicircular canals also detect angular acceleration that is created by a sudden rotation, like spinning in a circle. Each canal is located in a plane that is 90 degrees to the other two semicircular canals. The hair cells are located within an enlargement at the base of each canal called the ampulla. The hair cells within the ampulla are attached to the crista, which is analogous to the organ of Corti in the cochlea. The cilia of the hair cells extend into a membrane called the cupula. When there is a head rotation, the walls of the canal and the cupula move, but the fluid movement lags behind due to inertia. The opposing movement between the fluid and the cupula bends the cilia of the hair cells in the opposite direction of the head movement. The bending motion in one direction causes an excitation of the hair cells and a release of neurotransmitters. Moving in the opposite direction inhibits neurotransmitter release. The released neurotransmitters stimulate action potentials within the vestibular nerve. The on/off arrangement of the hair cells allows the brain to detect the orientation of the head at all times. The function of the semicircular canals is easily demonstrated by spinning rapidly in a circle for 15 to 30 seconds and then stopping. The sustained motion within the semicircular canals eventually stops bending the cupula and the sensation of spinning subsides. However, once the spinning motion ceases, the fluid causes the cupula to bend in the opposite direction, which gives the sensation of motion in the opposite direction.

The otolith organs are located between the semicircular canals and the cochlea; they contain a pair of large chambers called the saccule and the utricle. These two structures within the otolith detect changes in the angle of the head and linear acceleration, which are all responses to gravity. The utricle and saccule have a sensory epithelium called the macula that is vertical in the saccule and horizontal in the utricle when the head is upright. The vestibular macula contains hair cells with their cilia projecting into a gelatinous membrane called the otolith membrane. *Otolith* means "ear stone" in Greek, and within the otolith membrane are many tiny calcium carbonate stones (1–5 micrometers in diameter), the otoliths. These stones are heavier than the surrounding fluid and membrane, so gravity pulls them down. The weight of the otoliths being pulled down by gravity also causes the membrane to be pulled down and thus bends the cilia of the hair cells. Bending in one direction stimulates an action potential in the vestibular nerves, and bending in the opposite direction inhibits an action potential. The hair cells within the macula can detect head movement in any direction due to their respective orientation within the utricle and saccule. In addition, the otolith organs on each side of the head are mirror images of each other. This means that a head tilt will result in the activation of hair cells on one side of the head, while the corresponding location on the opposite side of the head will be inactivated. Any head tilt or acceleration will result in the activation of certain hair cells and the inactivation of others. Collectively the brain can interpret these activation/inactivation patterns for all forms of head orientations unambiguously. A great example of the otolith organs at work is being on a moving sidewalk. A person will experience a sudden acceleration stepping onto the walkway and then feel a deceleration stepping off.

Lynelle Smith

See also: Auditory System; Autonomic Nervous System; Balance; Cochlea; Dizziness; Meniere's Disease; Nystagmus; Vestibulocochlear Nerve

Further Reading

Bear, Mark F., Barry W. Connors, & Michael A. Paradiso. (2007). *Neuroscience exploring the brain* (3rd ed.). Baltimore, MD: Lippincott Williams & Wilkins.

Gray, Lincoln. (2013).*Vestibular system: Structure and function* (Chap. 10). Retrieved from http://neuroscience.uth.tmc.edu/s2/chapter10.html

Watson, Mary Ann, & F. Owen Black. (2013). *The human balance system*. Retrieved from http://vestibular.org/understanding-vestibular-disorder/human-balance-system

VESTIBULOCOCHLEAR NERVE

The vestibulocochlear nerve is a cranial nerve that supplies both hearing and balance information to the brain. All cranial nerves are paired, meaning one nerve supplies the right side and the other nerve supplies the left. The vestibulocochlear nerve is the eighth of 12 paired cranial nerves and is called cranial nerve VIII. The vestibulocochlear nerves are purely sensory and have two divisions: vestibular and cochlear. The vestibular portion deals with the sensation of balance, while the cochlear division is used for auditory information.

Anatomy and Physiology

Within the skull and deep to the external ear, the vestibulocochlear nerve's sensory receptors are located in the membranous labyrinth. This is a very delicate small structure that is tubular, filled with endolymph, and connected to a series of tunnels within the petrous portion of the temporal bone. The tunnel walls are called the bony labyrinth, which is connected to the inner ear by two openings, the oval window with the stapes bone and the round window with a flexible membrane called the round window membrane. The stapes vibrates when a sound wave hits it, resulting in a pressure wave into both the bony and membranous labyrinths. This pressure wave travels through the channels and makes the round window membrane vibrate. In turn, the endolymph moves, resulting in the sound wave being propagated.

The sensory receptors in the cochlea and vestibular structures are small and can be easily damaged. The outputs of these sensory receptors travel a short distance to their receiving neurons, which are located in the cochlea and the semicircular canals. The cells in the cochlea make up the spinal ganglion, while the neurons in the base of the semicircular canals make up the vestibular ganglion. These neurons' axons bundle and travel together, making up cranial nerve VIII. The nerve travels through the internal auditory meatus with the facial nerve. Both the vestibulocochlear and facial nerves then enter the brainstem at the junction of the pons and medulla. This is where the two divisions of the vestibulocochlear nerve begin to diverge from each other.

Vestibular Component of the Nerve

The fibers from the vestibular division terminate in the vestibular nuclear complex within the floor of the fourth ventricle. This makes up the vestibulocerebellar tract. The axons from the vestibular nuclear complex terminate in several nuclei within the brainstem and spinal cord to affect the muscles used for maintaining balance. The lateral vestibulospinal tract is made of ipsilateral fibers from the lateral vestibular nucleus to terminate down the spinal cord onto neurons that control extensor muscles. The medial and inferior vestibular nuclei have shared connections to the cerebellum to control and coordinate balance while the body is moving. Finally, all vestibular complex nuclei project to the three cranial nerve nuclei used to control the muscles of the eyes. This makes up the medial longitudinal fasciculus, which is critical in maintaining the body's orientation in space as well as maintaining fixation of an object during head movement. These fibers terminate onto both the left and right nuclei of cranial nerves III, IV, and VII. These interconnections show how the vestibular division is highly integrated with vision.

Cochlear Component of the Nerve

The fibers from the cochlear division terminate in the dorsal and ventral cochlear nuclei. The dorsal cochlear nucleus receives high-frequency information, while the ventral cochlear nucleus receives information about low frequencies. The pathway to the cerebral cortex from here is not well understood. However, a few synapses have been studied in patients with cortical deafness, as described in the following. The outputs of the dorsal and ventral cochlear nuclei cross to the other side of the brainstem and ascend toward the brain. This forms the lateral lemniscus, a tract of ascending axons to the cerebral cortex. Some axons cross over and synapse in the contralateral trapezoid body or superior olivary nucleus before joining the lateral lemniscus. There are few fibers that do not cross over and terminate in the ispilateral superior olivary nucleus and ascend in the ipsilateral lateral lemniscus. From here, axons of both the left and right lateral lemnisci terminate in the inferior colliculus. The inferior colliculus axons terminate into the thalamus, which sends its axons to the transverse temporal gyrus. It is here where sound is interpreted in the brain.

Clinical Symptoms and Treatment

If the vestibular component of the nerve is damaged, the result is reduction or complete loss of balance. In particular, patients will feel dizzy, may fall more often, and have abnormal eye movements. Patients may also have nausea, causing them to vomit. The most common lesion to the vestibulocochlear nerve is a tumor of the Schwann cells surrounding the nerve. Removal of the tumor may be necessary for balance function to return. Finally, patients may be trained to overcome their balance deficit by using their eyes more effectively, as vision can override vestibular issues. This is because the eyes can see the horizon and realize that it is stable and not truly moving.

If the cochlear component of the nerve is damaged, the result is reduction or complete loss of hearing. This usually occurs from skull fractures or ear infections. Tumors can occur in the internal auditory meatus, which can damage both divisions of the vestibulocochlear nerve as well as the facial nerve. Finally, lesions to the lateral lemniscus typically result in a characteristically partial deafness on the contralateral side. This is because the small amount of ipsilateral fibers is spared on the affected side and can carry the auditory information to the brain. Treatment may include antibiotics to heal the infection or hearing aids.

Jennifer L. Hellier

See also: Auditory System; Balance; Cochlea; Cranial Nerves; Dizziness; Nerves; Vestibular System

Further Reading

Liang, Barbara. (2012). *The 12 cranial nerves.* Retrieved from http://www.wisc-online.com/objects/ViewObject.aspx?ID=AP11504
Yale University School of Medicine. (1998). *Cranial nerves.* Retrieved from http://www.yale.edu/cnerves/

VIBRATION SENSATION

Animals and particularly humans can sense touch via several different modalities such as two-point discrimination touch, flutter, pressure, and vibration to name a few. Vibration is an oscillatory, mechanical waveform that can be periodic like a pendulum on a grandfather clock or random such as tires moving on a dirt road. Either form will produce a wave that alternates between increasing and decreasing in length, which can be felt by the sense of vibration.

Derived from a Greek word meaning to "shake," *pallesthesia* is the medical term for the sensation of mechanical vibration on or near the body. Vibrations can be conducted by the bones in the middle ear for the sense of hearing, which in turn results in movement of the hair cells in the cochlea. Additionally, vibrations can be detected by touch receptors in the skin and by nerves near bones, which are able to conduct vibrations. The sensory pathway that is used to detect vibration sensation is the dorsal columns/medial lemniscus system, which transmits the signal from the periphery to the spinal cord, brainstem, and sensory cortices of the brain.

Testing Vibration Sense in a Neurological Exam

Health care providers, particularly neurologists, will test vibration sense to determine (1) hearing ability, (2) deafness, (3) general exteroception ability, and

(4) peripheral neuropathies of the extremities in patients. A tuning fork, a metal instrument with two prongs of equal length and a handle, is used to test vibration sensations.

To determine hearing ability, the neurologist will hit the prongs against his or her hand to cause the fork to vibrate and then place the fork next to the person's ear or on the bones of the skull behind the ear. This is to test the two categories of deafness—conductive and sensorineural. Conductive hearing loss is the result of a disruption in sound wave conduction within the outer and middle ear. Sensorineural deafness, on the other hand, is the result of damage or injury to the cochlea or the auditory nerve that prevents the transduction of the electrical impulse created by sound waves. A combination of both conductive and sensorineural hearing loss is called mixed deafness. Deafness can be unilateral, affecting one ear, or bilateral, affecting both ears. Tuning fork tests, such as the Weber's test and the Rinne's test, are used to distinguish between the type of hearing loss, the extent of the loss, as well as the differentiation between unilateral and bilateral deafness.

To determine general exteroception and nerve conduction abilities of the body, the health care provider will place a vibrating tuning fork first on the sternum of the patient and then on each extremity (arms and legs). Placing the tuning fork on the sternum allows the person to identify the sensation and understand what he or she should feel. To test the lower body, the vibrating fork is placed on the ball of the individual's right or left big toe. If the patient can feel the vibration, then it suggests that nerve conduction from the furthest distance of the leg is working normally. If the patient cannot feel the vibration, then the health care provider will move the vibrating tuning fork to the next bony prominence: the malleolus of the ankle, the tibial shaft, the tibial tuberosity, and then the anterior iliac crest. The lack of vibration sense can tell the neurologist where nerve damage or peripheral neuropathies are located on the leg. The test is repeated on the other lower extremity and then on each upper extremity, starting with the pads of the fingers and then moving superiorly to the shoulder.

Jennifer L. Hellier

See also: Discriminative Touch; Exteroception; Interoception; Senses of Animals; Touch

Further Reading

Dougherty, Patrick, & Chieyeko Tsuchitani. (2015). Somatosensory pathways. In John H. Byrne (Ed.), *Neuroscience Online, an electronic textbook for the neurosciences* (Chap. 4). Retrieved from http://neuroscience.uth.tmc.edu/s2/chapter04.html

Swenson, Rand. (2006). Chapter 7: Somatosensory Systems. In *Review of clinical and functional neuroscience*. Dartmouth College. Retrieved from https://www.dartmouth.edu/~rswenson/NeuroSci/chapter_7A.html

VISCERAL SENSATION

Visceral sensation, also known as visceral pain, is pain that results from the activation of nociceptors of areas including but not limited to the thoracic, pelvic, or abdominal organs (the viscera). Visceral organs that are most often associated with visceral sensations are the lungs, heart, stomach, kidneys, and bladder. Visceral pain is diffuse and usually very difficult to localize. In fact, visceral pain may have referred sensations that are localized relatively far from the actual cause of the pain or sensation. Symptoms accompanying visceral pain can include but are not limited to nausea, vomiting, and changes in vital signs like blood pressure and heart rate.

Previously, the viscera were considered to be insensitive to pain, but today it is well documented that pain from internal organs is a true sensation. This pain can be widespread and could cause a social burden in one's life. For example, myocardial (heart muscle) ischemia (death) is the most frequent cause of cardiac pain and is the most common cause of death in the United States. Other conditions that start with visceral pain include but are not limited to appendicitis (inflammation of the appendix), cholecystitis (inflammation of the gallbladder), and nephrolithiasis (kidney stones). Visceral pain from these conditions can be very localized to a specific position and move toward the organ (like that found in appendicitis), or one can experience what is called referred pain. Referred pain is common with presentation of gallstones in the gallbladder. Patients often complain of pain in the right shoulder, which is not near where the gallbladder is located. Another example of referred pain is when one is having a myocardial infarction (heart attack) and experiences pain in the left jaw and pain traveling down the left arm. It is very common that the autonomic nervous system plays a role in visceral sensations.

Transmission of Visceral Sensation in the Body

In the past, there were two ideas of how visceral sensation was transmitted: (1) viscera are innervated by separate classes of sensory receptors including pain receptors, and (2) internal organs are innervated by a single and homogenous class of sensory receptors that at low frequencies of activation send normal regulatory signals and at high frequencies of activation signal pain. High threshold receptors have been found in places including but not limited to the heart, lungs, small intestine, and urinary bladder. Damage to the viscus (singular form of viscera) affects the normal pattern of motility for that organ, and secretion produces drastic changes in the environment that surrounds nociceptor endings.

Treatment

Two goals in the treatment of visceral sensation are (1) to alleviate pain and (2) to address the underlying pathology of the pain. Sometimes identifying the underlying pathology is not possible. In cases like this, symptomatic treatment can be administered. Symptomatic treatment includes medications like analgesics

(NSAIDs and opiates), antidepressants (SSRIs), and antispasmodics (loperamide). Nerve blocks, local anesthetics, and steroid injections are more invasive therapies, but these generally have a limited number of treatments. These injections may only offer temporary relief, but permanent nerve blocks can be done by destruction of nerve tissue.

Research

Research by Drs. Fernando Cervero and Jennifer Laird (2004) describes many aspects of visceral sensation, which includes how visceral pain is transmitted throughout the body, the biochemistry of visceral pain, new techniques used to study visceral pain, and how their research can be integrated into clinical practice. Many specialists still continue to treat visceral pain as just a symptom instead of as a distinct neurological entity. However, Cervero and Laird (2004) have shown that the most effective treatment of visceral pain includes electrophysiological and imaging techniques. For instance, when microstimulation of the thalamus was used to evoke visceral pain experiences like angina or labor pain, it significantly altered the sensation even in individuals who experienced these pains years before. Their research highlights the role of the thalamus in processing memories of pain and the existence of long-lived neural mechanisms that are capable of storing the results of previously painful experiences even for years after the fact.

Renee Johnson

See also: Autonomic Nervous System; Nociception; Nociceptors; Phantom Pain

Further Reading

Cervero, Fernando, & Jennifer M. A. Laird. (2004). Understanding the signaling and transmission of visceral nociceptive events. *Journal of Neurobiology, 61*(1), 45–54.

Collett, Beverly. (2013). Visceral pain: The importance of pain management services. *British Journal of Pain, 7*(1), 6–7. Retrieved from http://bjp.sagepub.com/content/7/1/6.full .pdf+html

International Association for the Study of Pain. (2012). Acute vs. chronic presentation of visceral pain. Retrieved from http://iasp-pain.org/files/Content/ContentFolders/Global YearAgainstPain2/VisceralPainFactSheets/3-AcuteVsChronic.pdf

VISION-TOUCH SYNESTHESIA: *See* Mirror-Touch Synesthesia

VISUAL FIELDS

The visual system is a complex assortment of neurons that allows animals and humans to see the world around them. This system is made of a series of different tracts and nuclei much like the "tracks" and "ports or stations" on a railroad system.

Each part of the track is important, and when there is damage to any one part, it ultimately affects the visual field.

History

Hippocrates (460–377 BCE) was one of the first to recognize the visual field. The first documented testing, in fact, was performed by asking the patient to cover one eye while watching a fixed point. The tester would then ask the patient to identify objects held in the sides and outer edges of the visual field, usually at four points. This type of testing is called confrontation visual field evaluation. British ophthalmologist Jannik Bjerrum (1851–1920) expanded this testing in the 19th century. Bjerrum mapped visual fields by holding a white object in front of a black screen known as the tangent screen.

Over time, several additional tests were developed, such as the Amsler grid, which measures a person's central visual field, to a kinetic perimetry test that tests the perimeter of the visual field. Many of these tests are still used today during a routine eye exam. Because vision is critical to humans, it is important for everyone to have an annual eye exam to maintain a healthy visual system.

Anatomy and Physiology

When a person looks at an object, the total amount of area that can be seen is known as the visual field. Health care providers test the visual field by having individuals focus on an object directly in front of them without moving their eyes or their head. Because the eye is a sphere, the resulting visual field is divided into the size of the angle seen both vertically and horizontally from a single eye. Thus, the typical dimensions for a human's visual field is 60 degrees superiorly, 75 degrees inferiorly, 60 degrees nasally, and 100 degrees temporally.

The visual field is divided into two halves: the nasal and temporal fields. Both of these fields are then further divided into superior and inferior sections, thus giving the visual field four distinct quadrants. Because animals have two eyes, there are two visual fields.

Vision Loss

When damage occurs to the optic pathway, an individual's ability to see the world around him or her changes. The location in which the visual field is affected determines what portion of the vision or visual field is compromised. This may manifest as blind spots in vision, blurred or hazy vision, or even total blindness. Injury to the visual tract can be caused by infections, diabetes, and congenital defects, to name a few.

A person's visual field can be compromised in five basic areas: (1) the optic nerve, (2) optic chiasm, (3) optic tract, (4) optic radiation, or (5) visual cortex.

Starting at the optic nerve, before the optic chiasm, an injury here causes a break in the visual pathway. This stops all information from being sent to the visual cortex, resulting in monocular blindness.

The optic chiasm is where the information from both eyes meets before proceeding down the optic tract. Only the information from the nasal visual field crosses here while the temporal tract proceeds to the optic tract. The optic chiasm is positioned anterior to the pituitary gland. Thus, pituitary gland tumors can press on the optic chiasm, causing injury and loss of both temporal visual fields. This condition is called bitemporal hemianopsia. The optic chiasm splits and becomes two optic tracts. Damage to the optic tract will manifest as a condition called homonymous hemianopsia. This is due to damage of the ipsilateral nasal visual field and damage to the contralateral temporal visual field.

The optic radiation is a network of neurons that takes visual information from the lateral geniculate nucleus to the primary visual cortex. When the optic radiation is damaged, it results in a condition called quadrantanopsia. Persons with this injury show decreased visual sensation in the ipsilateral nasal field and contralateral temporal field either in the superior or inferior portion of the visual field.

Finally, the visual cortex is the end point for the visual tract. When there is damage to this brain region, it can result in a condition called homonymous hemianopsia with macular sparing. This means that all vision is lost in the ipsilateral nasal visual field and the contralateral temporal visual field, except for a small portion in the center of both visual fields that projects to the macula.

Adam K. Mills

See also: Blind Spot; Occipital Lobe; Optic Nerve; Retina; Tunnel Vision; Visual Perception; Visual System

Further Reading

Carroll, Joy N., & Chris A. Johnson. (2013). *Visual field testing: From one medical student to another.* University of Iowa Health Care Ophthalmology & Visual Sciences. Retrieved from http://EyeRounds.org/tutorials/VF-testing/

Purves, Dale, et al. (Eds.). (2001). Visual field deficits. In *Neuroscience* (2nd ed.). Sunderland, MA: Sinauer Associates. Retrieved from http://www.ncbi.nlm.nih.gov/books/NBK10912/

VISUAL MOTOR SYSTEM

The ability to have "eye-hand coordination" is an essential process of the visual motor system. In animals, this ability is necessary for survival, particularly when trying to eat, drink, and make shelter. The visual motor system in humans also allows us to write, craft (e.g., draw, color, cut, glue), build, drive, dress, cook, play sports, and play video games. Vision is used to bring information about the external environment to the brain. When an individual moves, vision provides the brain with feedback information about how accurate and successful the person's intentional (voluntary) movements were. The brain will then use this information to adjust the person's actions to correct errors and to improve eye-hand coordination.

There are three main steps necessary for successful and efficient eye-hand coordination: (1) strong visual skills that are developed by the ocular motor system, which in turn are interpreted by the brain (also termed visual perception skills); (2) well-defined fine motor skills; and (3) integration of visual and fine motor skills together to perform the visual motor task.

Anatomy and Physiology

The ocular motor system controls eye movements as well as eyelid closure, the amount of light that enters the eyes via the extraocular muscles, and the refractive properties of the eye via the intraocular muscles. Together these muscles work in concert to guide vision and to maintain a stable image of an object on the retina. There are six extraocular muscles (three pairs for each eye) that contract or relax to control eye movement, while the levator palpebrae muscle is used to close the eyelid.

Since only a small part of the retina is responsible for visual acuity (sharp vision)—called the fovea centralis—it is essential for the eyeball to move so that it can track an object and maintain its clarity on the retina. Thus, the eye must move quickly as well as have very precise movements. For example, as you are reading this entry, your eyes are moving across the page and at the same time the words stay in focus. This shifting of gaze is produced by the extraocular muscles. Some of these movements are intentional (voluntary) and others are automatic (involuntary). However, research is needed to better understand how voluntary and involuntary eye movements are integrated by the ocular motor system to perform these actions. It is known that the vestibular system does play a role in involuntary eye movements through the vestibulo-ocular reflex.

Fine motor skills is a term describing coordinated actions of small muscle groups. Most often the term is used to describe the coordination of the wrists, hands, and fingers in completing very specific tasks, such as holding a knife and fork, catching a ball, or writing with a pen. Fine motor skills depend on (1) the core strength of the hand and fingers, and (2) proprioceptive processing skills, which determine the location of the fingers in space and the strength needed by the hand and fingers to manipulate objects to perform the precision of a task like buttoning a jacket.

Integrating visual skills with fine motor skills is a task that begins around three months of age in humans. This is when infants begin to grasp a caretaker's finger with their hand. However, at this young age it is more of a reflex than a voluntary action. Over time the reflex becomes voluntary and intentional in reaching and grabbing for toys or other objects. Using vision, infants will begin to determine how far away an object is and how to adjust their reach to grab the item. By age three, children will have been working on their eye-hand coordination and begin to improve their fine motor skills with prewriting. Drawing lines and shapes and coloring will help toddlers integrate their ocular motor skills (following the shape of a circle with their eyes) with their fine motor skills (drawing or copying a circle on paper).

Visual Motor Activities

There are many activities that one can perform daily to improve one's visual motor system and skills. Some include: (1) practice making shapes with different media—pipe cleaners, toothpicks, or string; (2) color—outline the picture to help see where to keep the crayon for coloring; (3) put jigsaw puzzles together—looking at the shape and color of the puzzle piece will help improve ocular motor skills, while putting the pieces together will improve fine motor skills; and (4) cut out shapes and paste them together to make a picture.

Jennifer L. Hellier

See also: Proprioception; Retina; Visual Perception; Visual System

Further Reading

Dragoi, Valentin. (2015). Ocular motor system. In John H. Byrne (Ed.), *Neuroscience Online, an electronic textbook for the neurosciences* (Chap. 7). Retrieved from http://neuro science.uth.tmc.edu/s3/chapter07.html

Phelan, Shannon. (2015). Visual motor integration: What is it and how to develop this skill. *North Shore Pediatric Therapy*. Retrieved from http://nspt4kids.com/parenting /visual-motor-integration-develop-skill/

VISUAL PERCEPTION

The visual system is a sensory system that is responsible for the sense of sight or vision. Visual perception, however, consists of the psychological process of how an animal or person sees a visual image. Specifically, visual perception is how the brain interprets the external environment and surroundings that are contained by visible light, and that interpretation can vary from person to person based on their previous experiences. Because of this difference, the visual system is a separate entry in this encyclopedia. Finally, sight is the combination of the visual system, visual processing, and visual perception.

History

For thousands of years, people have realized that the eye and brain are intimately interconnected. The visual pathway from the eyes to the brain was first documented and described by Galen of Pergamon (130–200 CE). Considering the technology of the time, scientists are still amazed at Galen's accuracy in many of his anatomical drawings and physiological understandings of the visual system. However, he did make a few mistakes that are now better understood with modern scientific tools.

Our understanding of particularly the neurophysiology of the visual system is attributed to Canadian neurophysiologist David H. Hubel (1926–2013) and Swedish neurophysiologist Torsten N. Wiesel (1924–). Together, Hubel and Wiesel won the 1981 Nobel Prize in Physiology or Medicine for their contributions to neuroscience about vision and are considered the fathers of the visual system.

Visual Processing

Once an object's image hits the retina, the neuronal signals for that image are carried from the optic nerve and terminate in the visual cortex. It is here where the signal is processed and then passed on to visual association cortices to be translated into visual perception. The visual cortex is found at the posterior part of the brain called the occipital lobe. There are two occipital lobes, one on each brain hemisphere, and they each receive information from the opposite visual fields (what the eye sees when it is fixed and looking straight ahead).

The signals are then relayed to the V1 region of the visual cortex. This is the first of the hierarchy for visual processing. The V1 region is also called the primary visual cortex, Brodmann area 17, and the striate cortex. The striate cortex is named as such due to the striped nature of myelinated fiber within the cortex. The visual cortex is responsible for the initial processing of image information. In humans, it makes up the largest of all sensory systems that are represented in the brain. The neurons located in V1 send their axons to three main brain regions: (1) the extrastriate visual cortices (regions V2, V3, V3a, and V4) for additional processing of the visual signal; (2) the superior colliculus to modulate eye movements; and (3) the lateral geniculate nucleus (LGN) to have central control of the sensory input.

Neurons in the extrastriate cortex will then project to the medial temporal, inferotemporal, and posterior parietal cortices. From the output cells of the retina a represented map is found not only in the LGN but also in the striate and the extrastriate cortices. In fact, there are six retinotopic maps in the occipital lobe with one each in V1, V2, V3, V3a, V4, and in the middle temporal area that borders the temporal and occipital lobes (called V5, which is important for the perception of movement). In addition, the retinal representations are found in the inferotemporal and posterior parietal cortices. The posterior parietal cortex is responsible for integrating both somatic and visual sensations together. These topographical maps of the retina throughout the visual system show how the visual signals are conserved and organized so that the object's information is preserved in the brain.

In humans, neurons in the striate and extrastriate cortices process the most basic information, such as light intensity, colors, lines and edges making "bars," and orientation. As visual information passes through the hierarchy of the visual cortex, the processing becomes more and more complex, making the image more realistic. When an object's visual signal reaches the visual association cortices, the neurons will respond to complete objects that were seen in the visual field. This means, for example, that cells in the visual association cortex will be activated when a specific type of bird, like an adult bald eagle, is seen. This information is then moved into two different pathways of the brain, called the ventral and dorsal streams, to identify "what" the object is and "where" it is in space compared to the person.

Visual Perception

Visual perception takes the information from visual processing and attempts to "make sense" of the object. Additionally, visual perception is important for the perception of movement, the perception of depth, and figure-ground perception. These three types of visual perception are based in Gestalt psychology, which tries to understand how the human eye sees objects first as a whole and then as a sum of its individual parts. It also looks at how the entire object is anticipated even when the parts are not integrated, such as filling in the "blind spots" of the visual field to complete the entire image.

To perceive movement, the neurons located in region V5 are activated when the speed and direction of an object are seen. In humans, the vestibular system is also necessary for understanding motion perception. This is because the system compares the speed of the person against the speed of the object to determine the motion. There are some people who cannot perceive movement. This rare condition is called akinetopsia. Persons with akinetopsia see the world in several "still" pictures instead of fluid actions. Research has shown that these individuals have a lesion in V5, thus confirming the location of motion perception.

Seeing the world in three dimensions (3D) and seeing how far an object is from a person is called depth perception. This perception is best with binocular vision as well as utilizing depth cues such as stereopsis, parallax, and convergence of the eyes. Stereopsis is the impression of depth by viewing a 3D scene (or external environment) with both eyes. The different locations of each eye on the head present a disparity in what is seen, which is then processed by the brain to perceive depth. Parallax is used to determine distance by looking at an object along two different lines of sight and measuring it against the angle made by the two lines. Closer objects have a larger parallax compared to far objects. Using parallax is how ancient astronomers determined the distance of the moon, sun, and stars. Finally, the inward movement of both eyes (looking toward the center) is called convergence. This helps in focusing the object onto the retina and producing binocular vision and stereopsis.

Figure-ground perception is the process of determining a "figure" from the "background." For example, it is how you are reading this entry and seeing each letter and word as its own figure and not part of the white background. Specifically, figure-ground perception looks at edges (or borders) of the figure as well as its shape, so that it can be perceived in the brain as a singular object. One of the most famous figure-ground perception examples comes from Danish psychologist Edgar Rubin (1886–1951). It is a vase-face drawing that is also considered an optical illusion. The vase is white and in the middle of a black background. However, the black area looks like two faces looking at each other with a white space between them. This drawing—called the Rubin vase—focuses on the edges of the vase, which are also the edges of the two faces. If the person focuses on the white side of the border, the brain will see a white vase. But if the person focuses on the black sides of the edges, the brain will interpret the image as two faces. The visual system will go back and forth between the two images and the two interpretations.

For the brain to determine which to look at as the "figure" and the "ground," it uses other cues that are based on the size, the shape, the color, and the movement of the object. Generally, the object is smaller than the background, the shape tends to be curved—particularly convex, the color is more distinct and varied for an object compared to the "monotone" color of the background, and the movement of the object is faster than the "static" background.

Jennifer L. Hellier

See also: Blind Spot; Color Blindness; Color Perception; Hubel, David H.; Occipital Lobe; Optic Nerve; Perception; Retina; Sensory Receptors; Tunnel Vision; Visual Fields; Visual System; Wiesel, Torsten N.

Further Reading

Bear, Mark F., Barry W. Connors, & Michael A. Paradiso. (2007). *Neuroscience exploring the brain* (3rd ed.). Baltimore, MD: Lippincott Williams & Wilkins.

Dragoi, Valentin, & Chieyeko Tsuchitani. (1997). Visual processing: Cortical pathways. In *Neuroscience Online, an electronic textbook for the neurosciences* (Chap. 15). Retrieved from http://neuroscience.uth.tmc.edu/s2/chapter15.html

Kandel, Eric R., James H. Schwartz, Thomas M. Jessell, Steven A. Siegelbaum, & A. J. Hudspeth (Eds.). (2012). *Principles of neural science* (5th ed.). New York, NY: McGraw-Hill.

VISUAL PROCESSING: *See* Visual Perception

VISUAL SYSTEM

The visual system is responsible for the sense of sight or vision. Animals are highly visual, particularly humans and other mammals, as this sensory system helps them see their prey, see their food, and see their surroundings. The visual system is one of the most well-studied central nervous system processes as vision is extremely important to humans. Visual perception, however, consists of the psychological process of how a person sees a visual image. Because of this difference, visual perception is a separate entry in this encyclopedia.

Anatomy and Physiology

The visual system is made up of several anatomical structures: the eye—and its retina; optic nerves—the output of the retina, which are the second pair of cranial nerves; optic chiasm; optic tract; lateral geniculate nucleus (LGN); optic radiation; visual cortex; and visual association cortex. Since mammals have two eyes, all of the aforementioned structures are found in both the left and right sides of the brain, except for the optic chiasm. There is only one optic chiasm, as this is where the left and right optic nerves come together and cross some of their fibers.

Eye

The eye is a complex organ that acts like a camera as it uses the laws of optics. The eye uses light from an external object to focus an image onto its photoreceptors. These photoreceptors are found at the posterior portion of the eye in the retina. To help focus the light and project the image, the eye refracts the incoming light first through the cornea—a transparent structure at the anterior portion of the eye that covers the iris, pupil, and anterior chamber. The light then passes through the pupil and is refracted again via the lens. Together, the cornea and the lens act like a compound lens to project the image upside down on the retina.

Retina

The retina is made up of 10 distinct layers of neurons that modulate the light stimulus. The neural processing of the retina is very complex but can be reduced to four main stages: photoreception, transmission to bipolar cells, transmission to ganglion cells, and transmission to the optic nerve. Of all the different neurons within the retina, there are only two types of photoreceptor cells: the rods and the cones. The rods respond to dim light (such as moonlight) and produce black-and-white vision; the cones respond to bright light and produce color vision. Surrounding neurons within the other layers of the retina modulate the output signals from the rods and cones and then transfer this information to the bipolar cells. Further modulation of the signals is performed, and the bipolar cells transmit this information to the ganglion cells, the outermost layer of the retina. Finally, the ganglion cells' axons produce action potentials that travel along the optic nerve into the brain.

Optic Nerves

The output of the retina consists of ganglion cells and their axons, which make up the optic nerves. The optic nerves travel along the underside of the brain. The representation of the visual world travels within the optic nerves all the way to the back of the brain. These brain regions are called the occipital lobes. But before the signals reach their final destinations, they are processed by relaying the information to other brain structures. The majority of the axons terminate within the LGN. The remaining axons travel to the superior colliculus, which is important for moving the head when something "catches the eye" and for controlling eye movements called saccades.

Optic Chiasm

The optic chiasm is found at the base of the hypothalamus. It looks like a large white "X" because of the large number of myelinated axons. This crossing of information is important because it takes specific halves of the visual fields and projects them to specific halves of the brain. This means that the left halves of the visual fields of both eyes are crossed over and projected to the right cerebral hemisphere, while the right halves of the visual field of both eyes are sent to the left cerebral hemisphere. Small portions of the optic nerve axons that arrive from the centers of both visual fields are projected to both hemispheres for redundancy purposes.

Optic Tract

The optic tract begins immediately after the optic chiasm and eventually splits into two divisions: the left and right optic tracts. The information carried within these tracts is exclusive to the same side as its visual field. This means that images seen in the left half of the visual field will flow into the left optic tract and the right visual field halves enter the right optic tract. These tracts follow the posterior portion of the thalamus ending in the LGN.

LGN

The term *geniculate* means to bend as this nucleus wraps to the lateral side of the posterior part of the thalamus and is ellipsoid in shape. The LGN is separated into six distinct layers with each layer receiving certain visual information. These layers have either parvocellular or magnocellular neurons, which are the target neurons for specific axons within the optic tract. Parvocellular neurons are commonly called P cells and are necessary for processing color and edges of an image; magnocellular neurons or M cells are important for depth perception and motion. Additionally, K cells (neurons within the retina that help with color vision) terminate on small neurons lying between the six layers. Layers 1, 4, and 6 receive information from the contralateral temporal visual field, while layers 2, 3, and 5 receive information from the ipsilateral nasal visual field. The output of the P, M, and K cells make the optic radiation and end in the primary visual cortex.

Optic Radiation

From the left and right LGN, visual information is sent to the V1 region of the occipital lobe via the left and right optic radiations. V1 of the occipital lobe is also called the primary visual cortex and has six layers of neurons. The optic radiations move posteriorly and medially to the most posterior portion of the occipital lobe. P cell axons terminate in layer 4Cβ, while the M cell axons end in layer 4Cα. Finally, the K cells connect to blobs (large neurons) located in layers 2 and 3 of V1. Up to now, visual signals have been processed relatively straightforwardly. This will change once the signal enters the visual cortex.

Visual Cortex

The visual cortex is responsible for processing image information. In humans, it makes up the largest of the sensory systems that are represented in the brain. The visual cortex has a hierarchy of regions starting with V1, which is the primary visual cortex or the striate cortex. This region's input comes directly from the LGN. The extrastriate visual cortices are regions V2, V3, V4, and V5. These secondary visual areas are necessary for processing the most basic information, such as light intensity, colors, lines and edges making "bars," and orientation. For example, neurons in V1 and V2 are activated when specific orientations of bars or combinations of bars are seen in a specific region of the visual field. It is thought that this helps with identifying corners and edges of an image. As visual information passes through the hierarchy of the visual cortex, the processing becomes more and more complex, making the image more realistic.

Visual Association Cortex

Finally, the visual association cortex receives information from the hierarchy of the visual cortex. Here, the neurons respond to complete objects that were seen in the visual field. For example, cells in the visual association cortex are activated when a specific type of car, like a red Toyota Prius, is seen. This information is then moved into two different pathways of the brain, called the ventral and dorsal streams, to identify "what" the object is and "where" it is in space. The ventral stream moves toward the temporal lobe, while the dorsal stream moves toward the parietal lobe. The ventral stream is used in first recognizing that the object is a "vehicle," then identifying the object as a "red car," and then applying it to a specific category: "a red Toyota Prius." The dorsal stream will take the surrounding environment of the red Toyota Prius to help place its location in reference to the person. This is called spatial attention.

Jennifer L. Hellier

See also: Blind Spot; Hubel, David H.; Occipital Lobe; Optic Nerve; Retina; Sensory Receptors; Visual Fields; Visual Perception; Visual Threshold; Wiesel, Torsten N.

Further Reading

Bear, Mark F., Barry W. Connors, & Michael A. Paradiso. (2007). *Neuroscience exploring the brain* (3rd ed.). Baltimore, MD: Lippincott Williams & Wilkins.
Kandel, Eric R., James H. Schwartz, Thomas M. Jessell, Steven A. Siegelbaum, & A. J. Hudspeth (Eds.). (2012). *Principles of neural science* (5th ed.). New York, NY: McGraw-Hill.

VISUAL THRESHOLD

The medical definition for visual threshold is the lowest or minimal level of light intensity evoking a visual sensation. However, the absolute threshold has been redefined by signal detection theory. This theory states that visual threshold is the level at which a stimulus will be detected at least 50 percent of the time. This threshold for a person, however, can be influenced by adaption to the light stimulus, attention and expectation of the stimulus, and cognitive processes.

Anatomy and Physiology

The human eye senses light via specialized nerve cells called photoreceptor cells. There are two types of photoreceptor cells: rods and cones. Together these photoreceptor cells have the ability to sense light, color, movement, and other visual stimuli. Rods function best at low levels of light and are responsible for night (scotopic) vision. These cells are incredibly sensitive and under optimal conditions a single unit of light, or photon, may activate rod photoreceptors. This property of having high sensitivity allows rods to have fine light and motion detection. Cones process color perception and details of an object, while rods are used for night and peripheral visions. Cones are named by their size and shape, and they are more prominent in humans and other diurnal animals compared to nocturnal animals. Because cones identify details of an object, they need plenty of light to be activated. This is called photopic vision.

Testing Absolute Visual Threshold

Since vision is dependent on light stimulus, threshold of vision can be difficult to determine. For this reason, testing absolute visual threshold requires that the person must be adapted to a dark room, which will optimize the sensitivity of the individual's rod photoreceptors. Typically it takes about 40 minutes for a person to adapt to the dark. The light stimulus is then presented to a region of the retina with the highest concentration of rods—generally the peripheral portion of the eye. The duration of the light stimulus begins at a short length (1 millisecond) and then increases until the stimulus is correctly identified 50 percent of the time.

Although this test is very accurate, it is not practical to have each person sit in a dark room for 40 minutes prior to the exam. Thus, a faster test has been developed, but instead this test determines a person's threshold of visual processing. Absolute threshold in this test is the presentation speed where an individual correctly detects a word 50 percent of the time, which is the same as chance (the person either sees or does not see the word). Only those who can read are able to complete this exam.

Testing Absolute Visual Processing

The stimulus in this test is a word that is presented between two nonsense words. For instance, the word "garden" is presented between "wzltyp" and "qambcx." The duration of the word presentation is extremely fast, about 33 milliseconds long. If the individual does not see the word, then a new word is presented between two nonsense words for twice as long, 66 milliseconds. The duration of the word presentation continues to increase until the individual sees the word 50 percent of the time.

Jennifer L. Hellier

See also: Cones; Optic Nerve; Retina; Rods; Visual Perception; Visual System

Further Reading

Blake, R. Randolph, & Robert Fox. (1969). Visual form recognition threshold and the psychological refractory period. *Perception & Psychophysics, 5*(1), 46–48.

Crozier, W. J. (1940). The theory of the visual threshold: I. Time and intensity. *Proceedings of the National Academy of Sciences USA, 26*(1), 54–60. Retrieved from http://www.ncbi.nlm.nih.gov/pmc/articles/PMC1078006/

Hecht, Selig, Simon Shlaer, & Maurice H. Pirenne. (1942). Energy, quanta, and vision. *Journal of General Physiology, 25*(6), 819–840. Retrieved from https://www.ncbi.nlm.nih.gov/pmc/articles/PMC2142545/pdf/819.pdf

VOMERONASAL ORGAN

Most animals have a very strong sense of smell, as it is important for finding food and potential mates as well as determining the presence of nearby predators. Thus, nonhuman mammals and reptiles have two systems: the main olfactory system to detect volatile odors (chemical stimuli) and an accessory olfactory system to detect fluid-phase stimuli as well as volatile odors. Fluid-phase stimuli are commonly known as pheromones, and it is important to note that some pheromones can be detected via the main olfactory system. The accessory olfactory system has a special organ to sense the fluid-phase stimuli. This structure is a bone that separates the left and right nasal cavities (between the nose and the mouth) and is called the vomeronasal organ. This organ specifically lies between the vomer and nasal bones and was first critically described by Dutch surgeon Ludwig Lewin Jacobson (1783–1843), thus the organ is often referred to as Jacobson's or Jacobsonian's organ. Mammals curl back their upper lip (flehmen) to stimulate the vomeronasal organ, while snakes stick out their tongue, simultaneously touching the vomeronasal organ, to detect prey.

There has been quite a bit of controversy between scientists about whether or not humans have a truly functioning vomeronasal organ. Popular culture and popular science literature speculate that there is a functioning human vomeronasal organ that is stimulated by pheromones, but basic scientists have argued against that notion, particularly since the definition of pheromone includes: "chemical substances released by one member of a species as communication with another member, to their mutual benefit" (Meredith, 2001).

Anatomy and Physiology

The vomeronasal organ is the peripheral sensory organ of the accessory olfactory system. In animals—nonhuman mammals, amphibians, and reptiles—it is a paired organ found at the roof of the mouth. In 90 percent of humans, however, it is found unilaterally at the base of the nasal septum (Meredith, 2001). The vomeronasal system is involved in both chemical and pheromone communications. It consists of an epithelium with microvillar vomeronasal sensory neurons and a lamina propria that lies below the epithelium. The vomeronasal sensory neurons have axons that exit the epithelium through the lamina propria as an axon bundle, which in turn enters the brain for perception. In mice and hamsters, studies have shown that testosterone and luteinizing hormone levels increase when males are exposed to female mice or hamster chemosensory stimuli. This process occurs through the vomeronasal system. Similarly, female prairie voles will enter estrus (or their uterus will enlarge) when their vomeronasal organ is stimulated by the scent of a nearby male. Such responses have not been observed in humans.

In human embryos, the vomeronasal organ is very similar to those of other species such that it contains bipolar cells and generates luteinizing hormone-releasing hormone (LHRH)–producing cells. However, as the embryo matures (by 30 weeks of age), the vomeronasal organ becomes more simplified compared to other species. In adults, the vomeronasal organ is found in the nasal septum; however, it does not have large blood vessels to supply the cells or any supporting cartilage. Furthermore, following nasal surgery where the septum is removed, studies have shown that the human vomeronasal organ consists of a blind-ending tube that is lined with a pseudostratified epithelium with submucosal glands. However, no clear axon bundles have been observed penetrating the lamina propria in the same way it is seen in vomeronasal epithelia of other species. As this is very different from other species, it appears that this blind-ending tube is the remnant of the vomeronasal organ in adult humans.

In animals with a well-developed vomeronasal organ, the sensory neurons' axons bundle together and synapse in the accessory olfactory bulb's primary neurons, called mitral cells. Here, the signal is then passed on to the amygdala and the hypothalamus for perception. It has a direct involvement with sex hormone activities that include the start of mating behaviors as well as influencing aggressiveness.

Jennifer L. Hellier

See also: Olfactory Mucosa; Olfactory System; Pheromones; Senses of Animals

Further Reading

Dénes, Lorand, Zsuzsanna Pap, Annamaria Szántó, Istvan Gergely, & Tudor Sorin Pop. (2015). Human vomeronasal epithelium development: An immunohistochemical overview. *Acta microbiologica et immunologica Hungarica, 62*(2), 167–181. http://dx.doi .org/10.1556/030.62.2015.2.7

Meredith, Michael. (2001). Human vomeronasal organ function: A critical review of best and worst cases. *Chemical Senses, 26*(4), 433–445. Retrieved from http://chemse .oxfordjournals.org/content/26/4/433.full

Shigeru Takami, Maiko Yukimatsu, George Matsumura, Sawa Horie, & Fumiaki Nishiyama. (2016). Morphological analysis for neuron-like cells in the vomeronasal organ of human fetuses at the middle of gestation. *Anatomical Record* (Hoboken), *299*(1), 88–97. http://dx.doi.org/10.1002/ar.23290.

VOMITING: *See* Emesis

W

WIESEL, TORSTEN N.

Torsten N. Wiesel is a Nobel laureate and earned this award for his pioneering work in the visual system. In 1981, Dr. Wiesel shared the Nobel Prize in Physiology or Medicine with David Hubel for their work investigating how visual information is transmitted to and processed in the brain's visual cortex. Their investigations studied specialized functions and mapping of the functional architecture of individual cells within the visual cortex. Their efforts further examined the development of the visual cortex and the role of innate and experiential factors. This work analyzed the flow of nerve impulses from the eye to the visual cortex and described structural and functional details of that part of the brain. Wiesel and Hubel's work lent strong support to the view that prompt surgery is imperative in correcting certain eye defects that are detectable in newborn children, such as congenital cataracts (cloudiness in the lens of the eye).

Dr. Wiesel was born in Uppsala, Sweden, in 1924, and received his medical degree from Karolinska Institute in 1954. His academic career spans the Karolinska Institute, Johns Hopkins University Medical School, and a 24-year position at Harvard Medical School where he did much of his neurophysiological research work in the Department of Neurobiology. After earning his medical degree, Dr. Wiesel became a postdoctoral fellow at the Wilmer Institute, Johns Hopkins Medical School where he met his colleague, Dr. David Hubel. This began their 20-year scientific collaboration and led to their Nobel Prize. In addition, Drs. Wiesel and Hubel have written a book together describing their research and collaborative work, titled *Brain and Visual Perception: The Story of a 25-Year Collaboration* (2004).

Torsten Wiesel has received numerous awards for his work in neuropsychological research including, most recently, the 1996 Helen Keller Prize for Vision Research, the 1998 Society for Neuroscience Presidential Award, the 2005 Institute of Medicine David Rall Medal, the 2005 National Medal of Science Award (USA), the 2006 Spanish National Research Council Gold Medal, and the 2007 Marshall M. Parks MD Medal of Excellence Children's Eye Foundation Award, which he shared with colleague David Hubel.

Dr. Wiesel's work includes serving on the Committee of Human Rights of the National Academies of Science (USA) and the International Human Rights Network of Academies and Scholarly Societies. He is a founding member of the Israeli-Palestinian Science Organization (IPSO). Furthermore, Dr. Wiesel has served as chair of the board of the Aaron Diamond AIDS Research Center (1995–2001), president of the International Brain Research Organization, IBRO (1998–2004), chair of the Board of Governors of the New York Academy of Sciences (2001–2006), and on the board of directors of the Population Council (1999–2008).

In 2007, Wiesel's efforts to support research on eye diseases were recognized when the Torsten Wiesel Research Institute was established as part of the World Eye Organization, based in Chengdu, China. This institute allows scientists to engage in basic and clinical research on eye diseases prevalent in Asian populations.

Karen Savoie

See also: Hubel, David H.; Visual System

Further Reading

Hubel, David H., & Torsten N. Wiesel. (2004). *Brain and visual perception: The story of a 25-year collaboration.* New York, NY: Oxford University Press.

Appendix

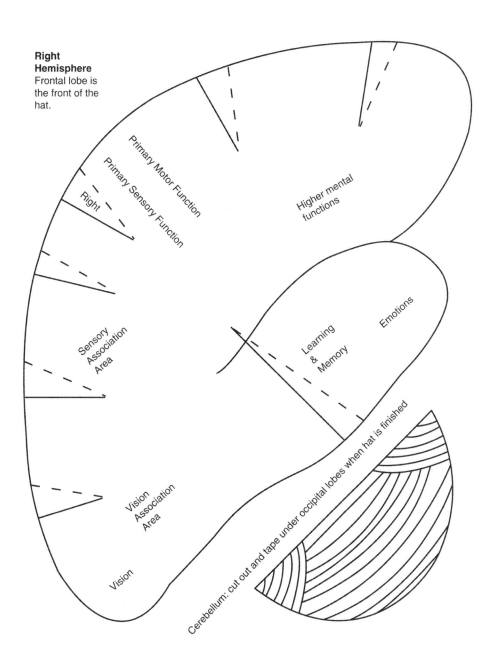

Right Hemisphere Frontal lobe is the front of the hat.

Primary Motor Function

Primary Sensory Function

Right

Higher mental functions

Sensory Association Area

Learning & Memory

Emotions

Vision Association Area

Vision

Cerebellum: cut out and tape under occipital lobes when hat is finished

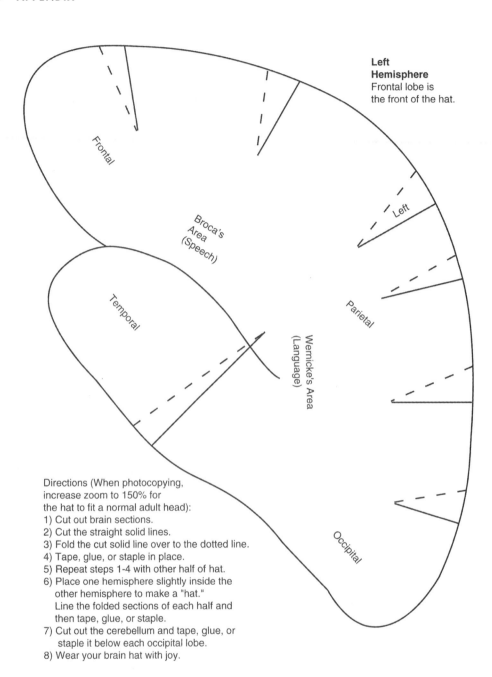

**Left
Hemisphere**
Frontal lobe is
the front of the hat.

Frontal

Broca's
Area
(Speech)

Temporal

Left

Parietal

Wernicke's Area
(Language)

Occipital

Directions (When photocopying,
increase zoom to 150% for
the hat to fit a normal adult head):
1) Cut out brain sections.
2) Cut the straight solid lines.
3) Fold the cut solid line over to the dotted line.
4) Tape, glue, or staple in place.
5) Repeat steps 1-4 with other half of hat.
6) Place one hemisphere slightly inside the
   other hemisphere to make a "hat."
   Line the folded sections of each half and
   then tape, glue, or staple.
7) Cut out the cerebellum and tape, glue, or
   staple it below each occipital lobe.
8) Wear your brain hat with joy.

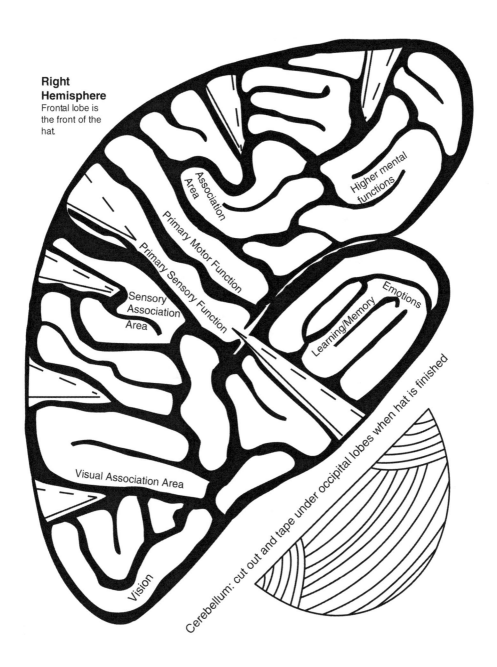

Right Hemisphere
Frontal lobe is the front of the hat.

Association Area

Higher mental functions

Primary Motor Function

Primary Sensory Function

Sensory Association Area

Learning/Memory

Emotions

Visual Association Area

Vision

Cerebellum: cut out and tape under occipital lobes when hat is finished

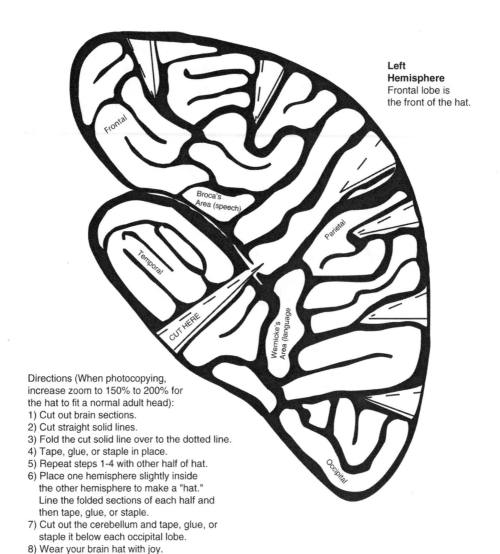

**Left
Hemisphere**
Frontal lobe is
the front of the hat.

Directions (When photocopying,
increase zoom to 150% to 200% for
the hat to fit a normal adult head):
1) Cut out brain sections.
2) Cut straight solid lines.
3) Fold the cut solid line over to the dotted line.
4) Tape, glue, or staple in place.
5) Repeat steps 1-4 with other half of hat.
6) Place one hemisphere slightly inside
   the other hemisphere to make a "hat."
   Line the folded sections of each half and
   then tape, glue, or staple.
7) Cut out the cerebellum and tape, glue, or
   staple it below each occipital lobe.
8) Wear your brain hat with joy.

Glossary

Afferent—fibers, particularly sensory, that travel toward the central nervous system.

Aneurism—an unusually large expansion in the wall of an artery that causes weakness and possibly tears in the arterial wall.

Anions—negatively charged ions.

Axons—the output of a brain cell or neuron that transmits an action potential and connects to other neurons; the wire-like parts of neurons along which electrical signals travel.

Cations—positively charged ions.

Caudal—of, at, or toward the tail; toward the posterior end of a body.

Congenital defects—the abnormal anatomy a person is born with.

Contralateral—of or pertaining to the opposite side.

Cranium—the skull of a vertebrate; the part of the skull that encloses the brain.

Cytosol—the fluid within a cell; the water-soluble components of the cytoplasm.

Demyelination—damage to the myelin sheath where the myelin is removed from the axon.

Dendrites or **dendritic arbors**—branches or fine branches that extend from the neuron's cell body and that receive input signals for the neuron.

Depolarization—the movement of chemicals that may contribute to the development of an action potential in a neuron. Specifically, when the membrane potential becomes less negative and closer to threshold to generate an action potential.

Efferent—fibers, particularly motor pathways, that travel away from the central nervous system.

Efflux—the act of flowing outward; flow out of a neuron or glial cell.

Endolymph—a special fluid found in the inner ear used for sensing balance and for transmitting sound waves.

Equilibrium—the sense of balance; the ability to perceive directions such as up and down.

Etiology—the causes of a disease or condition, or how that disease or condition comes about.

Ganglion (singular); **Ganglia** (plural)—a collection of cell bodies that is located outside of the central nervous system.

Glia or **Glial cells**—types of brain cells that support neurons or nerve cells; cells in the nervous system that lack the ability to communicate by sending electrical signals.

Gustatory—of or relating to taste or tasting; the sense of taste.

Gyrus (singular); **Gyri** (plural)—a ridge or fold in brain tissue. The combination of gyri and sulci is what gives the brain its convoluted and folded appearance.

Hyperpolarization—the movement of chemicals that contribute to the cessation of an action potential in a neuron.

Influx—the act of flowing inward; to flow into a neuron or glial cell.

Innervate—to communicate by neurons; stimulating through nerves or axons.

Ion channel—a protein in the cell membrane that forms a pore and lets certain ions through when open.

Ipsilateral—Latin meaning "same side."

Ischemia—insufficient blood supply caused by vasoconstriction or a local obstacle to the arterial flow.

Limbic system—the emotional circuit of the brain.

Macula—a region of the retina that has the greatest ability to sense light.

Myelin—a protective covering of a neuron's axon that helps transmit nerve impulses faster.

Nerves—bundles of axons that exist outside of the central nervous system and are part of the peripheral nervous system.

Neurons or **Nerve cells**—specialized brain cells that allow communication and transmission of information among one another and with target cells and tissues throughout the body.

Neuroscience—the study of structure, function, development, physiology, pharmacology, and pathology of the nervous system.

Neurotransmitters—chemicals used to activate neurons and begin the process of depolarization.

Nucleus (singular); **Nuclei** (plural)—a collection of cell bodies that is located within the central nervous system.

Olfaction—the sense of smell; the act of smelling.

Pathophysiology—the abnormal functioning of a body component as a result of disease, injury, or some other medical condition.

Photoreceptors—specialized proteins that respond to light.

Physiology—the normal functions of a particular organ, tissue, cell, or other bodily component.

Primary visual cortex—also called the striate cortex of the occipital lobe because it looks striped. It is the location where vision begins to be integrated.

Propagate—to transmit an action potential; how an action potential travels toward its target cell.

Proprioception—the sense of where one's body is in space, particularly for identifying limb position.

Receptor fields—areas or regions that receive external stimuli such as touch.

Retina—the photosensitive lining of the back of the eye where images are focused.

Rostral—of or relating to the rostrum; toward the nose or beak.

Somatosensation—body senses, such as temperature, pressure, and pain.

Sulcus (singular); **Sulci** (plural)—a trough or groove in brain tissue. The combination of gyri and sulci is what gives the brain its convoluted and folded appearance.

Synapse—a physical connection of two neurons where a chemical signal is released from an action potential; the communication points between two neurons.

Tracts—a long group of fibers (axons) that transmits information electrically within the central nervous system.

Vesicles—small membranous sacs containing signaling molecules known as neurotransmitters.

Viscera—organs that are found in the body, especially those located in the abdominal cavity of an animal or human.

Index

Note: Page numbers in **bold** indicate the location of main entries.

205–206, 377–378; Meniere's disease affecting, 57, 224–226, 411; misophonia associated with, 231–232; Mosquito machine impacting, 235–236; otoacoustic emissions in, 293–294; sound localization in, 39, 41, 367; stereocilia in, 372–373; thalamus interaction with, 43, 401; tinnitus in, 38, 57, 224, 232, 410–412; tonotopic map of, 412–413; vestibulocochlear nerve in, 43, 81, 123, 412, 433–435; vibration sensation associated with, 435–436

Auditory-Tactile Synesthesia, **44–45**; applications of, 45; hearing-touch connection in, 46, 387; types of, 44–45

Auditory Threshold, **45–47**; classical auditory testing for, 45–46; types of auditory tests for, 46

Aura, **47–49**; epilepsy/seizures associated with, 47, 48, 49, 352; evidence of, 48; historical views of, 47–48; types of, 48–49

Autism Spectrum Disorders, 119, 325, 371

Autonomic Nervous System (ANS), **49–51**; adrenaline in, 4–6; amygdala interaction with, 22; anatomy of, 49–50; autonomic ganglia in, 169–170; baroreceptors in, 58–60, 200, 201, 291; chemoreception controlled by, 98; familial dysautonomia affecting, 160; glossopharyngeal nerve interaction with, 172; heightened senses affected by, 179; Horner syndrome involving, 185; neurologist studying, 253; noradrenaline affecting, 261–262; olfactory nerve associated with, 277; parasympathetic nervous system in, 49, 306–307, 429; peripheral nervous system including, 306–307; physiology of, 50–51; sympathetic nervous system in, 4–6, 49–50, 185, 261–262, 306–307; thermal sense response via, 406; vagus nerve role in, 307, 429

Axel, Richard (1946–), **51–52**; Buck's work with, 52, 85, 272

Axon, **52–54**; action potential transmission via, 2–4, 52–54; anatomy and physiology of, 53–54; ganglia and, 169; history and function of, 53; nerves as bundles of, 249–250; peripheral nervous system communication via, 52–53, 305–306; peripheral neuropathy affecting, 309

Balance, **55–58**; diseases affecting, 55, 57, 161, 224; dizziness affecting, 55, 57, 135–137; exteroception with, 154–155; muscles and joint position for, 55, 56; Romberg test for, 56; semicircular canal affecting, 57, 154, 354; sensory inputs for, 55; vestibular sense affecting, 55, 56, 57, 154–155, 354; vestibulocochlear nerve affecting, 433, 434–435; visual input for, 55, 56, 57

Ballot, Christophorus Henricus Diedericus Buys (1817–1890), 137

Bancroft, Anne (1931–2005), 378

Barbier, Charles (n.d.), 75

Baroreceptors, **58–60**; anatomy and physiology of, 58–59; blood pressure regulation via, 58–60, 291; diseases affecting, 59; history of, 58; interoception involving, 200, 201

Bartoshuk, Linda (1938–), **60–61**, 382

Basal Ganglia, 78, 103, 104, 170

Bell, Alexander Graham, 205

Bell, Charles (1774–1842), 62, 324

Bell's Palsy, **61–63**; ageusia associated with, 12; diagnosis and symptoms of, 62; facial nerve impairment in, 61–63, 158, 382; history of, 61–62; Melkersson-Rosenthal syndrome related to, 220; peripheral neuropathy in, 308; superior salivatory nucleus affected by, 382; treatment for, 63

Benedict, Lily, 363

Benign Joint Hypermobility Syndrome (BJHS), 325

Benign Paroxysmal Positional Vertigo (BPPV), 55, 57, 135–136, 296
Bernard, Claude (1813–1878), 58
Bernstein, Leonard (1918–1990), 101
Bietti, G. B. (n.d.), 64
Bietti's Crystalline Dystrophy (BCD), **63–65**; cause of, 64; diagnosis and treatment of, 65; future research and developments in, 65; inheritance of, 64; symptoms of, 64–65
Bipolar Disorder, 37
Bitter Sensation, **65–67**; supertaster's intensity of, 382, 383; taste buds with, 394; taste system including, 398; Type II taste cell role in, 421–422
Bjerrum, Jannik (1851–1920), 439
Blige, Mary J. (1971–), 387
Blind Spot, **67–69**; anatomy and physiology of, 67–68; diseases, disorders, and treatments related to, 68; history of, 67
Blindness, **69–71**; anophthalmia as lack of eyes causing, 25–27; Bietti's crystalline dystrophy leading to, 64–65; Braille use with, 74–76, 133, 218; cone dystrophy leading to, 116; cortical blindness as, 265, 266; echolocation with, 355; heightened senses with, 179, 180; history of, 69; hyperopia and, 192; Keller with, 205–206, 377; occipital lobe damage leading to, 265, 266; optic nerve hypoplasia causing, 289–291; prevention and research on, 70–71; retinopathy leading to, 340; Sullivan with, 377–378; treatments and outcomes of, 70; types and symptoms of, 69–70
Blink Reflex, **71–72**; anatomy of, 72; function and purpose of, 71–72
Blood Pressure. *See also* Hypertension: baroreceptors regulating, 58–60, 291, emesis affecting, 230; fainting and changes in, 159; glossopharyngeal nerve interaction with, 172; noradrenaline affecting, 261, 262; orthostatic hypotension

affecting, 159, 161, 291–293; retinopathy affected by, 339; vagus nerve control of, 430; visceral sensation affecting, 437
Bonaparte, Napoleon (1769–1821), 75
Bowlby, John, 212
Bowman, William (1816–1892), 73
Bowman's Glands, **72–74**; anatomy and physiology of, 73; history of, 73; olfactory mucosa location of, 275; research on, 73–74
Braille, **74–76**; components of, 75–76; discriminative touch for, 133; history of, 74–75; Meissner's corpuscles role in reading, 218
Braille, Louis (1809–1852), 69, 74–75
Brain Anatomy, **76–79**. *See also specific brain structures*; amygdala, 21–23, 78; basal ganglia, 78; brain building with clay, 77; brain cut-out hat activity, 301; brain divisions in, 76; brainstem, 76, 77, 78, 79–81, 94; central nervous system including, 76, 77, 78, 93–94; cerebellum, 76, 77, 78, 94; cerebral cortex, 77, 78, 95–97; cerebrum, 76, 77, 78; chronoception associated with, 103; corpus callosum, 78; damage to brain impacting, 78–79, 94 (*see also* Brain Damage/Injury/Trauma); forebrain in, 76; frontal lobe, 77, 78, 93; hindbrain in, 76; hippocampus, 78, 94; hypothalamus, 76, 78, 94; limbic system comprised of, 211; midbrain in, 76, 78, 94; occipital lobe, 77, 78, 94; parietal lobe, 77, 78, 93–94; pituitary gland, 78; Ramón y Cajal research on, 149–150, 329–330; structures in, 78; temporal lobe, 77, 78, 94; thalamus, 76, 78, 94, 399–402
Brain Awareness Week, 362
Brain Damage/Injury/Trauma. *See also* Brain Lesions; Brain Tumors; Strokes: agnosia associated with, 13, 14, 15; anosmia associated with, 27, 28; auditory-tactile synesthesia associated with, 44–45; auras associated with, 47;

as, 321; musky smells as, 321; pepperminty smells as, 321; pungent smells as, 321; putrid smells as, 321

Proprioception, **322–324**; balance affected by, 55, 56; exteroception with, 154; further research in, 323–324; golgi tendon organs for, 323; joint position sense in, 322–323; joint receptors for, 322; loss of, 323; muscle spindles for, 322–323; neurological examination of, 252; proprioception deficit disorders affecting, 323, 324–326

Proprioception Deficit Disorders (PDD), **324–326**; applications and impairment from, 324–325; history of, 324; loss of proprioception via, 323; research on, 325

Prosopagnosia, 14

Pryse-Phillips, William (n.d.), 278

Ptosis, **326–327**; causes of, 326–327; myasthenia gravis associated with, 239; signs and symptoms of, 326; treatment for, 327

Pure Amusia, 14

Pure Auditory Nonverbal Agnosia, 14

Pure Word Deafness, 14, 196

Ramón y Cajal, Santiago (1852–1934), **329–330**; entorhinal cortex research by, 149–150

Ranvier, Louis-Antoine, 53

Rare Diseases: list of, 245 (see also specific diseases); National Organization for Rare Disorders for, 245–247; Rare Disease Day for, 245

Ravel, Maurice (1875–1937), 14

Reagan, Ronald (1911–2004), 19, 246

Reflex, **330–334**; anatomy and physiology of, 330, 332–333; Babinski (plantar) reflex as, 331; biceps-jerk reflex as, 331; blink reflex as, 71–72; consensual pupillary light reflex as, 120–121; disease and injury affecting, 333–334; golgi tendon organs role in, 174; neurological examination assessing, 252, 331; otolith reflexes as, 295; patellar

(knee-jerk) reflex as, 330, 331, 332–333; peripheral nervous system role in, 306; prosthetics and, 334; reflex syncope and, 159; reflex test, 331

Refractive Amblyopia, 16

Rehabilitation Act of 1973, 29

Renal Failure, 12

Repolarization. See Hyperpolarization

Restless Legs Syndrome (RLS), **334–336**; diagnosis and management of, 336; etiology of, 335; symptoms of, 335–336

Restricted Environmental Stimulation Therapy, 357

Retina, **337–339**; accommodation via, 1–2, 318; age-related macular degeneration affecting, 69, 70, 163, 338; anatomy of, 337–338; astigmatism affecting, 33–34, 129–130, 319, 327; auras and retinal fatigue, 48; Bietti's crystalline dystrophy affecting, 63–65; blind spot and, 67–68; blink reflex protecting, 72; circadian rhythm associated with, 105; color blindness and, 111–112; color perception and, 113–114, 305; cones in (see Cones); consensual pupillary light reflex associated with, 120; detachment of, 338; diabetes affecting, 134; diplopia associated with, 129–130; disease affecting, 338–339 (see also specific diseases); fovea centralis in, 162–164, 337, 343–344, 441; glaucoma affecting, 69–70, 192, 288, 289, 418, 419; Holmes-Adie syndrome affecting, 181; hyperopia affecting, 33, 191–192, 319; lateral inhibition in, 199; microphthalmia affecting, 228; myopia affecting, 33, 241, 319; neuropil in, 255; ocular dominance columns and, 267, 268; optic nerve interaction with, 123, 287, 338; physiology of, 338; presbyopia affecting, 33, 318; retinitis pigmentosa in, 418, 419; retinopathy affecting, 339–341; rods in (see

About the Editor and Contributors

Editor

Jennifer L. Hellier, PhD, is an Assistant Professor in the Departments of Family Medicine and Cell & Developmental Biology, the Director of the Colorado Health Professions Development (Co-HPD) program, and the Associate Director of Pre-Health Programs in the Colorado Area Health Education Centers (AHEC) Program Office. Dr. Hellier earned her doctoral degree in neuroscience from Colorado State University, Fort Collins, Colorado, and completed her baccalaureate of science at the University of Southern California, Los Angeles. Previous to her leadership and development of the Co-HPD pipeline programs, Dr. Hellier performed peer-reviewed scientific research in schizophrenia, olfaction, and epilepsy in a neuroscience lab on the University of Colorado Anschutz Medical Campus. Earlier in her career, Dr. Hellier was an Instructor in the Neurology Department at Harvard Medical School, and a postdoctoral fellow at the University of Colorado Health Science Campus. Dr. Hellier is a native of Colorado and loves hiking and camping in Colorado's beautiful mountains.

Contributors

Simi Abraham is a student at the University of Colorado, Denver, majoring in biology with minors in chemistry and in multidisciplinary research methods through the Honors and Leadership Program. She works at Anschutz Medical Campus in the Division of Hematology and volunteers as an undergraduate researcher at National Jewish.

Carolyn Johnson Atwater has a BA in psychology from the University of Colorado at Boulder.

Riannon C. Atwater has a BS in biology from the University of Colorado, Denver, with minors in multidisciplinary research methods and leadership studies. She plans on continuing to medical school.

Dianna Bartel, PhD, is an Associate Research Scientist in the Spiegel Lab where she coordinates research communications across academic and business platforms to advance novel therapeutics into the clinic. Previously she was a postdoctoral research associate in the department of neurosurgery at Yale University School of Medicine. Her research primarily focuses on the glial cells of the brain.

B. Dnate' Baxter, BS, MS, is a research associate at the University of Colorado Anschutz Medical Campus and a member of the Rocky Mountain Taste and Smell Center.

Patricia A. Bloomquist, BS, is a retiree from AT&T and Ball Aerospace. She currently is the owner of Compass Real Estate and enjoys volunteering for different organizations.

Emma Boxer is a graduate of the University of Colorado, Denver. She currently has an internship at the Denver Museum of Nature & Science where she has researched the genetics of the bitter taste of PTC and PROP and is currently researching the genetics of a possible sixth taste: fatty acids.

Nicholas Breitnauer, MD, is an internal medicine/pediatrics resident at the University of Colorado.

Jeremy E. Brothers, PharmD, is a graduate of the University of Colorado Skaggs School of Pharmacy and Pharmaceutical Sciences. He has continued his education with a residency in critical care–based pharmacy. He did his undergraduate work at Virginia Tech and is originally from the Washington, D.C., area.

Lin Browning, MA, is the Executive Director at Central Colorado Area Health Education Center (CCAHEC). She has a master's degree in education with emphasis on curriculum and instruction. She has taught students in grades K–8 and has experience in special education and working with students with communicative disabilities.

James Danahey is an undergraduate student at the University of Colorado, Boulder. He is double majoring in biochemistry and classics, and is determined to pursue a career in medicine.

Kendra DeHay, BA, is currently studying for her master of science in biomedical science and biotechnology from the University of Colorado Anschutz Medical Campus. She earned her bachelor of arts in integrative physiology at the University of Colorado at Boulder in 2014.

Stephanie Dunlap, PharmD, is a 2014 graduate of the University of Colorado Skaggs School of Pharmacy and Pharmaceutical Sciences. She received a bachelor of arts in the field of molecular and cellular biology from the University of Illinois, Urbana-Champaign, in 2010.

Charles A. Ferguson, PhD, is a Professor in the Department of Integrative Biology at the University of Colorado, Denver. While his academic interests focus on neurobiology and neurotoxicology, his primary research today focuses on the transition of high school students pursuing STEM disciplines to college.

Michael Freer, BS, is a graduate of Fort Lewis College, Durango, Colorado. He is currently a member of the U.S. Navy Reserves and is assigned to the reserve command in Spokane, Washington.

Michael S. Harper, PhD, is a senior medical student at the University of Colorado. He earned his BS in neuroscience at the College of William and Mary, and his PhD in immunology at the University of Colorado through the Medical Scientist Training Program.

Paul Hong, BS, was born in Seoul, South Korea, and came to Colorado at the age of 12. He was educated at the University of Colorado at Colorado Springs, majoring in biochemistry. There, he has studied anatomical and biological sciences, as well as other health care–related issues in America.

Renee Johnson, BS, is a graduate student in the Biomedical Forensic Sciences Program at Boston University Medical campus. She plans on becoming a forensic toxicologist and working in a lab to identify new drugs that are being synthesized and used illicitly.

Aaron Jones, BS, is a second-year medical student at Rocky Vista University. He is a graduate of the University of Colorado, Denver, with a major in biology and a minor in ethnic studies.

Cynthia M. Joseph, BS, is a second-year medical student at Boonshoft School of Medicine. She is a graduate of the University of Colorado, Denver, with a major in biology and a minor in multidisciplinary research methods. Additionally, she was a member of the University Honors and Leadership Program.

Jonathon Keeney, PhD, earned his honors BA in molecular, cellular, and developmental biology at the University of Colorado, Boulder, and his PhD in neuroscience from the University of Colorado Anschutz Medical Campus. His research explores genomic mechanisms by which human brain size has increased, and how these mechanisms influence disease.

Christopher Knoeckel, BA, is an MD/PhD student in the Neuroscience Program at the University of Colorado Anschutz Medical Campus. His research focuses on the role of activity in the development of the peripheral nervous system.

Lisa M. J. Lee, PhD, is an assistant professor in the department of cell and developmental biology at University of Colorado School of Medicine. She teaches embryology, histology, and anatomy, and her research focus is in educational technology and human–computer interaction.

Roberto Lopez is currently a fourth-year medical student at Rocky Vista University and earned his undergraduate degree from the University of Colorado, Denver. Previously, he worked in a neuroscience research laboratory on the University of Colorado Anschutz Medical Campus. He is a published author in the field of olfaction and olfactory activity maps.

Stephen Mazurkivich, BS, is a second-year medical student at The Commonwealth Medical College. He received his undergraduate degree in biology at Fort Lewis College in Durango, Colorado.

Shannen McNamara graduated from Colorado Mesa University with a BS in biology. She earned her Emergency Medical Technician (EMT) Certification in 2014. She currently works in research and plans to pursue further medical education.

Robin Michaels, PhD, received her doctorate from the University of Minnesota, Minneapolis, and completed postdoctoral training at Washington University in St. Louis. She is an Associate Professor in the Department of Biomedical Sciences and serves as Associate Dean of Student Affairs and Admissions, University of Minnesota Medical School, Duluth.

Adam K. Mills, DC, is a graduate of Parker University where he received a doctorate in chiropractic and a bachelor's in anatomy; in addition, he received a bachelor's in biology from Colorado State University, Pueblo. He practices chiropractic in rural Colorado.

Eric B. Moore is a biology undergraduate with a premedical focus at the University of Colorado at Denver.

Mario J. Perez, BS, is a fourth-year medical student at the University of Colorado Anschutz Medical Campus. Previously he was the lead research associate in the Division of Pulmonary Sciences and Critical Care Medicine at the University of Colorado Anschutz Medical Campus.

Vidya Pugazhenthi, PharmD, graduated in 2014 from the University of Colorado Skaggs School of Pharmacy and Pharmaceutical Sciences. She previously studied at the University of Denver with a focus in biochemistry.

Lisa A. Rabe, PhD, is a lecturer in the Department of Craniofacial Biology at the University of Colorado School of Dental Medicine where she teaches medical microbiology and immunology. After conducting research for several years in the field of immunology, she now devotes her energy to teaching and sharing her passion for science.

Michael Romani, DDS, is a California native who received his bachelor of science degree in biology from California State University, Fresno. He is continuing his education and is completing a residency in periodontics.

Ernesto Salcedo, PhD, is a faculty member in the Department of Cell and Developmental Biology at the University of Colorado School of Medicine. He received his bachelor's degree from Duke University and his doctorate degree from the University of Texas Health Sciences Center at San Antonio. Dr. Salcedo serves as a Research Associate at the Denver Museum of Nature & Science, providing talks on olfaction and neuroscience to public audiences.

C. J. Saunders, PhD, is a postdoctoral researcher in the Department of Otorhinolaryngology at the University of Pennsylvania. He is a recent graduate of the Neuroscience Program at the University of Colorado, where his dissertation research focused on the role of airway chemosensory cells in mediating sensations of irritation and inflammation.

Karen Savoie, RDH, BS, is a graduate of Louisiana State University Health Sciences Center and has been a registered dental hygienist for more than 30 years. Her primary focus is improving oral health and access to care for vulnerable populations.

Lauren C. Seeberger, MD, is a board-certified neurologist specializing in movement disorders. She provides treatment and care for patients with Parkinson's disease, Parkinson-plus syndromes, Lewy body disease, Huntington's disease, dystonia, Tourette, tics, chorea, ataxia, restless legs syndrome, myoclonus, drug-induced movement disorders, essential tremor, and tremor.

Elizabeth Shick, DDS, MPH, is a pediatric dentist and received her degrees in dentistry and public health from the University of North Carolina at Chapel Hill. She specializes in infant oral health, perinatal oral health, and global oral health. She currently lives in Denver, Colorado, and is an Assistant Professor at the University of Colorado School of Dental Medicine.

Darin T. Sisneros, BS, is a medical student attending the University of Colorado Anschutz Medical Campus. Previously, he graduated from Adams State University, earning his bachelor of science in cellular and molecular biology. With a passion for science, he has performed research as an undergraduate.

Drake E. Sisneros, BS, is a medical student attending the University of Colorado Anschutz Medical Campus. He graduated with a BS in cellular and molecular biology from Adams State University. Etiology, pathology, and research promoting human health pique his interest. He became fascinated with the olfactory system after doing independent research involving the development of anosmia.

Erin Slocum, RN, is a graduate of the University of Colorado at Boulder and received her BSN from the University of Northern Colorado. She is currently nursing in northern Colorado.

Lynelle Smith, BS, is a medical student at the University of Colorado Anschutz Medical Campus. Previously she was a research assistant in the Department of Pulmonary Science and Critical Care Medicine at the University of Colorado Anschutz Medical Campus.

Danielle Stutzman, PharmD, graduated in 2014 from Skaggs School of Pharmacy and Pharmaceutical Sciences, University of Colorado Anschutz Medical Campus. She is a graduate of the University of Colorado, Boulder, and received a bachelor of arts in molecular cellular developmental biology and psychology.

Melissa Tjandra, BA, is a master's student studying biomedical science and biotechnology at the University of Colorado Anschutz Medical Campus.

Vivian Vu, BS, is a graduate student in cardiovascular science at the University of Glasgow. Previously, she majored in biological sciences with minors in chemistry and business administration at the University of Denver.

Alyssa M. Wienecke is a pre–health care undergraduate student at Biola University, La Mirada, California. She is majoring in human biology and planning to pursue a career in neurology after graduating. In her studies, she is working to better understand autism and find better treatments or therapies for the autistic.

Gage Williamson obtained his BS in biomedical sciences from the University of Colorado, Colorado Springs. He has research experience in molecular oncology, exploring the role of the yeast gene Rad26^{ATRIP} in microtubule damage response pathways to determine the function of the human ATRIP gene in patients with microcephalic primordial dwarfism.

Courtney E. Wilson is currently a PhD student in the neuroscience program at the University of Colorado Anschutz Medical Campus. She works in Dr. Sue Kinnamon's laboratory and focuses on Type III cell signaling in the mammalian taste bud.

Audrey S. Yee, MD, earned her medical degree from the University of Kansas School of Medicine, and then completed an adult neurology residency and three fellowships—basic neurophysiology, clinical neuromuscular/neurodiagnostics, and clinical research—at the University of Colorado School of Medicine.